Role Development

in Professional Nursing Practice

FOURTH EDITION

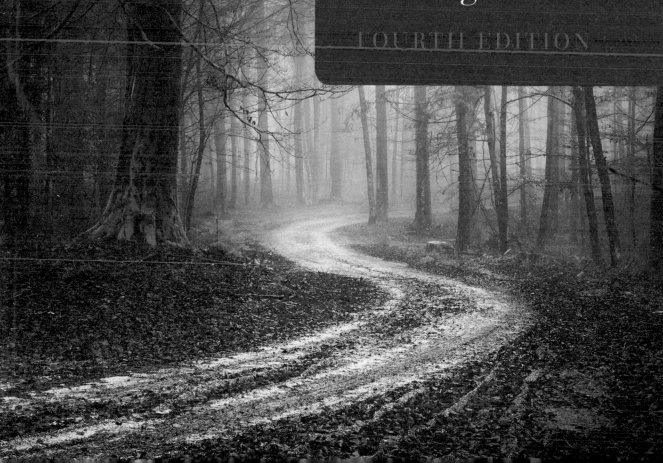

The Pedagogy

Role Development in Professional Nursing Practice, Fourth Edition drives comprehension through various strategies that meet the learning needs of students, while also generating enthusiasm about the topic. This interactive approach addresses different learning styles, making this the ideal text to ensure mastery of key concepts. The pedagogical aids that appear in most chapters include the following:

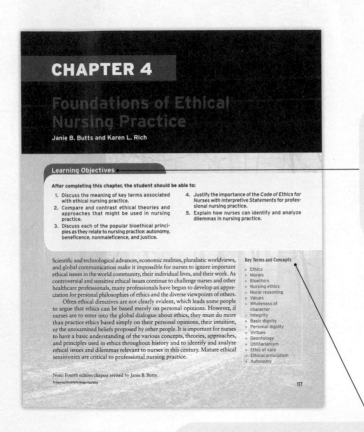

Learning Objectives
These objectives provide instructors and students with a snapshot of the key information they will encounter in each chapter. They serve as a checklist to help guide and focus study.

Key Terms and Concepts Found in a list at the beginning of each chapter, these terms will create an expanded vocabulary.

of change. There are five steps included in the framework: knowledge, persuasion, decision, implementation/trial, and confirmation. During the knowledge step, the innovation is described so that the decision-making unit develops an understanding of the suggested change. Next, the change agent works to develop favorable attitudes toward the innovation and subsequently a decision is made to adopt or reject the innovation. During the implementation or trial step, the innovation is in place and adjustments may occur. Finally, during the step of confirmation, the decision-making unit seeks reinforcement that the decision was correct, or they may choose to reverse the decision (Sellers & McCrea, 2014, p. 360).

Conclusion

Numerous models are available in the literature to guide nurses in the use of evidence-based practice. The models share similarities and differences but do have a common foundation because all use a planned action approach to moving knowledge to practice. The steps taken together provide a process for locating and synthesizing knowledge, and systematically using the change process for integrating and sustaining evidence-based changes in practice (Tracy & Barnsteiner, 2014).

Currently, the greatest challenge we face in fully implementing evidence-based practice in nursing as a profession is how to get the evidence to the practicing nurse. Nurses are very busy taking care of patients. From the perspective of the individual, it can indeed be daunting, especially when many practicing nurses are not knowledgeable about evidence-based nursing practice. Nevertheless, daunting or not, the impetus for evidence-based practice will continue to grow. As healthcare costs continue to climb, consistent, data-based answers to patient care problems are an expectation.

CASE STUDY 10-1 • MR. P.

Mr. P. is a 52-year-old, married, Hispanic male who is approximately 100 pounds overweight. Mr. P. has developed hypertension and adult-onset diabetes. He is currently being followed in a clinic setting. As a nurse working in the clinic setting, you have noticed that many of the patients you see in the clinic that are demographically similar to Mr. P. experience poorer health outcomes as compared with your patients who are members of different patient populations.

Case Study Questions

1. What PICO(T) questions can you ask to generate evidence for the patient population and patient problem(s) represented in the case study?
2. Based on a search of the literature, your expertise, and what you know about the preferences of this patient population, what are some evidence-based nursing interventions that you might want to translate into clinical practice in this clinic setting?

> *Case Studies* Case studies encourage active learning and promote critical thinking skills in learners. Students can read about real-life scenarios, and then analyze the situation they are presented with.

Strategies for overcoming barriers and increasing adoption of evidence-based practice within an organization include:

- Specific identification of the facilitators and barriers to evidence-based practice. This will require administrative support by providing the time and the funds for necessary resources as well as enhancement of job descriptions to include criteria related to evidence-based practice.
- Education and training to improve knowledge and strengthen beliefs related to the benefits of evidence-based practice. This may require offering incentives such as a paid registration to a conference for the best clinical question in a unit-wide contest.
- Creation of an environment that encourages an inquisitive approach to patient care. Achievement of this environment may require the development of a center of evidence-based practice, access to electronic resources in the workplace, providing opportunities for nurses to collaborate with nurse researchers or faculty with nursing research expertise, and providing opportunities to disseminate the results of evidence-based practice projects (Houser, 2011, p. 12).

Whichever strategies are incorporated, it is important to note that multifaceted interventions are much more likely to be effective in facilitating evidence-based practice within an organization. It is also important to note that once evidence-based practice projects are complete, passive dissemination of results within an organization is ineffective in changing practice.

Searching for Evidence

Competencies expected of the nurse include reading original research and evidence reports related to the practice area and the ability to locate relevant evidence reports and guidelines (QSEN, 2015). In order to find the evidence, the nurse must learn to ask clinical questions and search electronic indexes and other resources.

Asking the Question

Nurses must learn to ask questions in a format that facilitates searching for evidence. Developing a question that accurately reflects the practice to be evaluated, in a format that focuses the search for evidence, is a good place to begin (Tracy & Barnsteiner, 2014). It has been suggested that all nurses should learn how to use the PICO(T) format to ask clinical questions. PICO(T) is simply an acronym that assists in the formatting of clinical questions. Using this format helps the nurse to ask pertinent clinical questions, focus on asking the right questions, and choose relevant guidelines.

CRITICAL THINKING QUESTIONS

How is new evidence disseminated to the bedside nurse in the organization in which you practice as a nursing student? How does the organization promote evidence-based practice? Do the nurses in the organization use current evidence in practice?

> *Critical Thinking Questions* Review key concepts with these questions in each chapter.

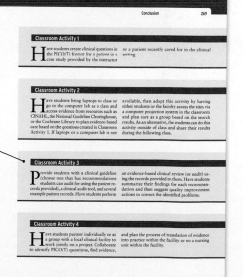

Classroom Activity 1

Have students create clinical questions in the PICO(T) format for a patient in a case study provided by the instructor or a patient recently cared for in the clinical setting.

Classroom Activity 2

Have students bring laptops to class or go to the computer lab as a class and access evidence from resources such as CINAHL, the National Guideline Clearinghouse, or the Cochrane Library to plan evidence-based care based on the questions created in Classroom Activity 1. If laptops or a computer lab is not available, then adapt this activity by having either students or the faculty access the sites via a computer projection system in the classroom and plan care as a group based on the search results. As an alternative, the students can do this activity outside of class and share their results during the following class.

Classroom Activity 3

Provide students with a clinical guideline (choose one that has recommendations students can audit for using the patient records provided), a clinical audit tool, and several example patient records. Have students perform an evidence-based clinical review (or audit) using the records provided to them. Have students summarize their findings for each recommendation and then suggest quality improvement actions to correct the identified problems.

Classroom Activity 4

Have students partner individually or as a group with a local clinical facility to work jointly on a project. Collaborate to identify PICO(T) questions, find evidence, and plan the process of translation of evidence into practice within the facility or on a nursing unit within the facility.

> *Classroom Activities* Each chapter includes classroom activities that focus on how the information in the text applies to everyday practice. Students can answer questions in a group or as individuals.

Edited by

KATHLEEN MASTERS, DNS, RN

Professor
University of Southern Mississippi
College of Nursing
Hattiesburg, Mississippi

Role Development
in Professional
Nursing Practice

FOURTH EDITION

JONES & BARTLETT
LEARNING

World Headquarters
Jones & Bartlett Learning
5 Wall Street
Burlington, MA 01803
978-443-5000
info@jblearning.com
www.jblearning.com

Jones & Bartlett Learning books and products are available through most bookstores and online booksellers. To contact Jones & Bartlett Learning directly, call 800-832-0034, fax 978-443-8000, or visit our website, www.jblearning.com.

Substantial discounts on bulk quantities of Jones & Bartlett Learning publications are available to corporations, professional associations, and other qualified organizations. For details and specific discount information, contact the special sales department at Jones & Bartlett Learning via the above contact information or send an email to specialsales@jblearning.com.

08323-1

Production Credits
VP, Executive Publisher: David D. Cella
Executive Editor: Amanda Martin
Acquisitions Editor: Teresa Reilly
Editorial Assistant: Danielle Bessette
Production Editor: Vanessa Richards
Senior Marketing Manager: Jennifer Scherzay
VP, Manufacturing and Inventory Control: Therese Connell

Composition: Integra Software Services Pvt. Ltd.
Cover Design: Kristin E. Parker
Rights & Media Specialist: Wes DeShano
Media Development Editor: Shannon Sheehan
Cover Image: © robertiez/iStock/Getty Images Plus/Getty
Printing and Binding: RR Donnelley
Cover Printing: RR Donnelley

Library of Congress Cataloging-in-Publication Data
Role development in professional nursing practice / [edited by] Kathleen Masters. – Fourth edition.
      p. ; cm.
   Includes bibliographical references and index.
   ISBN 978-1-284-07832-9 (pbk.)
   I. Masters, Kathleen, editor.
   [DNLM: 1. Nursing–standards. 2. Nursing–trends. 3. Nurse's Role. 4. Philosophy, Nursing.
   5. Professional Practice. WY 16]
   RT82
   610.73–dc23
                                                    2015022040
6048

Printed in the United States of America
20 19 18 17 16   10 9 8 7 6 5 4 3 2

Dedication

This book is dedicated to my Heavenly Father and to my loving family: my husband, Eddie, and my two daughters, Rebecca and Rachel. Words cannot express my appreciation for their ongoing encouragement and support throughout my career.

CONTENTS

PREFACE

Although the process of professional development is a lifelong journey, it is a journey that begins in earnest during the time of initial academic preparation. The goal of this book is to provide nursing students with a road map to help guide them along their journey as a professional nurse.

This book is organized into two units. The chapters in the first unit focus on the foundational concepts that are essential to the development of the individual professional nurse. The chapters in Unit II address issues related to professional nursing practice and the management of patient care, specifically in the context of quality and safety. In the fourth edition, the chapter content is conceptualized, when applicable, around nursing competencies, professional standards, and recommendations from national groups, such as Institute of Medicine reports.

The chapters included in Unit I provide the student nurse with a basic foundation in areas such as nursing history, theory, philosophy, ethics, socialization into the nursing role, and the social context of nursing. All chapters have been updated, and several chapters in Unit I have been expanded in this edition. Revisions to the chapter on nursing history include the addition of contributions of prominent nurses and achievements related to nursing in the United Kingdom, Canada, and Australia. The theory chapter now includes additional nursing theorists as well as a brief overview of several non-nursing theories frequently used in nursing research and practice. The social context of nursing chapter now incorporates not only societal trends, but also trends in nursing practice and education. The chapter related to professional career development in nursing has been completely rewritten for this edition.

The chapters in Unit II are more directly related to patient care management. In the fourth edition, Unit II chapter topics are presented in the context of quality and safety. Chapter topics include the role of the nurse in patient safety, the role of the nurse in quality improvement, evidence-based nursing practice, the role of the nurse in patient-centered care, informatics in nursing practice, the role of the nurse related to teamwork and collaboration, ethical issues in nursing practice, and the law as it relates to patient care and nursing. Most Unit II chapters have undergone major revisions with a refocus of the content on recommended nursing and healthcare competencies.

The fourth edition continues to incorporate the *Nurse of the Future: Nursing Core Competencies* throughout each chapter. The *Nurse of the Future: Nursing Core Competencies* "emanate from the foundation of nursing knowledge" (Massachusetts Department of Higher Education, 2010, p. 4) and are based on the American Association of Colleges of Nursing's *Essentials of Baccalaureate Education for Professional Nursing Practice*, National League for Nursing Council of Associate Degree Nursing competencies, Institute of Medicine recommendations, Quality and Safety Education for Nurses (QSEN) competencies, and American Nurses Association standards, as well as other professional organization standards and recommendations. The 10 competencies included in the model are patient-centered care, professionalism, informatics and technology, evidence-based practice, leadership, systems-based practice, safety, communication, teamwork and collaboration, and quality improvement. Essential knowledge, skills, and attitudes (KSA)

BOARD OF HIGHER EDUCATION NURSING INITIATIVE
NURSING CORE COMPETENCIES
The science and practice of nursing

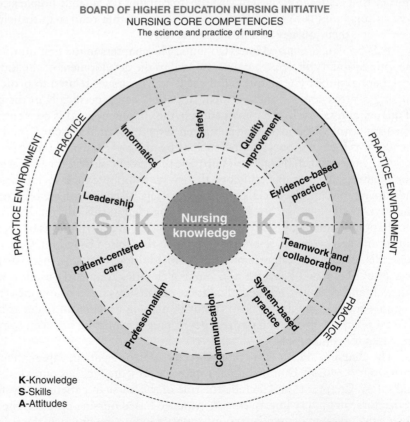

K-Knowledge
S-Skills
A-Attitudes

Source: Modified from Massachusetts Department of Higher Education. (2010). *Nurse of the future: Nursing core competencies* (p. 5). Retrieved from http://www.mass.edu/currentinit /documents/NursingCoreCompetencies.pdf. Used with permission of the Massachusetts Department of Higher Education Nurse of the Future Competency Committee, Boston, MA, October 2015.

reflecting cognitive, psychomotor, and affective learning domains are specified for each competency. The KSA identified in the model reflect the expectations for initial nursing practice following the completion of a prelicensure professional nursing education program (Massachusetts Department of Higher Education, 2010, p. 4).

The *Nurse of the Future: Nursing Core Competencies* graphic illustrates through the use of broken lines the reciprocal and continuous relationship between each of the competencies and nursing knowledge, that the competencies can overlap and are not mutually exclusive, and that all competencies are of equal importance. In addition, nursing knowledge is placed as the core in the graphic to illustrate that nursing knowledge reflects the overarching art and science of professional nursing practice (Massachusetts Department of Higher Education, 2010, p. 4).

This new edition has competency boxes throughout the chapters that link examples of the KSA appropriate to the chapter content to *Nurse of the Future: Nursing Core Competencies* required of entry-level professional nurses. The competency model in its entirety is available online at www.mass .edu/currentinit/documents/NursingCoreCompetencies.pdf.

This new edition continues to use case studies, congruent with Benner, Sutphen, Leonard, and Day's (2010) Carnegie Report recommendations that nursing educators teach for "situated cognition" using narrative strategies to lead to "situated action," thus increasing the clinical connection in our teaching or that we teach for "clinical salience." In addition, critical thinking questions are included throughout each chapter to promote student reflection on the chapter concepts. Classroom activities are also provided based on chapter content. Additional resources not connected to this text, but applicable to the content herein, include a toolkit focused on the nursing core competencies available at www.mass.edu/nahi/documents/Toolkit-First%20Edition -May%202014-r1.pdf and teaching activities related to nursing competencies available on the QSEN website at www.qsen.org/teaching-strategies/.

Although the topics included in this textbook are not inclusive of all that could be discussed in relationship to the broad theme of role development in professional nursing practice, it is my prayer that the subjects herein make a contribution to the profession of nursing by providing the student with a solid foundation and a desire to grow as a professional nurse throughout the journey that we call a professional nursing career. Let the journey begin.

—*Kathleen Masters*

References

Benner, P., Sutphen, M., Leonard, V., & Day, L. (2010). *Educating nurses: A call for radical transformation*. San Francisco, CA: Jossey-Bass.

Massachusetts Department of Higher Education. (2010). *Nurse of the future: Nursing core competencies*. Retrieved from http://www.mass.edu/currentinit/documents /NursingCoreCompetencies.pdf

CONTRIBUTORS

Janie B. Butts, PhD, RN
University of Southern Mississippi
College of Nursing
Hattiesburg, Mississippi

Cynthia Chatham, DSN, RN
University of Southern Mississippi
College of Nursing
Long Beach, Mississippi

Mary Louise Coyne, DNSc, RN
University of Southern Mississippi
College of Nursing
Long Beach, Mississippi

Kathleen Driscoll, JD, MS, RN
University of Cincinnati
College of Nursing
Cincinnati, Ohio

Rowena W. Elliott, PhD, RN, FAAN
University of Southern Mississippi
College of Nursing
Hattiesburg, Mississippi

Melanie Gilmore, PhD, RN
University of Southern Mississippi
College of Nursing
Hattiesburg, Mississippi

Cathy K. Hughes, DNP, RN
University of Southern Mississippi
College of Nursing
Hattiesburg, Mississippi

Karen Saucier Lundy, PhD, RN, FAAN
Professor Emeritus
University of Southern Mississippi
College of Nursing
Hattiesburg, Mississippi

Evadna Lyons, PhD, RN
East Central Community College
School of Nursing
Decatur, Mississippi

Katherine Elizabeth Nugent, PhD, RN
Dean, College of Nursing
University of Southern Mississippi
Hattiesburg, Mississippi

Karen L. Rich, PhD, RN
University of Southern Mississippi
College of Nursing
Long Beach, Mississippi

Jill Rushing, MSN, RN
University of Southern Mississippi
College of Nursing
Hattiesburg, Mississippi

Mary W. Stewart, PhD, RN
Director of PhD Program
University of Mississippi Medical Center
School of Nursing
Jackson, Mississippi

Sharon Vincent, DNP, RN, CNOR
University of North Carolina
College of Nursing
Charlotte, North Carolina

Foundations of Professional Nursing Practice

CHAPTER 1

A History of Health Care and Nursing

Karen Saucier Lundy and Kathleen Masters

Learning Objectives

After completing this chapter, the student should be able to:

1. Identify social, political, and economic influences on the development of professional nursing practice.

2. Identify important leaders and events that have significantly affected the development of professional nursing practice.

Although no specialized nurse role per se developed in early civilizations, human cultures recognized the need for nursing care. The truly sick person was weak and helpless and could not fulfill the duties that were normally expected of a member of the community. In such cases, someone had to watch over the patient, nurse him or her, and provide care. In most societies, this nurse role was filled by a family member, usually female. As in most cultures, the childbearing woman had special needs that often resulted in a specialized role for the caregiver. Every society since the dawn of time had someone to nurse and take care of the mother and infant around the childbearing events. In whatever form the nurse took, the role was associated with compassion, health promotion, and kindness (Bullough & Bullough, 1978).

Classical Era

More than 4,000 years ago, Egyptian physicians and nurses used an abundant pharmacological repertoire to cure the ill and injured. The Ebers Papyrus lists more than 700 remedies for ailments ranging from snakebites to puerperal fever (Kalisch & Kalisch, 1986). Healing appeared in

Key Terms and Concepts

» Greek era
» Roman era
» Deaconesses
» Florence Nightingale
» Reformation
» Chadwick Report
» Shattuck Report
» William Rathbone
» Ethel Fenwick
» Jeanne Mance
» Mary Agnes Snively
» Goldmark Report
» Brown Report
» Isabel Hampton Robb
» American Nurses Association (ANA)
» Lavinia Lloyd Dock
» *American Journal of Nursing (AJN)*
» Margaret Sanger
» Lillian Wald
» Jane A. Delano
» Annie Goodrich

Note: This chapter is adapted from Lundy, K. S., & Bender, K. W. (2009). History of community health and public health nursing. In K. S. Lundy & S. Janes (Eds.), *Community health nursing: Caring for the public's health* (2nd ed., 62–99). Sudbury, MA: Jones and Bartlett.

the Egyptian culture as the successful result of a contest between invisible beings of good and evil (Shryock, 1959). Around 1000 B.C., the Egyptians constructed elaborate drainage systems, developed pharmaceutical herbs and preparations, and embalmed the dead. The Hebrews formulated an elaborate hygiene code that dealt with laws governing both personal and community hygiene, such as contagion, disinfection, and sanitation through the preparation of food and water. The Jewish contribution to health is greater in sanitation than in their concept of disease. Garbage and excreta were disposed of outside the city or camp, infectious diseases were quarantined, spitting was outlawed as unhygienic, and bodily cleanliness became a prerequisite for moral purity. Although many of the Hebrew ideas about hygiene were Egyptian in origin, the Hebrews were the first to codify them and link them with spiritual godliness (Bullough & Bullough, 1978).

Disease and disability in the Mesopotamian area were considered a great curse, a divine punishment for grievous acts against the gods. Experiencing illness as punishment for a sin linked the sick person to anything even remotely deviant. Not only was the person suffering from the illness, but he or she also was branded by all of society as having deserved it. Those who obeyed God's law lived in health and happiness, and those who transgressed the law were punished with illness and suffering. The sick person then had to make atonement for the sins, enlist a priest or other spiritual healer to lift the curse, or live with the illness to its ultimate outcome (Bullough & Bullough, 1978). Nursing care by a family member or relative would be needed, regardless of the outcome of the sin, curse, disease-atonement-recovery, or death cycle. This logic became the basis for explanation of why some people "get sick and some don't" for many centuries and still persists to some degree in most cultures today.

The Greeks and Health

In Greek mythology, the god of medicine, Asclepias, cured disease. One of his daughters, Hygeia, from whom we derive the word *hygiene*, was the goddess of preventive health and protected humans from disease. Panacea, Asclepias' other daughter, was known as the all-healing "universal remedy," and today her name is used to describe any ultimate cure-all in medicine. She was known as the "light" of the day, and her name was invoked and shrines built to her during times of epidemics (Brooke, 1997).

During the **Greek era**, Hippocrates of Cos emphasized the rational treatment of sickness as a natural rather than god-inflicted phenomenon. Hippocrates (460–370 B.C.) is considered the father of medicine because of his arrangements of the oral and written remedies and diseases, which had long been secrets held by priests and religious healers, into a textbook of medicine that was used for centuries (Bullough & Bullough, 1978).

In Greek society, health was considered to result from a balance between mind and body. Hippocrates wrote a most important book, *Air, Water and Places*, which detailed the relationship between humans and the environment. This is considered a milestone in the eventual development of the science of epidemiology as the first such treatise on the connectedness of the web of life. This topic of the relationship between humans and their environment did not reoccur until the development of bacteriology in the late 1800s (Rosen, 1958).

Perhaps the idea that most damaged the practice and scientific theory of medicine and health for centuries was the doctrine of the four humors, first spoken of by Empedocles of Acragas (493–433 B.C.). Empedocles was a philosopher and a physician, and as a result, he synthesized his cosmological ideas with his medical theory. He believed that the same four elements that made up the universe were found in humans and in all animate beings (Bullough & Bullough, 1978). Empedocles believed that man was a microcosm, a small world within the macrocosm, or external environment. The four humors of the body (blood, bile, phlegm, and black bile) corresponded to the four elements of the larger world (fire, air, water, and earth) (Kalisch & Kalisch, 1986). Depending on the prevailing humor, a person was sanguine, choleric, phlegmatic, or melancholic. Because of this strongly held and persistent belief in the connection between the balance of the four humors and health status, treatment was aimed at restoring the appropriate balance of the four humors through the control of their corresponding elements. Through manipulating the two sets of opposite qualities—hot and cold, wet and dry—balance was the goal of the intervention. Fire was hot and dry, air was hot and wet, water was cold and wet, and earth was cold and dry. For example, if a person had a fever, cold compresses would be prescribed; for a chill the person would be warmed. Such doctrine gave rise to faulty and ineffective treatment of disease that influenced medical education for many years (Taylor, 1922).

Plato, in *The Republic*, details the importance of recreation, a balanced mind and body, nutrition, and exercise. A distinction was made among gender, class, and health as early as the Greek era; only males of the aristocracy could afford the luxury of maintaining a healthful lifestyle (Rosen, 1958).

In *The Iliad*, a poem about the attempts to capture Troy and rescue Helen from her lover Paris, 140 different wounds are described. The mortality rate averaged 77.6%, the highest as a result of sword and spear thrusts and the lowest from superficial arrow wounds. There was considerable need for nursing care, and Achilles, Patroclus, and other princes often acted as nurses to the injured. The early stages of Greek medicine reflected the influences of Egyptian, Babylonian, and Hebrew medicine. Therefore, good medical and nursing techniques were used to treat these war wounds: The arrow was drawn or cut out, the wound washed, soothing herbs applied, and the wound bandaged. However, in sickness in which no wound occurred, an evil spirit was considered the cause. The Greeks applied rational causes and cures to external injuries, while internal ailments continued to be linked to spiritual maladies (Bullough & Bullough, 1978).

Roman Era

During the rise and the fall of the **Roman era** (31 B.C.–A.D. 476), Greek culture continued to be a strong influence. The Romans easily adopted Greek culture and expanded the Greeks' accomplishments, especially in the fields of engineering, law, and government. For Romans, the government had an obligation to protect its citizens, not only from outside aggression such as warring neighbors, but from inside the civilization, in the form of health laws. According to Bullough and Bullough (1978), Rome was essentially a "Greek cultural colony" (p. 20).

Galen of Pergamum (A.D. 129–199), often known as the greatest Greek physician after Hippocrates, left for Rome after studying medicine in Greece and Egypt and gained great fame as a medical practitioner, lecturer, and experimenter. In his lifetime, medicine evolved into a science; he submitted traditional healing practices to experimentation and was possibly the greatest medical researcher before the 1600s (Bullough & Bullough, 1978). He was considered the last of the great physicians of antiquity (Kalisch & Kalisch, 1986).

The Greek physicians and healers certainly made the most contributions to medicine, but the Romans surpassed the Greeks in promoting the evolution of nursing. Roman armies developed the notion of a mobile war nursing unit because their battles took them far from home where they could be cared for by wives and family. This portable hospital was a series of tents arranged in corridors; as battles wore on, these tents gave way to buildings that became permanent convalescent camps at the battle sites (Rosen, 1958). Many of these early military hospitals have been excavated by archaeologists along the banks of the Rhine and Danube Rivers. They had wards, recreation areas, baths, pharmacies, and even rooms for officers who needed a "rest cure" (Bullough & Bullough, 1978). Coexisting were the Greek dispensary forms of temples, or the *iatreia*, which started out as a type of physician waiting room. These eventually developed into a primitive type of hospital, places for surgical clients to stay until they could be taken home by their families. Although nurses during the Roman era were usually family members, servants, or slaves, nursing had strengthened its position in medical care and emerged during the Roman era as a separate and distinct specialty.

The Romans developed massive aqueducts, bathhouses, and sewer systems during this era. At the height of the Roman Empire, Rome provided 40 gallons of water per person per day to its 1 million inhabitants, which is comparable to our rates of consumption today (Rosen, 1958).

Middle Ages

Many of the advancements of the Greco-Roman era were reversed during the Middle Ages (A.D. 476–1453) after the decline of the Roman Empire. The Middle Ages, or the medieval era, served as a transition between ancient and modern civilizations. Once again, myth, magic, and religion were explanations and cures for illness and health problems. The medieval world was the result of a fusion of three streams of thought, actions, and ways of life—Greco-Roman, Germanic, and Christian—into one (Donahue, 1985). Nursing was most influenced by Christianity with the beginning of **deaconesses**, or female servants, doing the work of God by ministering to the needs of others. Deacons in the early Christian churches were apparently available only to care for men, while deaconesses cared for the needs of women. The role of deaconesses in the church was considered a forward step in the development of nursing and in the 1800s would strongly influence the young **Florence Nightingale**. During this era, Roman military hospitals were replaced by civilian ones. In early Christianity, the *Diakonia*, a kind of combination outpatient and welfare office, was managed by deacons and deaconesses and served as the equivalent of a hospital. Jesus served as the example of charity and compassion for the poor and marginal of society.

Communicable diseases were rampant during the Middle Ages, primarily because of the walled cities that emerged in response to the paranoia and isolation of the populations. Infection was next to impossible to control. Physicians had little to offer, deferring to the church for management of disease. Nursing roles were carried out primarily by religious orders.

The oldest hospital (other than military hospitals in the Roman era) in Europe was most likely the *Hôtel-Dieu* in Lyons, France, founded about 542 by Childebert I, king of France. The *Hôtel-Dieu* in Paris was founded around 652 by Saint Landry, bishop of Paris. During the Middle Ages, charitable institutions, hospitals, and medical schools increased in number, with the religious leaders as caregivers. The word *hospital*, which is derived from the Latin word *hospitalis*, meaning service of guests, was most likely more of a shelter for travelers and other pilgrims as well as the occasional person who needed extra care (Kalisch & Kalisch, 1986). Early European hospitals were more like hospices or homes for the aged, sick pilgrims, or orphans. Nurses in these early hospitals were religious deaconesses who chose to care for others in a life of servitude and spiritual sacrifice.

Black Death

During the Middle Ages, a series of horrible epidemics, including the Black Death or bubonic plague, ravaged the civilized world (Diamond, 1997). In the 1300s, Europe, Asia, and Africa saw nearly half their populations lost to the bubonic plague. Worldwide, more than 60 million deaths were attributed to this horrible plague. In some parts of Europe, only one-fourth of the population survived, with some places having too few survivors alive to bury the dead. Families abandoned sick children and the sick were often left to die alone (Cartwright, 1972).

Nurses and physicians were powerless to avert the disease. Black spots and tumors on the skin appeared, and petechiae and hemorrhages gave the skin a darkened appearance. There was also acute inflammation of the lungs, burning sensations, unquenchable thirst, and inflammation of the entire body. Hardly anyone afflicted survived the third day of the attack. So great was the fear of contagion that ships carrying bodies of infected persons were set to sail without a crew to drift from port to port through the North, Black, and Mediterranean Seas with their dead passengers (Cohen, 1989).

Medieval people knew that this disease was in some way communicable, but they were unsure of the mode of transmission (Diamond, 1997); hence the avoidance of victims and a reliance on isolation techniques. During this time, the practice of quarantine in city ports was developed as a preventive measure that is still used today (Bullough & Bullough, 1978; Kalisch & Kalisch, 1986).

The Renaissance

During the rebirth of Europe, political, social, and economic advances occurred along with a tremendous revival of learning. Donahue (1985) contends that the Renaissance has been "viewed as both a blessing and a curse" (p. 188). There was a renewed interest in the arts and sciences, which helped advance medical science (Boorstin, 1985; Bullough & Bullough, 1978). Columbus and other explorers discovered new worlds, and belief in a sun-centered rather than an Earth-centered universe was promoted by Copernicus (1473–1543). Sir Isaac Newton's (1642–1727) theory of gravity changed the world forever. Gunpowder was introduced, and social and religious upheavals resulted in the American and French Revolutions at the end of the 1700s. In the arts and sciences, Leonardo da Vinci, known as one of "the greatest geniuses of all time," made a number of anatomic drawings based on dissection experiences. These drawings have become classics in the progression of knowledge about the human anatomy. Many artists of this time left an indelible mark and continue to exert influence today, including Michelangelo, Raphael, and Titian (Donahue, 1985).

The Reformation

Religious changes during the Renaissance influenced nursing perhaps more than any other aspect of society. Particularly important was the rise of Protestantism as a result of the reform movements of Martin Luther (1483–1546) in Germany and John Calvin (1509–1564) in France and Switzerland. Although the various sects were numerous in the Protestant movement, the agreement among the leaders was almost unanimous on the abolition of the monastic or cloistered career. The effects on nursing were drastic: Monastic-affiliated institutions, including hospitals and schools, were closed, and orders of nuns, including nurses, were dissolved. Even in countries where Catholicism flourished, royal leaders seized monasteries frequently.

Religious leaders, such as Martin Luther, who led the **Reformation** in 1517, were well aware of the lack of adequate nursing care as a result of these sweeping changes. Luther advocated that each town establish something akin to a "community chest" to raise funds for hospitals and nurse visitors for the poor (Dietz & Lehozky, 1963). Thus, the closures of the monasteries eventually resulted in the creation of public hospitals where laywomen performed nursing care. It was difficult to find laywomen who were willing to work in these hospitals to care for the sick, so judges began giving prostitutes, publically intoxicated women, and poverty-stricken women the option of going to jail, going to the poorhouse, or working in the public hospital. Unlike the sick wards in monasteries, which were generally considered to be clean and well managed, the public hospitals were filthy, disorganized buildings where people went to die while being cared for by laywomen who were not trained, motivated, or qualified to care for the sick (Sitzman & Judd, 2014a).

In England, where there had been at least 450 charitable foundations before the Reformation, only a few survived the reign of Henry VIII, who closed most of the monastic hospitals (Donahue, 1985). Eventually, Henry VIII's son, Edward VI, who reigned from 1547 to 1553, endowed some hospitals, namely, St. Bartholomew's Hospital and St. Thomas' Hospital, which would eventually house the Nightingale School of Nursing later in the 1800s (Bullough & Bullough, 1978).

The Dark Period of Nursing

The last half of the period between 1500 and 1860 is widely regarded as the "dark period of nursing" because nursing conditions were at their worst (Donahue, 1985). Education for girls, which had been provided by the nuns in religious schools, was lost. Because of the elimination of hospitals and schools, there was no one to pass on knowledge about caring for the sick. As a result, the hospitals were managed and staffed by municipal authorities; women entering nursing service often came from illiterate classes, and even then, there were too few to serve (Dietz & Lehozky, 1963). The lay attendants who filled the nursing role were illiterate, rough, inconsiderate, and often immoral and alcoholic. Intelligent women and men could not be persuaded to accept such a degraded and low-status position in the offensive municipal hospitals of London. Nursing slipped back into a role of servitude as menial, low-status work. According to Donahue (1985), when a woman could no longer make it as a gambler, prostitute, or thief, she might become a nurse. Eventually, women serving jail sentences for crimes such as prostitution and stealing were ordered to care for the sick in the hospitals instead of serving their sentences in the city jail (Dietz & Lehozky, 1963). The nurses of this era took bribes from clients, became inappropriately involved with them, and survived the best way they could, often at the expense of their assigned clients.

Nursing had, during this era, virtually no social standing or organization. Even Catholic sisters of the religious orders throughout Europe "came to a complete standstill" professionally because of the intolerance of society (Donahue, 1985, p. 231). Charles Dickens, in *Martin Chuzzlewit* (1844), created the enduring characters of Sairey Gamp and Betsy Prig. Sairey Gamp was a visiting nurse based on an actual hired attendant whom Dickens had met in a friend's home. Sairey Gamp was hired to care for sick family members but was instead cruel to her clients, stole from them, and ate their rations; she was an alcoholic and has been immortalized forever as a reminder of the world in which Florence Nightingale came of age (Donahue, 1985).

In the New World, the first hospital in the Americas, the *Hospital de la Purísima Concepción*, was founded some time before 1524 by Hernando Cortez, the conqueror of Mexico. The first hospital in the continental United States was erected in Manhattan in 1658 for the care of sick soldiers and slaves. In 1717, a hospital for infectious diseases was built in Boston; the first hospital established by a private gift was the Charity Hospital in New Orleans. A sailor, Jean Louis, donated the endowment for the hospital's founding (Bullough & Bullough, 1978).

During the 1600s and 1700s, colonial hospitals with little resemblance to modern hospitals were often used to house the poor and downtrodden. Hospitals called "pesthouses" were created to care for clients with contagious diseases; their primary purpose was to protect the public at large, rather than to treat and care for the clients. Contagious diseases were rampant during the early years of the American colonies, often being spread by the large number of immigrants who brought these diseases with them on their long journey to America. Medicine was not as developed as in Europe, and nursing remained in the hands of the uneducated. By 1720, average life expectancy at birth was only around 35 years. Plagues were a constant nightmare, with outbreaks of smallpox and yellow fever. In 1751, the first true hospital in the new colonies, Pennsylvania Hospital, was erected in Philadelphia on the recommendation of Benjamin Franklin (Kalisch & Kalisch, 1986).

By today's standards, hospitals in the 1800s were disgraceful, dirty, unventilated, and contaminated by infections; to be a client in a hospital actually increased one's risk of dying. As in England, nursing was considered an inferior occupation. After the sweeping changes of the Reformation, educated religious health workers were replaced with lay people who were "down and outers," in prison, or had no option left but to work with the sick (Kalisch & Kalisch, 1986).

The Industrial Revolution

During the mid-1700s in England, capitalism emerged as an economic system based on profit. This emerging system resulted in mass production, as contrasted with the previous system of individual workers and craftsmen. In the simplest terms, the Industrial Revolution was the application of machine power to processes formerly done by hand. Machinery was invented during this era and ultimately standardized quality; individual craftsmen were forced to give up their crafts and lands and become factory laborers for the capitalist owners. All types of industries were affected; this new-found efficiency produced profit for owners of the means of production. Because of this, the era of invention flourished, factories grew, and people moved in record numbers to the work in the cities. Urban areas grew, tenement housing projects emerged, and overcrowding in cities seriously threatened individuals' well-being (Donahue, 1985).

Workers were forced to go to the machines, rather than the other way around. Such relocations meant giving up not only farming, but a way of life that had existed for centuries. The emphasis on profit over people led to child labor, frequent layoffs, and long workdays filled with stressful, tedious, unfamiliar work. Labor unions did not exist, and neither was there any legal protection against exploitation of workers, including children (Donahue, 1985). All these rapid changes and often threatening conditions created the world of Charles Dickens, where, as in his book *Oliver Twist*, children worked as adults without question.

According to Donahue (1985), urban life, trade, and industrialization contributed to these overwhelming health hazards, and the situation was confounded by the lack of an adequate means of social control. Reforms were desperately needed, and the social reform movement emerged in response to the unhealthy by-products of the Industrial Revolution. It was in this world of the 1800s that reformers such as John Stuart Mill (1806–1873) emerged. Although the Industrial Revolution began in England, it quickly spread to the rest of Europe and to the United States (Bullough & Bullough, 1978). The reform movement is critical to understanding the emerging health concerns that were later addressed by Florence Nightingale. Mill championed popular education, the emancipation of women, trade unions, and religious toleration. Other reform issues of the era included the abolition of slavery and, most important for nursing, more humane care of the sick, the poor, and the wounded (Bullough & Bullough, 1978). There was a renewed energy in the religious community with the reemergence of new religious orders in the Catholic Church that provided service to the sick and disenfranchised.

Epidemics had ravaged Europe for centuries, but they became even more serious with urbanization. Industrialization brought people to cities, where they worked in close quarters (as compared with the isolation of the farm), and contributed to the social decay of the second half of the 1800s. Sanitation was poor or nonexistent, sewage disposal from the growing population was lacking, cities were filthy, public laws were weak or nonexistent, and congestion of the cities inevitably brought pests in the form of rats, lice, and bedbugs, which transmitted many pathogens. Communicable diseases continued to plague the population, especially those who lived in these unsanitary environments. For example, during the mid-1700s typhus and typhoid fever claimed twice as many lives each year as did the Battle of Waterloo (Hanlon & Pickett, 1984). Through foreign trade and immigration, infectious diseases were spread to all of Europe and eventually to the growing United States.

The Chadwick Report

Edwin Chadwick became a major figure in the development of the field of public health in Great Britain by drawing attention to the cost of the unsanitary conditions that shortened the life span of the laboring class and threatened the wealth of Britain. Although the first sanitation legislation, which established a National Vaccination Board, was passed in 1837, Chadwick found in his classic study, *Report on an Inquiry into the Sanitary Conditions of the Labouring Population of Great Britain*, that death rates were high in large industrial cities such as Liverpool. A more startling finding, from what is often referred to simply as the **Chadwick Report**, was that more than half the children of labor-class workers died by age 5, indicating poor living conditions that affected the health of the most vulnerable. Laborers lived only half as long as the upper classes.

One consequence of the report was the establishment in 1848 of the first board of health, the General Board of Health for England (Richardson, 1887). More legislation followed that initiated social reform in the areas of child welfare, elder care, the sick, the mentally ill, factory health, and education. Soon sewers and fireplugs, based on an available water supply, appeared as indicators that the public health linkages from the Chadwick Report had an impact.

The Shattuck Report

In the United States during the 1800s, waves of epidemics of yellow fever, smallpox, cholera, typhoid fever, and typhus continued to plague the population as in England and the rest of the world. As cities continued to grow in the industrialized young nation, poor workers crowded into larger cities and suffered from illnesses caused by the unsanitary living conditions (Hanlon & Pickett, 1984). Similar to Chadwick's classic study in England, Lemuel Shattuck, a Boston bookseller and publisher who had an interest in public health, organized the American Statistical Society in 1839 and issued a census of Boston in 1845. Shattuck's census revealed high infant mortality rates and high overall population mortality rates. In 1850, in his *Report of the Massachusetts Sanitary Commission*, Shattuck not only outlined his findings on the unsanitary conditions, but also made recommendations for public health reform that included the bookkeeping of population statistics and development of a monitoring system that would provide information to the public about environmental, food, and drug safety and infectious disease control (Rosen, 1958). He also called for services for well-child care, school-age children's health, immunizations, mental health, health education for all, and health planning. The **Shattuck Report** was revolutionary in its scope and vision for public health, but it was virtually ignored during Shattuck's lifetime. Nineteen years later, in 1869, the first state board of health was formed (Kalisch & Kalisch, 1986).

And Then There Was Nightingale...

Florence Nightingale was named one of the 100 most influential persons of the last millennium by *Life* magazine (The 100 people who made the millennium, 1997). She was one of only eight women identified as such. Of those eight women, including Joan of Arc, Helen Keller, and Elizabeth I, Nightingale was identified as a true "angel of mercy," having reformed military health care in the Crimean War and used her political savvy to forever change the way society views the health of the vulnerable, the poor, and the forgotten. She is probably one of the most written about women in history (Bullough & Bullough, 1978). *Florence Nightingale* has become synonymous with modern nursing.

Florence Nightingale was the second child born on May 12, 1820, to the wealthy English family of William and Frances Nightingale in her namesake city, Florence, Italy. As a young child, Florence displayed incredible curiosity and intellectual abilities not common to female children of the Victorian age. She mastered the fundamentals of Greek and Latin, and she studied history, art, mathematics, and philosophy. To her family's dismay, she believed that God had called her to be a nurse. Nightingale was keenly aware of the suffering that industrialization created; she became obsessed with the plight of the miserable and suffering people. Conditions of general starvation accompanied the Industrial Revolution, prisons and workhouses overflowed, and persons in all sections of British life were displaced. She wrote in the spring of 1842, "My mind is absorbed with the sufferings of man; it besets me behind and before.... All that the poets sing of the glories of this world seem to me untrue. All the people that I see are eaten up with care or poverty or disease" (Woodham-Smith, 1951, p. 31).

For Nightingale, her entire life would be haunted by this conflict between the opulent life of gaiety that she enjoyed and the plight and misery of the world, which she was unable to alleviate. She was, in essence, an "alien spirit in the rich and aristocratic social sphere of Victorian England" (Palmer, 1977, p. 14). Nightingale remained unmarried, and at the age of 25, she expressed a desire to be trained as a nurse in an English hospital. Her parents emphatically denied her request, and for the next 7 years, she made repeated attempts to change their minds and allow her to enter nurse training. She wrote, "I crave for some regular occupation, for something worth doing instead of frittering my time away on useless trifles" (Woodham-Smith, 1951, p. 162). During this time, she continued her education through the study of math and science and spent 5 years collecting data about public health and hospitals (Dietz & Lehozky, 1963). During a tour of Egypt in 1849 with family and friends, Nightingale spent her 30th year in Alexandria with the Sisters of Charity of St. Vincent de Paul, where her conviction to study nursing was only reinforced (Tooley, 1910). While in Egypt, Nightingale studied Egyptian, Platonic, and Hermetic philosophy; Christian scripture; and the works of poets, mystics, and missionaries in her efforts to understand the nature of God and her "calling" as it fit into the divine plan (Calabria, 1996; Dossey, 2000).

The next spring, Nightingale traveled unaccompanied to the Kaiserwerth Institute in Germany and stayed there for 2 weeks, vowing to return to train as a nurse. In June 1851, Nightingale took her future into her own hands and announced to her family that she planned to return to Kaiserwerth and study nursing. According to Dietz and Lehozky (1963, p. 42), her mother had "hysterics" and scene followed scene. Her father "retreated into the shadows," and her sister, Parthe, expressed that the family name was forever disgraced (Cook, 1913).

In 1851, at the age of 31, Nightingale was finally permitted to go to Kaiserwerth, and she studied there for 3 months with Pastor Fliedner. Her family insisted that she tell no one outside the family of her whereabouts, and her mother forbade her to write any letters from Kaiserwerth. While there, Nightingale learned about the care of the sick and the importance of discipline and commitment of oneself to God (Donahue, 1985). She returned to England and cared for her then ailing father, from whom she finally gained some support for her intent to become a nurse—her lifelong dream.

In 1852, Nightingale wrote the essay "Cassandra," which stands today as a classic feminist treatise against the idleness of Victorian women. Through her voluminous journal writings, Nightingale reveals her inner struggle throughout her adulthood with what was expected of a woman and what she could accomplish with her life. The life expected of an aristocratic woman in her day was one she grew to loathe; throughout her writings, she poured out her detestation of the life of an idle woman (Nightingale, 1979, p. 5). In "Cassandra," Nightingale put her thoughts to paper, and many scholars believe that her eventual intent was to extend the essay to a novel. She wrote in "Cassandra," "Why have women passion, intellect, moral activity—these three—in a place in society where no one of the three can be exercised?" (Nightingale, 1979, p. 37). Although uncertain about the meaning of the name Cassandra, many scholars believe that it came from the Greek goddess Cassandra, who was cursed by Apollo and doomed to see and speak the truth but never to be believed. Nightingale saw the conventional life of women as a waste of time and abilities. After receiving a generous yearly endowment from her father, Nightingale moved to London and worked briefly as the superintendent of the Establishment for Gentlewomen During Illness hospital, finally realizing her dream of working as a nurse (Cook, 1913).

The Crimean Experience: "I Can Stand Out the War with Any Man"

Nightingale's opportunity for greatness came when she was offered the position of female nursing establishment of the English General Hospitals in Turkey by the secretary of war, Sir Sidney Herbert. Soon after the outbreak of the Crimean War, stories of the inadequate care and lack of medical resources for the soldiers became widely known throughout England (Woodham-Smith, 1951). The country was appalled at the conditions so vividly portrayed in the *London Times*. Pressure increased on Sir Herbert to react. He knew of one woman who was capable of bringing order out of the chaos and wrote a letter to Nightingale on October 15, 1854, as a plea for her service. Nightingale took the challenge from Sir Herbert and set sail with 38 self-proclaimed nurses with varied training and experiences, of whom 24 were Catholic and Anglican nuns. Their journey to the Crimea took a month, and on November 4, 1854, the brave nurses arrived at Istanbul and were taken to Scutari the same day. Faced with 3,000 to 4,000 wounded men in a hospital designed to accommodate 1,700, the nurses went to work (Kalisch & Kalisch, 1986). The nurses were faced with 4 miles of beds 18 inches apart. Most soldiers were lying naked with no bedding or blanket. There were no kitchen or laundry facilities. The little light present took the form of candles in beer bottles. The hospital was literally floating on an open sewage lagoon filled with rats and other vermin (Donahue, 1985).

By taking the newly arrived medical equipment and setting up kitchens, laundries, recreation rooms, reading rooms, and a canteen, Nightingale and her team of nurses proceeded to clean the barracks of lice and filth. Nightingale was in her element. She set out not only to provide humane health care for the soldiers but to essentially overhaul the administrative structure of the military health services (Williams, 1961).

Florence Nightingale and Sanitation

Although Nightingale never accepted the germ theory, she demanded clean dressings; clean bedding; well-cooked, edible, and appealing food; proper sanitation; and fresh air. After the other nurses were asleep, Nightingale made her famous solitary rounds with a lamp or lantern to check on the soldiers. Nightingale had a lifelong pattern of sleeping few hours, spending many nights writing, developing elaborate plans, and evaluating implemented changes. She seldom believed in the "hopeless" soldier, only one who needed extra attention. Nightingale was convinced that most of the maladies that the soldiers suffered and died from were preventable (Williams, 1961).

Before Nightingale's arrival and her radical and well-documented interventions based on sound public health principles, the mortality rate from the Crimean War was estimated to be from 42% to 73%. Nightingale is credited with reducing that rate to 2% within 6 months of her arrival at Scutari. She did this through careful, scientific epidemiological research (Dietz & Lehozky, 1963). Upon arriving at Scutari, Nightingale's first act was to order 200 scrubbing brushes. The death rate fell dramatically once Nightingale discovered that the hospital was built literally over an open sewage lagoon (Andrews, 2003).

According to Palmer (1982), Nightingale possessed the qualities of a good researcher: insatiable curiosity, command of her subject, familiarity with methods of inquiry, a good background of statistics, and the ability to discriminate and abstract. She used these skills to maintain detailed and copious notes and to codify observations. Nightingale relied on statistics and attention to detail to back up her conclusions about sanitation, management of care, and disease causation. Her now-famous "cox combs" are a hallmark of military health services management by which she diagrammed deaths in the Army from wounds and from other diseases and compared them with deaths that occurred in similar populations in England (Palmer, 1977).

Nightingale was first and foremost an administrator: She believed in a hierarchical administrative structure with ultimate control lodged in one person to whom all subordinates and offices reported. Within a matter of weeks of her arrival in the Crimea, Nightingale was the acknowledged administrator and organizer of a mammoth humanitarian effort. From her Crimean experience on, Nightingale involved herself primarily in organizational activities and health planning administration. Palmer contends that Nightingale "perceived the Crimean venture, which was set up as an experiment, as a golden opportunity to demonstrate the efficacy of female nursing" (Palmer, 1982, p. 4). Although Nightingale faced initial resistance from the unconvinced and oppositional medical officers and surgeons, she boldly defied convention and remained steadfastly focused on her mission to create a sanitary and highly structured environment for her "children"—the British soldiers who dedicated their lives to the defense of Great Britain. Through her resilience and insistence on absolute authority regarding nursing and the hospital environment, Nightingale was known to send nurses home to England from the Crimea for suspicious alcohol use and character weakness.

It was through this success at Scutari that she began a long career of influence on the public's health through social activism and reform, health policy, and the reformation of career nursing. Using her well-publicized successful "experiment" and supportive evidence from the Crimea, Nightingale effectively argued the case for the reform and creation of military health care that would serve as the model for people in uniform to the present (D'Antonio, 2002). Nightingale's ideas about proper hospital architecture and administration influenced a generation of medical doctors and the entire world, in both military and civilian service. Her work in *Notes on Hospitals*, published in 1860, provided the template for the organization of military health care in the Union Army when the U.S. Civil War erupted in 1861. Her vision for health care of soldiers and the responsibility of the governments that send them to war continues today; her influence can be seen throughout the previous century and into this century as health care for the women and men who serve their country is a vital part of the well-being of not only the soldiers but for society in general (D'Antonio, 2002).

Returning Home a Heroine: The Political Reformer

When Nightingale returned to London, she found that her efforts to provide comfort and health to the British soldier succeeded in making heroes of both herself and the soldiers (Woodham-Smith, 1951). Both had suffered from negative stereotypes: The soldier was often portrayed as a drunken oaf with little ambition or honor, the nurse as a tipsy, self-serving, illiterate, promiscuous loser. After the Crimean War and the efforts of Nightingale and her nurses, both returned with honor and dignity, nevermore the downtrodden and disrespected.

After her return from the Crimea, Florence Nightingale never made a public appearance, never attended a public function, and never issued a public statement (Bullough & Bullough, 1978). She single-handedly raised nursing from, as she put it, "the sink it was" into a respected and noble profession (Palmer, 1977). As an avid scholar and student of the Greek writer Plato, Nightingale believed that she had a moral obligation to work primarily for the good of the community. Because she believed that education formed character, she insisted that nursing must go beyond care for the sick; the mission of the trained nurse must include social reform to promote the good. This dual mission of nursing—caregiver and political reformer—has shaped the profession as we know it today. LeVasseur (1998) contends that Nightingale's insistence on nursing's involvement in a larger political ideal is the historical foundation of the field and distinguishes us from other scientific disciplines, such as medicine.

How did Nightingale accomplish this? She effected change through her wide command of acquaintances: Queen Victoria was a significant admirer of her intellect and ability to effect change, and Nightingale used her position as national heroine to get the attention of elected officials in Parliament. She was tireless and had an amazing capacity for work. She used people. Her brother-in-law, Sir Harry Verney, was a member of Parliament and often delivered her "messages" in the form of legislation. When she wanted the public incited, she turned to the press, writing letters to the *London Times* and having others of influence write articles. She was not above threats to "go public" by certain dates if an elected official refused to establish a commission or appoint a committee. And when those commissions were formed, Nightingale was ready with her list of selected people for appointment (Palmer, 1982).

Nightingale and Military Reforms

The first real test of Nightingale's military reforms came in the United States during the Civil War. Nightingale was asked by the Union to advise on the organization of hospitals and care of the sick and wounded. She sent recommendations back to the United States based on her experiences and analysis in the Crimea, and her advisement and influence gained wide publicity. Following her recommendations, the Union set up a sanitary commission and provided for regular inspection of camps. She expressed a desire to help with the Confederate military also but, unfortunately, had no channel of communication with them (Bullough & Bullough, 1978).

The Nightingale School of Nursing at St. Thomas: The Birth of Professional Nursing

The British public honored Nightingale by endowing 50,000 pounds sterling in her name upon her return to England from the Crimea. The money had been raised from the soldiers under her care and donations from the public. This Nightingale Fund eventually was used to create the Nightingale School of Nursing at St. Thomas, which was to be the beginning of professional nursing (Donahue, 1985). Nightingale, at the age of 40, decided that St. Thomas' Hospital was the place for her training school for nurses. While the negotiations for the school went forward, she spent her time writing *Notes on Nursing: What It Is and What It Is Not* (Nightingale, 1860). The small book of 77 pages, written for the British mother, was an instant success. An expanded library edition was written for nurses and used as the textbook for the students at St. Thomas. The book has since been translated into many languages, although it is believed that Nightingale refused all royalties earned from the publication of the book (Cook, 1913; Tooley, 1910). The nursing students chosen for the new training school were handpicked; they had to be of good moral character, sober, and honest. Nightingale believed that the strong emphasis on morals was critical to gaining respect for the new "Nightingale nurse," with no possible ties to the disgraceful association of past nurses. Nursing students were monitored throughout their 1-year program both on and off the hospital grounds; their activities were carefully watched for character weaknesses, and discipline was severe and swift for violators. Accounts from Nightingale's journals and notes reveal instant dismissal of nursing students for such behaviors as "flirtation, using the eyes unpleasantly, and being in the company of unsavory persons." Nightingale contended that "the future of nursing depends on how these young women behave themselves" (Smith, 1934, p. 234). She knew that the experiment at St. Thomas to educate nurses and raise nursing to a moral and professional calling was a drastic departure from the past images of nurses and would take extraordinary women of high moral character and intelligence. Nightingale knew every nursing student, or probationer, personally, often having the students at her house for weekend visits. She devised a system of daily journal keeping for the probationers; Nightingale herself read the journals monthly to evaluate their character and work habits. Every nursing student admitted to St. Thomas had to submit an acceptable "letter of good character," and Nightingale herself placed graduate nurses in approved nursing positions.

One of the most important features of the Nightingale School was its relative autonomy. Both the school and the hospital nursing service were organized under the head matron. This was especially significant because it meant that nursing service began independently of the medical staff in selecting, retaining, and disciplining students and nurses (Bullough & Bullough, 1978).

Nightingale was opposed to the use of a standardized government examination and the movement for licensure of trained nurses. She believed that schools of nursing would lose control of educational standards with the advent of national licensure, most notably those related to moral character. Nightingale led a staunch opposition to the movement by the British Nurses' Association (BNA) for licensure of trained nurses, one the BNA believed critical to protecting the public's safety by ensuring the qualification of nurses by licensure exam. Nightingale was convinced that qualifying a nurse by examination tested only the acquisition of technical skills, not the equally important evaluation of character. She believed nursing involved "divergencies too great for a single standard to be applied" (Nutting & Dock, 1907; Woodham-Smith, 1951).

Taking Health Care to the Community: Nightingale and Wellness

Early efforts to distinguish hospital from community health nursing are evidence of Nightingale's views on "health nursing," which she distinguished from "sick nursing." She wrote two influential papers, one in 1893, "Sick Nursing and Health-Nursing" (Nightingale, 1893), which was read in the United States at the Chicago Exposition, and the second, "Health Teaching in Towns and Villages" in 1894 (Monteiro, 1985). Both papers praised the success of prevention-based nursing practice. Winslow (1946) acknowledged Nightingale's influence in the United States by being one of the first in the field of public health to recognize the importance of taking responsibility for one's health. She wrote in 1891 that "There are more people to pick us up and help us stand on our own two feet" (Attewell, 1996). According to Palmer (1982), Nightingale was a leader in the wellness movement long before the concept was identified. Nightingale saw the nurse as the key figure in establishing a healthy society. She saw a logical extension of nursing in acute hospital settings to the community. Clearly, through her *Notes on Nursing*, she visualized the nurse as "the nation's first bulwark in health maintenance, the promotion of wellness, and the prevention of disease" (Palmer, 1982, p. 6).

William Rathbone, a wealthy ship owner and philanthropist, is credited with the establishment of the first visiting nurse service, which eventually evolved into district nursing in the community. He was so impressed with the private duty nursing care that his sick wife had received at home that he set out to develop a "district nursing service" in Liverpool, England. At his own expense, in 1859, he developed a corps of nurses trained to care for the sick poor in their homes (Bullough & Bullough, 1978). He divided the community into 16 districts; each was assigned a nurse and a social worker that provided nursing and health education. His experiment in district nursing was so successful that he was unable to find enough nurses to work in the districts. Rathbone contacted Nightingale for assistance. Her recommendation was to train more nurses, and she advised Rathbone to approach the Royal Liverpool Infirmary with a proposal for opening another training school for nurses (Rathbone, 1890; Tooley, 1910). The infirmary agreed to Rathbone's proposal, and district nursing soon spread throughout England as successful "health nursing" in the community for the sick poor through voluntary agencies (Rosen, 1958). Ever the visionary, Nightingale contended that "Hospitals are but an intermediate stage of civilization. The ultimate aim is to nurse the sick poor in their own homes (1893)" (Attewell, 1996). She also wrote in regard to visiting families at home: "We must not talk to them or at them but with them (1894)" (Attewell, 1996). A similar service, health visiting, began in Manchester, England, in 1862 by the Manchester and Salford Sanitary Association. The purpose of placing "health visitors" in the home was to provide health information and instruction to families. Eventually, health visitors evolved to provide preventive health education and district nurses to care for the sick at home (Bullough & Bullough, 1978).

Although Nightingale is best known for her reform of hospitals and the military, she was a great believer in the future of health care, which she anticipated should be preventive in nature and would more than likely take place in the home and community. Her accomplishments in the field of "sanitary nursing" extended beyond the walls of the hospital to include workhouse reform and community sanitation reform. In 1864, Nightingale and William Rathbone once again worked together to lead the reform of the Liverpool Workhouse Infirmary, where more than 1,200 sick paupers were crowded into unsanitary and unsafe conditions. Under the British Poor Laws, the most desperately poor of the large cities were gathered into large workhouses. When sick, they were sent to the Workhouse Infirmary. Trained nursing care was all but nonexistent. Through legislative pressure and a well-designed public campaign describing the horrors of the Workhouse Infirmary, reform of the workhouse system was accomplished by 1867. Although not as complete as Nightingale had wanted, nurses were in place and being paid a salary (Seymer, 1954).

The Legacy of Nightingale

Scores have been written about Nightingale—an almost mythic figure in history. She truly was a beloved legend throughout Great Britain by the time she left the Crimea in July 1856, 4 months after the war. Longfellow immortalized this "Lady with the Lamp" in his poem "Santa Filomena" (Longfellow, 1857). However, when Nightingale returned to London after the Crimean War, she remained haunted by her experiences related to the soldiers dying of preventable diseases. She was troubled by nightmares and had difficulty sleeping in the years that followed (Woodham-Smith, 1983). Nightingale became a prolific writer and a staunch defender of the causes of the British soldier, sanitation in England and India, and trained nursing.

As a woman, she was not able to hold an official government post, nor could she vote. Historians have had varied opinions about the exact nature of the disability that kept her homebound for the remainder of her life. Recent scholars have speculated that she experienced post-traumatic stress disorder (PTSD) from her experiences in the Crimea; there is also considerable evidence that she suffered from the painful disease brucellosis (Barker, 1989; Young, 1995). She exerted incredible influence through friends and acquaintances, directing from her sick room sanitation and poor law reform. Her mission to "cleanse" spread from the military to the British Empire; her fight for improved sanitation both at home and in India consumed her energies for the remainder of her life (Vicinus & Nergaard, 1990).

According to Monteiro (1985), two recurrent themes are found throughout Nightingale's writings about disease prevention and wellness outside the hospital. The most persistent theme is that nurses must be trained differently and instructed specifically in district and instructive nursing. She consistently wrote that the "health nurse" must be trained in the nature of poverty and its influence on health, something she referred to as the "pauperization" of the poor. She also believed that above all, health nurses must be good teachers about hygiene and helping families learn to better care for themselves (Nightingale, 1893). She insisted that untrained, "good intended women" could not substitute for nursing care in the home. Nightingale pushed for an extensive orientation and additional training, including prior hospital experience, before one was hired as a district nurse. She outlined the qualifications in her paper "On Trained Nursing for the Sick Poor," in which she called for a month's "trial" in district nursing, a year's training in hospital nursing, and 3 to 6 months training in district nursing (Monteiro, 1985). She said, "There is no such thing as amateur nursing."

The second theme that emerged from her writings was the focus on the role of the nurse. She clearly distinguished the role of the health nurse in promoting what we today call self-care. In the past, philanthropic visitors in the form of Christian charity would visit the homes of the poor and offer them relief (Monteiro, 1985). Nightingale believed that such activities did little to teach the poor to care for themselves and further "pauperized" them—dependent and vulnerable—keeping them unhealthy, prone to disease, and reliant on others to keep them healthy. The nurse then must help the families at home manage a healthy environment for themselves, and Nightingale saw a trained nurse as being the only person who could pull off such a feat. She stated, "Never think that you have done anything effectual in nursing in London, till you nurse, not only the sick poor in workhouses, but those at home."

By 1901, Nightingale lived in a world without sight or sound, leaving her unable to write. Over the next 5 years, Nightingale lost her ability to communicate and most days existed in a state of unconsciousness. In November of 1907, Nightingale was honored with the Order of Merit by King Edward VII, the first time ever given to a woman. After 50 years, in May 1910, the Nightingale Training School of Nursing at St. Thomas celebrated its Jubilee. There were now more than a thousand training schools for nurses in the United States alone (Cook, 1913; Tooley, 1910).

Nightingale died in her sleep around noon on August 13, 1910, and was buried quietly and without pomp near the family's home at Embley, her coffin carried by six sergeants of the British Army. Only a small cross marks her grave at her request: "FN. Born 1820. Died 1910." (Brown, 1988). The family refused a national funeral and burial at Westminster Abbey out of respect for Nightingale's last wishes. She had lived for 90 years and 3 months.

Continued Development of Professional Nursing in the United Kingdom

Although Florence Nightingale opposed registration, based on the belief that the essential qualities of a nurse could not be taught, examined, or regulated, registration in the United Kingdom began in the 1880s. The Hospitals Association maintained a voluntary registry that was an administrative list. In an effort to protect the public led by **Ethel Fenwick**, the BNA was formed in 1887 with its charter granted in 1893 to unite British nurses and to provide registration as evidence of systematic training. Finally, in 1919, nurse registration became law. It took 30 years and the tireless efforts of Ethel Fenwick, who was supported by other nursing leaders such as Isla Stewart, Lucy Osbourne, and Mary Cochrane, to achieve mandated registration (Royal British Nurses' Association, n.d.).

Another milestone in British nursing history was the founding in 1916 of the College of Nursing as the professional organization for trained nurses. For a century, the organization has focused on professional standards for nurses in their education, practice, and working conditions. Although the principles of a professional organization and those of a trade union have not always fit together easily, the Royal College of Nursing has pursued its role as both the professional organization for nurses and the trade union for nurses (McGann, Crowther, & Dougall, 2009). Today the Royal College of Nursing is recognized as the voice of nursing by the government and the public in the United Kingdom (Royal College of Nursing, n.d.).

The Development of Professional Nursing in Canada

Marie Lollet Hebert, the wife of a surgeon-apothecary, is credited by many with being the first person in present-day Canada to provide nursing care to the sick as she assisted her husband after arriving in Quebec in 1617; however, the first trained nurses arrived in Quebec to care for the sick in 1639. These nurses were Augustine nuns who traveled to Canada to establish a medical mission to care for the physical and spiritual needs of their patients, and they established the first hospital in North America, the *Hôtel-Dieu de Québec*. These nuns also established the first apprenticeship program for nursing in North America. **Jeanne Mance** came from France to the French colony of Montreal in 1642 and founded the *Hôtel Dieu de Montréal* in 1645 (Canadian Museum of History, n.d.).

The hospital of the early 19th century did not appeal to the Canadian public. They were primarily homes for the poor and were staffed by those of a similar class, rather than by nurses (Mansell, 2004). The decades of the 1830s and 1840s in Canada were characterized by an influx of immigrants and outbreaks of diseases such as cholera. There is evidence that it was difficult, especially in times of outbreak, to find sufficient people to care for the sick. Little is known of the hospital "nurses" of this era, but the descriptions are unflattering and working in the hospital environment was difficult. Early midwives did have some standing in the community and were employed by individuals, although there is record of charitable organizations also employing midwives (Young, 2010).

During the Crimean War and American Civil War, nurses were extremely effective in providing treatment and comfort not only to battlefield casualties, but also to individuals who fell victim to accidents and infectious disease; however, it was in the North-West Rebellion of 1885 that Canadian nurses performed military service for the first time. At first, the nursing needs identified were for duties such as making bandages and preparing supplies. It soon became apparent that more direct participation by nurses was needed if the military was to provide effective medical field treatment. Seven nurses, under the direction of Reverend Mother Hannah Grier Coome, served in Moose Jaw and Saskatoon, Saskatchewan. Although their tour of duty lasted only 4 weeks, these women proved that nursing could, and should in the future, play a vital role in providing treatment to wounded soldiers. In 1899, the Canadian Army Medical Department was formed, followed by the creation of the Canadian Army Nursing Service. Nurses received the relative rank, pay, and allowances of an army lieutenant. Nursing sisters served thereafter in every military force sent out from Canada, from the South African War to the Korean War (Veterans Affairs Canada, n.d.).

In 1896, Lady Ishbel Aberdeen, wife of the governor-general of Canada, visited Vancouver. During this visit, she heard vivid accounts of the hardship and illness affecting women and children in rural areas. Later that same year at the National Council of Women, amid similar stories, a resolution was passed asking Lady Aberdeen to found an order of visiting nurses in Canada. The order was to be a memorial to the 60th anniversary of Queen Victoria's ascent to the throne of the British Empire; it received a royal charter in 1897. The first Victorian Order of Nurses (VON) sites were organized in the cities of Ottawa, Montreal, Toronto, Halifax, Vancouver, and Kingston. Today the VON delivers over 75 different programs and services such as prenatal education, mental health services, palliative care services, and visiting nursing through 52 local sites staffed by 4,500 healthcare workers and over 9,016 volunteers (VON, 2009).

By the mid to late 19th century, despite previous negativity, nursing came to be viewed as necessary to progressive medical interventions. To make the work of the nurse acceptable, changes had to be made to the prevailing view of nursing. In the 1870s, the ideas of Florence Nightingale were introduced in Canada. Dr. Theophilus Mack imported nurses who had worked with Nightingale and founded the first training school for nurses in Canada at St. Catharine's General Hospital in 1873. Many hospitals appeared across Canada from 1890 to 1910, and many of them developed training schools for nurses. By 1909, there were 70 hospital-based training schools in Canada (Mansell, 2004).

In 1908, **Mary Agnes Snively**, along with 16 representatives from organized nursing bodies, met in Ottawa to form the Canadian National Association of Trained Nurses (CNATN). By 1924, each of the nine provinces had a provincial nursing organization with membership in the CNATN. In 1924, the name of the CNATN was changed to the Canadian Nurses Association (CNA). CNA is currently a federation of 11 provincial and territorial nursing associations and colleges representing nearly 150,000 registered nurses (CNA, n.d.).

In 1944, the CNA approved the principle of collective bargaining. In 1946, the Registered Nurses Association of British Columbia became the first provincial nursing association to be certified as a bargaining agent. By the 1970s, other provincial nursing organizations gained this right. Between 1973 and 1987, nursing unions were created. Today, each of the 10 provinces has a nursing union in addition to a professional association (Ontario Nurses' Association, n.d.). One of the best known of these professional associations is the Registered Nurses' Association of Ontario (RNAO). Established in 1925 to advocate for healthy public policy, promote excellence in nursing practice, increase nursing's contribution to shaping the healthcare system, and influence decisions that affect nurses and the public they serve, the RNAO is the professional association representing registered nurses, nurse practitioners (NPs), and nursing students in Ontario (RNAO, n.d.). Through the RNAO, nurses in Canada have led the world in systematic implementation of evidence-based practice and have made their best practice guidelines available to all nurses to promote safe and effective care of patients.

As Canadians entered the decade of the 1960s, there was serious concern about the healthcare system. In 1961, all Canadian provinces signed on to the Hospital Insurance and Diagnostic Services Act. This legislation created a national, universal health insurance system. The same year, the Royal Commission on Health Services was established and presented four recommendations. One of the recommendations was to examine nursing education. Prior to this, the CNA had requested a survey of nursing schools across Canada with the goal of assessing how prepared the schools were for a national system of accreditation. The findings of this survey, paired with the commission's recommendation, led to the establishment of the Canadian Nurses Foundation (CNF) in 1962. The CNF provides funding for nurses to further their education and for research related to nursing care (CNF, 2014). The Canadian Association of Schools of Nursing is the organization that promotes national nursing education standards and is the national accrediting agency for university nursing programs in Canada (n.d.).

Nursing in Canada transformed itself to meet the needs of a changing Canadian society, and in doing so was responsible for a shift from nursing as a spiritual vocation to a secular but indispensable profession. Nurses' willingness to respond in times of need, whether economic, epidemic, or war, contributed to their importance in the healthcare system (Mansell, 2004). Canadian nursing associations agreed that starting in the year 2000, the basic educational preparation for the registered nurse would be the baccalaureate degree, and all provinces and territories launched a campaign known as EP 2000, which later became EP 2005. Currently, the baccalaureate degree earned from a university is the accepted entry level into nursing practice in Canada (Mansell, 2004).

The Development of Professional Nursing in Australia

In the earliest days of the colony, the care of the sick was performed by untrained convicts. Male attendants undertook the supervision of male patients and female attendants undertook duties with the female patients. Attention to hygiene standards was almost nonexistent. In 1885, the poor health and living conditions of disadvantaged sick persons in Melbourne prompted a group of concerned citizens to meet and form the Melbourne District Nursing Society. This society was formed to look after sick poor persons at home to prevent unnecessary hospitalization. Home visiting services also have a long history in Australia, with Victoria being the first state to introduce a district nursing service in 1885, followed by South Australia in 1894, Tasmania in 1896, New South Wales in 1900, Queensland in 1904, and Western Australia in 1905 (Australian Bureau of Statistics, 1985).

Australian nurses were involved in military nursing as civilian volunteers as early as the 1880s (The University of Melbourne, 2015); however, involvement of Australian women as nurses in war began in 1898 with the formation of the Australian Nursing Service of New South Wales, which was composed of 1 superintendent and 24 nurses. Based on the performance of the nurses, the Australian Army Nursing Service was formed in 1903 under the control of the federal government. The Royal Australian Army Nursing Corps (RAANC) had its beginnings in the Australian Army Nursing Service (RAANC, n.d.). Since that time, Australian nurses have dealt with war, the sick, the wounded, and the dead. They have served in Australia, in war zones around the world, in field hospitals, on hospital ships anchored off shore near battlefields, and on transports (Australian Government, 2009). Other military opportunities for nurses include the Royal Australian Navy and the Royal Australian Air Force.

Nursing registration in Australia began in 1920 as a state-based system. Prior to 1920, nurses received certificates from the hospitals where they trained, the Australian Trained Nurses Association (ATNA), or the Royal British Nurses' Association in order to practice. Today nurses and midwives are registered through the Nursing and Midwifery Board of Australia (NMBA), which is made up of member state and territorial boards of nursing and supported by the Australian Health Practitioner Regulation Agency. State and territorial boards are responsible for making registration and notification decisions related to individual nurses or midwives (NMBA, n.d.).

Around the turn of the 20th century, in order to create a formal means of supporting their role and improve nursing standards and education, the nurses of South Australia formed the South Australian branch of ATNA. It is from this organization that the Australian Nursing and Midwifery Federation in South Australia (ANMFSA) evolved (ANMFSA, 2012). The Australian Nursing and Midwifery Accreditation Council (ANMAC) is now the independent accrediting authority for nursing and midwifery under Australia's National Registration and Accreditation Scheme. The ANMAC is responsible for protecting and promoting the safety of the Australian community by promoting high standards of nursing and midwifery education through the development of accreditation standards, accreditation of programs, and assessment of internationally qualified nurses and midwives for migration (ANMAC, 2014).

In the late 1920s, two nurses, Evelyn Nowland and a Miss Clancy, began working separately on the idea of a union for nurses and were brought together by Jessie Street, who saw the improvement of nurses' wages and conditions as a feminist cause. What is now the New South Wales Nurses and Midwives' Association (NSWNMA) was registered as a trade union in 1931 (NSWNMA, 2014). Through the amalgamation of various organizations, there is now one national organization to represent registered nurses, enrolled nurses, midwives, and assistants doing nursing work in every state and territory throughout Australia: the Australian Nursing and Midwifery Federation (ANMF). The organization was established in 1924 and serves as a union for nurses with an ultimate goal of improving patient care. The ANMF is now composed of eight branches: the Australian Nursing and Midwifery Federation (South Australia branch), the NSWNMA, the Australian Nursing and Midwifery Federation Victorian Branch, the Queensland Nurses Union, the Australian Nursing and Midwifery Federation Tasmanian Branch, the Australian Nursing and Midwifery Federation Australian Capital Territory, the Australian Nursing and Midwifery Federation Northern Territory, and the Australian Nursing and Midwifery Federation Western Australian Branch (ANMF, 2015).

Early Nursing Education and Organization in the United States

Formal nursing education in the United States did not begin until 1862, when Dr. Marie Zakrzewska opened the New England Hospital for Women and Children, which had its own nurse training program (Sitzman & Judd, 2014b). Many of the first training schools for nursing were modeled after the Nightingale School of Nursing at St. Thomas in London. They included the Bellevue Training School for Nurses in New York City; the Connecticut Training School for Nurses in New Haven, Connecticut; and the Boston Training School for Nurses at Massachusetts General Hospital (Christy, 1975; Nutting & Dock, 1907). Based on the Victorian belief in the natural abilities of women to be sensitive, possess high morals, and be caregivers, early nursing training required that applicants be female. Sensitivity, high moral character, purity of character, subservience, and "ladylike" behavior became the associated traits of a "good nurse," thus setting the "feminization of nursing" as the ideal standard for a good nurse. These historical roots of gender- and race-based caregiving continued to exclude males and minorities from the nursing profession for many years and still influence career choices for men and women today. These early training schools provided a stable, subservient, white female workforce because student nurses served as the primary nursing staff for these early hospitals. Minority nurses found limited educational opportunities in this climate. The first African American nursing school graduate in the United States was Mary P. Mahoney. She graduated from the New England Hospital for Women and Children in 1879 (Sitzman & Judd, 2014b).

Nursing education in the newly formed schools was based on accepted practices that had not been validated by research. During this time in history, nurses primarily relied on tradition to guide practice, rather than engaging in research to test interventions; however, scientific advances did help to improve nursing practice as nurses altered interventions based on knowledge generated by scientists and physicians. During this time, a nurse, Clara Maass, gave her life as a volunteer subject in the research of yellow fever (Sitzman & Judd, 2014b).

CRITICAL THINKING QUESTIONS ✳

Some nurses believe that Florence Nightingale holds nursing back and represents the negative and backward elements of nursing. This view cites as evidence that Nightingale supported the subordination of nurses to physicians, opposed registration of nurses, and did not see mental health nurses as part of the profession. Wheeler (1999) has gone so far as to say, "The nursing profession needs to exorcise the myth of Nightingale, not necessarily because she was a bad person, but because the impact of her legacy has held the profession back too long." After reading this chapter, what do you think? Is Nightingale relevant in the 21st century to the nursing profession? Why or why not? ✳

A significant report, known simply as the **Goldmark Report**, *Nursing and Nursing Education in the United States*, was released in 1922 and advocated the establishment of university schools of nursing to train nursing leaders. The report, initiated by Nutting in 1918, was an exhaustive and comprehensive investigation into the state of nursing education and training resulting in a 500-page document. Josephine Goldmark, social worker and author of the pioneering research of nursing preparation in the United States, stated,

> From our field study of the nurse in public health nursing, in private duty, and as instructor and supervisor in hospitals, it is clear that there is need of a basic undergraduate training for all nurses alike, which should lead to a nursing diploma. (Goldmark, 1923, p. 35)

The first university school of nursing was developed at the University of Minnesota in 1909. Although the new nurse training school was under the college of medicine and offered only a 3-year diploma, the Minnesota program was nevertheless a significant leap forward in nursing education. *Nursing for the Future*, or the **Brown Report**, authored by Esther Lucille Brown in 1948 and sponsored by the Russell Sage Foundation, was critical of the quality and structure of nursing schools in the United States. The Brown Report became the catalyst for the implementation of educational nursing program accreditation through the National League for Nursing (Brown, 1936, 1948). As a result of the post–World War II nursing shortage, an Associate Degree in Nursing was established by Dr. Mildred Montag in 1952 as a 2-year program for registered nurses (Montag, 1959). In 1950, nursing became the first profession for which the same licensure exam, the State Board Test Pool, was used throughout the nation to license registered nurses. This increased mobility for the registered nurse resulted in a significant advantage for the relatively new profession of nursing (State board test pool examination, 1952).

The Evolution of Nursing in the United States: The First Century of Professional Nursing

The Profession of Nursing Is Born in the United States

Early nurse leaders of the 20th century included **Isabel Hampton Robb**, who in 1896 founded the Nurses' Associated Alumnae, which in 1911 officially became known as the **American Nurses Association (ANA)**; and **Lavinia Lloyd Dock**, who became a militant suffragist linking women's roles as nurses to the emerging women's movement in the United States.

Mary Adelaide Nutting, Lavinia L. Dock, Sophia Palmer, and Mary E. Davis were instrumental in developing the first nursing journal, the *American Journal of Nursing (AJN)* in October 1900. Through the ANA and the *AJN*, nurses then had a professional organization and a national journal with which to communicate with each other (Kalisch & Kalisch, 1986).

State licensure of trained nurses began in 1903 with the enactment of North Carolina's licensure law for nursing. Shortly thereafter, New Jersey, New York, and Virginia passed similar licensure laws for nursing. Over the next several years, professional nursing was well on its way to public recognition of practice and educational standards as state after state passed similar legislation.

Margaret Sanger worked as a nurse on the Lower East Side of New York City in 1912 with immigrant families. She was astonished to find widespread ignorance among these families about conception, pregnancy, and childbirth. After a horrifying experience with the death of a woman from a failed self-induced abortion, Sanger devoted her life to teaching women about birth control. A staunch activist in the early family planning movement, Sanger is credited with founding Planned Parenthood of America (Sanger, 1928).

By 1917, the emerging new profession saw two significant events that propelled the need for additional trained nurses in the United States: World War I and the influenza epidemic. Nightingale and the devastation of the Civil War had well established the need for nursing care in wartime. Mary Adelaide Nutting, now Professor of Nursing and Health at Columbia University, chaired the newly established Committee on Nursing in response to the need for nurses as the United States entered the war in Europe. Nurses in the United States realized early that World War I was unlike previous wars. It was a global conflict that involved coalitions of nations against nations and vast amounts of supplies and demanded the organization of all the nations' resources for military purposes (Kalisch & Kalisch, 1986). Along with **Lillian Wald** and **Jane A. Delano,** Director of Nursing in the American Red Cross, Nutting initiated a national publicity campaign to recruit young women to enter nurses' training. The Army School of Nursing, headed by **Annie Goodrich** as dean, and the Vassar Training Camp for Nurses prepared nurses for the war as well as home nursing and hygiene nursing through the Red Cross (Dock & Stewart, 1931). The committee estimated that there were at the most about 200,000 active "nurses" in the United States, both trained and untrained, which was inadequate for the military effort abroad (Kalisch & Kalisch, 1986).

At home, the influenza epidemic of 1917 to 1919 led to increased public awareness of the need for public health nursing and public education about hygiene and disease prevention. The successful campaign to attract nursing students focused heavily on patriotism, which ushered in the new era for nursing as a profession. By 1918, nursing school enrollments were up by 25%. In 1920, Congress passed a bill that provided nurses with military rank (Dock & Stewart, 1931). Following close behind, the passage of the Nineteenth Amendment to the U.S. Constitution granted women the right to vote.

Lillian Wald, Public Health Nursing, and Community Activism

The pattern for health visiting and district nursing practice outside the hospital was similar in the United States to that in England (Roberts, 1954). American cities were besieged by overcrowding and epidemics after the Civil War. The need for trained nurses evolved as in England, and schools throughout the United States developed along the Nightingale model. Visiting nurses were first sent to philanthropic organizations in New York City (1877), Boston (1886), Buffalo (1885), and Philadelphia (1886) to care for the sick at home. By the end of the century, most large cities had some form of visiting nursing program, and some headway was being made even in smaller towns (Heinrich, 1983). Industrial or occupational health nursing was first started in Vermont in 1895 by a marble company interested in the health and welfare of its workers and their families. Tuberculosis (TB) was a leading cause of death in the 1800s; nurses visited patients bedridden from TB and instructed persons in all settings about prevention of the disease (Abel, 1997).

Lillian Wald, a wealthy young woman with a great social conscience, graduated from the New York Hospital School of Nursing in 1891 and is credited with creating the title "public health nurse." After a year working in a mental institution, Wald entered medical school at Women's Medical College in New York. While in medical school, she was asked to visit immigrant mothers on New York's Lower East Side and instruct them on health matters. Wald was appalled by the conditions there. During one now famous home visit, a small child asked Wald to visit her sick mother. And the rest, as they say, is history (**Box 1-1**).

What Wald found changed her life forever and secured a place for her in American nursing history. Wald (1915) said, "All the maladjustments of our social and economic relations seemed epitomized in this brief journey" (p. 6). Wald was profoundly affected by her observations; she and her colleague, **Mary Brewster**, quickly established the **Henry Street Settlement** in this same neighborhood in 1893. She quit medical school and devoted the remainder of her life to "visions of a better world" for the public's health. According to Wald, "Nursing is love in action, and there is no finer manifestation of it than the care of the poor and disabled in their own homes" (Wald, 1915, p. 14).

The Henry Street Settlement was an independent nursing service where Wald lived and worked. This later became the Visiting Nurse Association of New York City, which laid the foundation for the establishment of public health nursing in the United States. The health needs of the population were met through addressing social, economic, and environmental determinants of health, in a pattern after Nightingale. These nurses helped educate families about disease transmission and emphasized the importance of good hygiene. They provided preventive, acute, and long-term care. As such, Henry Street

BOX 1-1 LILLIAN WALD TAKES A WALK

From the schoolroom where I had been giving a lesson in bed-making, a little girl led me one drizzling March morning. She had told me of her sick mother, and gathering from her incoherent account that a child had been born, I caught up the paraphernalia of the bed-making lesson and carried it with me.

The child led me over broken roadways … between tall, reeking houses whose laden fire-escapes, useless for their appointed purpose, bulged with household goods of every description. The rain added to the dismal appearance of the streets and to the discomfort of the crowds which thronged them, intensifying the odors, which assailed me from every side. Through Hester and Division Streets we went to the end of Ludlow; past odorous fish-stands, for the streets were a market-place, unregulated, un-supervised, unclean; past evil-smelling, uncovered garbage cans….

All the maladjustments of our social and economic relations seemed epitomized in this brief journey and what was found at the end of it. The family to which the child led me was neither criminal nor vicious. Although the husband was a cripple, one of those who stand on street corners exhibiting deformities to enlist compassion, and masking the begging of alms by a pretense of selling; although the family of seven shared their two rooms with boarders—who were literally boarders, since a piece of timber was placed over the floor for them to sleep on—and although the sick woman lay on a wretched, unclean bed, soiled with a hemorrhage two days old, they were not degraded human beings, judged by any measure of moral values.

In fact, it was very plain that they were sensitive to their condition, and when, at the end of my ministrations, they kissed my hands (those who have undergone similar experiences will, I am sure, understand), it would have been some solace if by any conviction of the moral unworthiness of the family I could have defended myself as a part of a society which permitted such conditions to exist. Indeed, my subsequent acquaintance with them revealed the fact that miserable as their state was, they were not without ideals for the family life, and for society, of which they were so unloved and unlovely a part.

That morning's experience was a baptism of fire. Deserted were the laboratory and the academic work of the college. I never returned to them. On my way from the sick-room to my comfortable student quarters, my mind was intent on my own responsibility. To my inexperience it seemed certain that conditions such as these were allowed because people did not know, and for me there was a challenge to know and to tell. When early morning found me still awake, my naive conviction remained that, if people knew things—and "things" meant everything implied in the condition of this family—such horrors would cease to exist, and I rejoiced that I had a training in the care of the sick that in itself would give me an organic relationship to the neighborhood in which this awakening had come.

Source: Wald, L. D. (1915). *The house on Henry Street*. New York, NY: Henry Holt.

went far beyond the care of the sick and the prevention of illness. It aimed at rectifying those causes that led to the poverty and misery. Wald was a tireless social activist for legislative reforms that would provide a more just distribution of services for the marginal and disadvantaged in the United States (Donahue, 1985). Wald began with 10 nurses in 1893, which grew to 250 nurses serving 1,300 clients a day by 1916. During this same period, the budget grew from nothing to more than $600,000 a year, all from private donations.

Wald hired African American nurse **Elizabeth Tyler** in 1906 as evidence of her commitment to cultural diversity. Although unable to visit white clients, Tyler made her own way by "finding" African American families who needed her service. In 3 months, Tyler had so many African American families within her caseload that Wald hired a second African American nurse, Edith Carter. Carter remained at Henry Street for 28 years until her retirement (Carnegie, 1991). During her tenure at Henry Street, Wald demonstrated her commitment to racial and cultural diversity by employing 25 African American nurses over the years, and she paid them salaries equal to white nurses and provided identical benefits and recognition to minority nurses (Carnegie, 1991). This was exceptional during the early part of the 1900s, a time when African American nurses were often denied admission to white schools of nursing and membership in professional organizations and were denied opportunities for employment in most settings. Because hospitals of this era often set quotas for African American clients, those nurses who managed to graduate from nursing schools found themselves with few clients who needed or could afford their services. African American nurses struggled for the right to take the registration examination available for white nurses.

Wald submitted a proposal to the city of New York after learning of a child's dismissal from a New York City school for a skin condition. Her proposal was for one of the Henry Street Settlement nurses to serve free for 1 month in a New York school. The results of her experiment were so convincing that salaries were approved for 12 school nurses. From this, school nursing was born in the United States and became one of many community specialties credited to Wald (Dietz & Lehozky, 1963). In 1909, Wald proposed a program to the Metropolitan Life Insurance Company to provide nursing visits to their industrial policyholders. Statistics kept by the company documented the lowered mortality rates of policyholders attributed to the nurses' public health practice and clinical expertise. The program demonstrated savings for the company and was so successful that it lasted until 1953 (Hamilton, 1988).

Wald's other significant accomplishments include the establishment of the Children's Bureau, set up in 1912 as part of the U.S. Department of Labor. She also was an enthusiastic supporter of and participant in women's suffrage, lobbied for inspections of the workplace, and supported her employee, Margaret Sanger, in her efforts to give women the right to birth control. She was active in the American Red Cross and International Red Cross and helped form the Women's Trade Union League to protect women from sweatshop conditions.

Wald first coined the phrase "public health nursing" and transformed the field of community health nursing from the narrow role of home visiting to the population focus of today's community health nurse (Robinson, 1946). According to Dock and Stewart (1931), the title of public health nurse was purposeful: The role designation was designed to link the public's health to governmental responsibility, not private funding. As state departments of health and local governments began to employ more and more public health nurses, their role increasingly focused on prevention of illness in the entire community. Discrimination developed between the visiting nurse, who was employed by the voluntary agencies primarily to provide home care to the sick, and the public health nurse, who concentrated on preventive measures (Brainard, 1922).

Early public health nurses came closer than hospital-based nurses to the autonomy and professionalism that Nightingale advocated. Their work was conducted in the unconfined setting of the home and community, they were independent, and they enjoyed recognition as specialists in preventive health (Buhler-Wilkerson, 1985). Public health nurses from the beginning were much more holistic in their practice than their hospital counterparts. They were involved with the health of industrial workers, immigrants, and their families and were concerned about exploitation of women and children. These nurses also played a part in prison reform and care of the mentally ill (Heinrich, 1983).

Considered the first African American public health nurse, **Jessie Sleet Scales** was hired in 1902 by the Charity Organization Society, a philanthropic organization, to visit African American families infected by TB. Scales provided district nursing care to New York City's African American families and is credited with paving the way for African American nurses in the practice of community health (Mosley, 1996).

Dorothea Lynde Dix

Dorothea Lynde Dix, a Boston schoolteacher, became aware of the horrendous conditions in prisons and mental institutions when asked to do a Sunday school class in the House of Correction at Cambridge, Massachusetts. She was appalled at what she saw and went about studying whether the conditions were isolated or widespread; she took 2 years off to visit every jail and almshouse from Cape Cod to Berkshire (Tiffany, 1890, p. 76). Her report was devastating. Boston was scandalized by the reality that the most progressive state in the Union was now associated with such appalling conditions. The shocked legislature voted to allocate funds to build hospitals. For the rest of her life, Dorothea Dix stood out as a tireless zealot for the humane treatment of the insane and imprisoned. She had exceptional savvy in dealing with legislators. She acquainted herself with the legislators and their records and displayed the "spirit of a crusader." For her contributions, Dix is recognized as one of the pioneers of the reform movement for mental health in the United States, and her efforts are felt worldwide to the present day (Dietz & Lehozky, 1963).

Dix was also known for her work in the Civil War, having been appointed superintendent of the female nurses of the Army by the secretary of war in 1861. Her tireless efforts led to the recruitment of more than 2,000 women to serve in the army during the Civil War. Officials had consulted with Nightingale concerning military hospitals and were determined not to make the same mistakes. Dix enjoyed far more sweeping powers than Nightingale in that she had the authority to organize hospitals, to appoint nurses, and to manage supplies for the wounded (Brockett & Vaughan, 1867). Among her most well-known nurses during the Civil War were the poet Walt Whitman and the author Louisa May Alcott (Donahue, 1985).

Clara Barton

The idea for the International Red Cross was the brainchild of a Swiss banker, J. Henri Dunant, who proposed the formation of a neutral international relief society that could be activated in time of war. The International Red Cross was ratified by the Geneva Convention on August 22, 1864. **Clara Barton**, through her work in the Civil War, had come to believe that such an organization was desperately needed in the United States. However, it was not until 1882 that Barton was able to convince Congress to ratify the Treaty of Geneva, thus becoming the founder of the American Red Cross (Kalisch & Kalisch, 1986). Barton also played a leadership role in the Spanish-American War in Cuba, where she led a group of nurses to provide care for both U.S. and Cuban soldiers and Cuban civilians. At the age of 76, Barton went to President McKinley and offered the help of the Red Cross in Cuba. The president agreed to allow Barton to go with Red Cross nurses, but only to care for the Cuban citizens. Once in Cuba, the U.S. military saw what Barton and her nurses were able to accomplish with the Cuban military, and American soldiers pressured military officials to allow Barton's help. Along with battling yellow fever, Barton was able to provide care to both Cuban and U.S. military personnel and eventually expanded that care to Cuban citizens in Santiago. One of Barton's most famous clients was young Colonel Teddy Roosevelt, who led his Rough Riders and who later became the president of the United States. Barton became an instant heroine both in Cuba and in the United States for her bravery, tenaciousness, and for organizing services for the military and civilians torn apart by war. On August 13, 1898, the Spanish-American War came to an end. The grateful people of Santiago, Cuba, built a statue to honor Clara Barton in the town square, where it stands to this day. The work of Barton and her Red Cross nurses spread through the newspapers of the United States and in the schools of nursing. A congressional committee investigating the work of Barton's Red Cross staff applauded the work of these nurses and recommended that the U.S. Medical Department create a permanent reserve corps of trained nurses. These reserve nurses became the Army Nurse Corps in 1901. Clara Barton will always be remembered both as the founder of the American Red Cross and the driving force behind the creation of the Army Nurse Corps (Frantz, 1998).

Birth of the Midwife in the United States

Women have always assisted other women in the birth of babies. These "lay midwives" were considered by communities to possess special skills and somewhat of a "calling." With the advent of professional nursing in England, registered nurses became associated with safer and more predictable childbirth practices. In England and in other countries where Nightingale nurses were prevalent, most registered nurses were also trained as midwives with a 6-month specialized training period. In the United States, the training of registered nurses in the practice of midwifery was prevented primarily by physicians. U.S. physicians saw midwives as a threat and intrusion into medical practice. Such resistance indirectly led to the proliferation of "granny wives" who were ignorant of modern practices, were untrained, and were associated with high maternal morbidity (Donahue, 1985).

The first organized midwifery service in the United States was the **Frontier Nursing Service** founded in 1925 by **Mary Breckinridge**. Breckinridge graduated from the St. Luke's Hospital Training School in New York in 1910 and received her midwifery certificate from the British Hospital for Mothers and Babies in London in 1925. She had extensive experience in the delivery of babies and midwifery systems in New Zealand and Australia. In rural Appalachia, babies had been delivered for decades by granny midwives, who relied mainly on tradition, myths, and superstition as the bases of their practice. For example, they might use ashes for medication and place a sharp axe, blade up, under the bed of a laboring woman to "cut" the pain. The people of Appalachia were isolated because of the terrain of the hollows and mountains, and roads were limited to most families. They had one of the highest birth rates in the United States. Breckinridge believed that if a midwifery service could work under these conditions, it could work anywhere (Donahue, 1985).

Breckinridge had to use English midwives for many years and only began training her own midwives in 1939 when she started the Frontier Graduate School of Nurse Midwifery in Hyden, Kentucky, with the advent of World War II. The nurse midwives accessed many of their families on horseback. In 1935, a small 12-bed hospital was built at Hyden and provided delivery services. The nurse midwives under the direction of Breckinridge were successful in lowering the highest maternal mortality rate in the United States (in Leslie County, Kentucky) to substantially below the national average. These nurses, as at Henry Street Settlement, provided health care for everyone in the district for a small annual fee. A delivery had an additional small fee. Nurse midwives provided primary care, prenatal care, and postnatal care, with an emphasis on prevention (Wertz & Wertz, 1977).

Armed with the right to vote, in the Roaring Twenties American women found the new freedom of the "flapper era"—shrinking dress hemlines, shortened hairstyles, and the increased use of cosmetics. Hospitals were used by greater numbers of people, and the scientific basis of medicine became well established because most surgical procedures were done in hospitals. Penicillin was discovered in 1928, creating a revolution in the prevention of infectious disease deaths (Donahue, 1985; Kalisch & Kalisch, 1986). The previously mentioned Goldmark Report recommended the establishment of college and university-based nursing programs.

Mary D. Osborne, who functioned as supervisor of public health nursing for the state of Mississippi from 1921 to 1946, had a vision for a collaboration with community nurses and granny midwives, who delivered 80% of the

African American babies in Mississippi. The infant and maternal mortality rates were both exceptionally high among African American families, and these granny midwives, who were also African American, were untrained and had little education.

Osborne took a creative approach to improving maternal and infant health among African American women. She developed a collaborative network of public health nurses and granny midwives; the nurses implemented training programs for the midwives, and the midwives in turn assisted the nurses in providing a higher standard of safe maternal and infant health care. The public health nurses used Osborne's book, *Manual for Midwives*, which contained guidelines for care and was used in the state until the 1970s. They taught good hygiene, infection prevention, and compliance with state regulations. Osborne's innovative program is credited with reducing the maternal and infant mortality rates in Mississippi and in other states where her program structure was adopted (Sabin, 1998).

The Nursing Profession Responds to the Great Depression and World War II

With the stock market crash of 1929 came the Great Depression, resulting in widespread unemployment of private-duty nurses and the closing of nursing schools with a simultaneous increase in need for charity health services for the population. Nursing students who had previously been the primary source to staff hospitals declined in number. Unemployed graduate nurses were hired to replace them for minimal wages, a trend that was to influence the profession for years to come (MacEachern, 1932).

Other nurses found themselves accompanying troops to Europe when the United States entered World War II. Military nurses provided care aboard hospital ships and were a critical presence at the invasion of Normandy in 1944, as well as in military operations in North Africa, Italy, France, and the Philippines. More than 100,000 nurses volunteered and were certified for military service in the Army and Navy Nurse Corps. The resulting severe shortage of nurses on the home front resulted in the development of the Cadet Nurse Corps. **Frances Payne Bolton**, congressional representative from Ohio, is credited with the founding of the Cadet Nurse Corps through the Bolton Act of 1945. By the end of the war, more than 180,000 nursing students had been trained through this act, while advanced practice graduate nurses in psychiatry and public health nursing had received graduate education to increase the numbers of nurse educators (Donahue, 1985; Kalisch & Kalisch, 1986).

Amid the Depression, many nurses found the expansion and advances in aviation as a new field for nurses. In efforts to increase the public's confidence in the safety of transcontinental air travel, nurses were hired in the promising new role of "nurse-stewardess" (Kalisch & Kalisch, 1986). Congress created an additional relief program, the Civil Works Administration, in 1933 that provided jobs to the unemployed, including placing nurses in schools, public hospitals and clinics, public health departments, and public health education community surveys and campaigns. The Social Security Act of 1935 was passed by Congress to provide old-age benefits, rehabilitation services, unemployment compensation administration, aid to dependent and/or disabled children and adults, and monies to state and local health services. The Social Security Act included Title VI, which authorized the use of federal funds for the training of public health personnel. This led to the placement of public health nurses in state health departments and the expansion of public health nursing as a viable career path.

While nursing was forging new paths for itself in various fields, during the 1930s Hollywood began featuring nurses in films. The only feature-length films to ever focus entirely on the nursing profession were released during this decade. *War Nurse* (1930), *Night Nurse* (1931), *Once to Every Woman* (1934), *The White Parade* (1934 Academy Award nominee for Best Picture), *Four Girls in White* (1939), *The White Angel* (1936), and *Doctor and Nurse* (1937) all used nurses as major characters. During the bleak years of the economic depression, young women found these nurse heroines who promoted idealism, self-sacrifice, and the profession of nursing over personal desires particularly appealing. No longer were nurses depicted as subservient handmaidens who worked as nurses only as a temporary pastime before marriage (Kalisch & Kalisch, 1986).

During the 1930s, the Association of Collegiate Schools of Nursing was formed to advance nursing education and promote research related to educational criteria in nursing. Goals were aimed at changing the professional level of the nurse with a focus on preparing nurses in the academic setting and thus preparing nurses for specialized roles such as faculty, administrators of schools of nursing, and supervisors (Judd, 2014).

Science and Health Care, 1945-1960: Decades of Change

Dramatic technological and scientific changes characterized the decades following World War II, including the discovery of sulfa drugs, new cardiac drugs, surgeries, and treatment for ventricular fibrillation (Howell, 1996). The Hill-Burton Act, passed in 1946, provided funds to increase the construction of new hospitals. A significant change in the healthcare system was the expansion of private health insurance coverage and the dramatic increase in the birth rate, called the "baby boom" generation. Clinical research, both in medicine and in nursing, became an expectation of health providers, and more nurses sought advanced degrees. The first ANA *Code of Ethics for Nurses* was adopted in 1950, and in 1953 the International Council of Nurses (ICN) adopted an international *Code of Ethics for Nurses*. In 1952, the first scholarly journal, *Journal of Nursing Research*, was first published in the United States (Kalisch & Kalisch, 2004).

As a result of increased numbers of hospital beds, additional financial resources for health care, and the post–World War II economic resurgence, nursing faced an acute shortage and nurses confronted increasingly stressful working conditions. Nurses began showing signs of the strain through debates about strikes and collective bargaining demands.

The ANA accepted African American nurses for membership, consequently ending racial discrimination in the dominant nursing organizations. The National Association of Colored Graduate Nurses was disbanded in 1951. Males entered nursing schools in record number, often as a result of previous military experience as medics. Prior to the 1950s and 1960s, male nurses also suffered minority status and were discouraged from nursing as a career. A fact seemingly forgotten by modern society, including Florence Nightingale and early U.S. nursing leaders, is that during medieval times more than one-half of the nurses were male. The Knights Hospitallers, Teutonic Knights, Franciscans, and many other male nursing orders had provided excellent nursing care for their societies. Saint Vincent de Paul had first conceived of the idea of social service. Pastor Theodor Fliedner, teacher and mentor of Florence Nightingale at Kaiserwerth in Germany; Ben Franklin; and Walt Whitman during the Civil War all either served as nurses or were strong advocates for male nurses (Kalisch & Kalisch, 1986).

Years of Revolution, Protest, and the New Order, 1961–2000

During the social upheaval of the 1960s, nursing was influenced by many changes in society, such as the women's movement, the organized protest against the Vietnam conflict, civil rights movement, President Lyndon Johnson's "Great Society" social reforms, and increased consumer involvement in health care. Specialization in nursing, such as cardiac intensive care unit, nurse anesthetist training, and the clinical specialist role for nursing became trends that affected both education and practice in the healthcare system. Medicare and Medicaid, enacted in 1965 under Title XVIII of the Social Security Act, provided access to health care for older adults, poor persons, and people with disabilities. The ANA took a courageous and controversial stand in that same year (1965) by approving its first position paper on nursing education, advocating for all nursing education for professional practice to take place in colleges and universities (ANA, 1965). Nurses returning from Vietnam faced emotional challenges in the form of PTSD that affected their postwar lives.

With increased specialization in medicine, the demand for primary care healthcare providers exceeded the supply (Christman, 1971). As a response to this need for general practitioners, Dr. Henry Silver, MD, and Dr. Loretta Ford, RN, collaborated to develop the first NP program in the United States at the University of Colorado (Ford & Silver, 1967). NPs were initially prepared in pediatrics with advanced role preparation in common childhood illness management and well-child care. Ford and Silver (1967) found that NPs could manage as much as 75% of the pediatric patients in community clinics, leading to the widespread use of and educational programs for NPs. The first state in 1971 to recognize diagnosis and treatment as part of the legal scope of practice for NPs was Idaho. Alaska and North Carolina were among the first states to expand the NP role to include prescriptive authority (Ford, 1979). By the turn of the century, NP programs were offered at the MSN level in family nursing; gerontology; and adult, neonatal, mental health, and maternal–child areas and have expanded to include the acute care practitioner as well (Huch, 2001). Currently, the preferred educational preparation for advanced practice nurse is the Doctor of Nursing Practice. Certification of NPs now occurs at the national level through the ANA and by many specialty organizations. NPs are licensed throughout the United States by state boards of nursing.

In the late 1980s, escalating healthcare costs resulting from the explosion of advanced technology and the increased life span of Americans led to the demand for healthcare reform. The nursing profession heralded healthcare reform with an unprecedented collaboration of more than 75 nursing associations, led by the ANA and the National League for Nursing, in the publication of *Nursing's Agenda for Health Care Reform*. In this document, the challenge of managed care was addressed in the context of cost containment and quality assurance of healthcare service for the nursing profession (ANA, 1991). Managed care is a market approach based on managed competition as a major strategy to contain healthcare costs, which is still the dominant approach used today (Lundy, Janes, & Hartman, 2001).

> **KEY COMPETENCY 1-1**
>
> Examples of Applicable *Nurse of the Future: Nursing Core Competencies*
>
> Professionalism:
>
> Knowledge (K8a) Understands responsibilities inherent in being a member of the nursing profession
>
> Skills (S8a) Understands the history and philosophy of the nursing profession
>
> Attitudes/Behaviors (A8a) Recognizes need for personal and professional behaviors that promote the profession of nursing
>
> *Source:* Massachusetts Department of Higher Education (2010). *Nurse of the future: Nursing core competencies* (p. 15). Retrieved from http://www.mass.edu/currentinit /documents/NursingCoreCompetencies.pdf

The New Century

The new century began with a renewed focus on quality and safety in patient care. The landmark publication from the Institute of Medicine (IOM) published in November 1999, *To Err Is Human*, was the launching pad from which this movement began in earnest. This report is best known for drawing attention to the scope of errors in health care; for the conclusion that most errors are related to faulty systems, processes, and conditions that allow error, rather than individual recklessness; and for the recommendation to design healthcare systems at all levels to make it more difficult to make errors. Subsequent reports followed focusing on quality through healthcare redesign and health professions education redesign (IOM, 2001, 2003).

With the roles of nurses in the healthcare system expected to continue to expand in the future, the focus is placed on raising the educational levels and competencies of nurses and fostering interdisciplinary collaboration to increase access, safety, and quality of patient care. For example, the latest Institute of Medicine (IOM, 2011) report, entitled *The Future of Nursing:*

Leading Change, Advancing Health, specifically calls for interdisciplinary education, decreasing barriers to nurses' scope of practice, and increasing the educational levels of nurses. The Robert Wood Johnson Foundation sponsored the Quality and Safety Education for Nurses (QSEN) initiative with the overall goal of "preparing future nurses who will have the knowledge, skills and attitudes (KSAs) necessary to continuously improve the quality and safety of the healthcare systems within which they work" (QSEN, 2007). The focus of QSEN is to develop the competencies of future nursing graduates in six key areas: patient-centered care, evidence-based practice, quality improvement, teamwork and collaboration, safety, and informatics.

In 2006, the Massachusetts Department of Higher Education (MDHE) and Massachusetts Organization of Nurse Executives convened a working session of stakeholders titled Creativity and Connections: Building the Framework for the Future of Nursing Education and Practice. From this beginning, the *Nurse of the Future: Nursing Core Competencies* (MDHE, 2010, p. 2) was developed in response to the goals of creating a seamless progression through all levels of nursing education and development of consensus on competencies. This movement to facilitate creation of a core set of entry-level nursing competencies and seamless transition in nursing education is not singular and reflects the current focus in the profession to increase the access, safety, and quality of health care.

U.S. healthcare system reform continues to be the topic of political debate with the primary focus on federal coverage, access, and control of healthcare costs. Healthcare organizations in a managed care environment see economic and quality outcome benefits of caring for patients and managing their care over a continuum of settings and needs. Patients are followed more closely within the system, during both illness and wellness. Hospital stays are shorter, and more healthcare services are provided in outpatient facilities and through community-based settings.

The Patient Protection and Affordable Care Act (PPACA) was signed into law on March 23, 2010, and was upheld as constitutional by the U.S. Supreme Court on June 28, 2012. The purpose of the PPACA is to provide affordable health care for all Americans. The law includes provisions for preventive care and protections for consumers that include ending preexisting exclusions for children, ending lifetime limits, and preventing companies from arbitrarily dropping coverage. It is predicted that this legislation will have results through 2029 and that during the next decade it will increase insurance coverage to 32 million additional people who are currently uninsured.

International Council of Nurses

A review of nursing history would not be complete without some discussion of the contributions of the International Council of Nurses (ICN). The ICN was founded in 1899 by women whose names are familiar to the student of nursing history—names such as Ethel Fenwick of Great Britain, Lavinia Dock of the United States, Mary Agnes Snively of Canada, and Agnes Karll of Germany—who believed in the link between women's rights and professional nursing. They advocated the creation of national nursing organizations that would allow women to self-govern the profession, and these early leaders from the United Kingdom, Canada, the United States, Germany, the Netherlands, and Scandinavia banded together in the ICN to encourage one another as they continued to build stronger national associations in their respective nations (Brush & Lynaugh, 1999, p. xi).

CRITICAL THINKING QUESTION *

What do you think would be the response of historical nursing leaders such as Florence Nightingale, Lillian Wald, and Mary Breckinridge if they could see what the profession of nursing looks like today? *

World War I and World War II presented threats to the organization, but the ICN emerged with greater participation from nurses in nations that had not previously participated in the organization. New members after World War I included China, Palestine, Brazil, and the Philippines. After World War II, there was again an influx of new membership that included nations from Africa, Asia, and South America. With an increasingly diverse membership, the ICN implemented a more global agenda. During the time of the Cold War when Russia, China, and nations in Eastern Europe did not participate, the ICN still defined the work of nurses worldwide and claimed the right to speak for nursing. During the decades that followed, the ICN forged closer links with the World Health Organization, added to its agenda the delivery of primary health care to people around the world, and actively supported the rights of nurses to fair employment and freedom from exploitation (Brush & Lynaugh, 1999, p. xii).

Currently located in Geneva, Switzerland, the ICN has grown into a federation of more than 130 national nurses associations, representing the more than 16 million nurses worldwide. ICN is the world's first and widest reaching international organization for health professionals, working to ensure quality nursing care for all, sound health policies globally, the advancement of nursing knowledge, and the presence worldwide of a respected nursing profession and a competent and satisfied nursing workforce (ICN, n.d.).

Conclusion

Contemplating the progression of nursing as a profession, it becomes evident from the preceding pages that similar issues, barriers, challenges, and opportunities were simultaneously present in locations around the globe. In each circumstance, nursing leaders arose to initiate change; whether related to nurse registration, standards for nursing education, or safe work environments, their ultimate goal was the provision of quality patient care. The history of professional nursing began with efforts to reach that goal, and we continue in this quest as our nursing organizations continue to develop and revise accreditation standards for programs of nursing, examine practice competencies, and review criteria for licensure.

Consensus regarding basic education and the entry level of registered nurses has not occurred in the United States, although progress has been made in neighboring Canada. Changes in the advanced practice role continue to challenge the nurse education and healthcare systems around the world as the primary healthcare needs of populations compete with acute care for scarce resources. A global community demands that nurses remain committed to cultural sensitivity in care delivery.

The history of health care and nursing provides ample examples of the wisdom of our forebears in the advocacy of nursing in challenging settings in an unknown future. By considering the lessons of our past, the nursing profession is positioned to lead the way in the provision of a full range of quality, cost-effective services required to care for patients in this century.

Classroom Activity 1

There are many theories about Nightingale's chronic illness, which caused her to be an invalid for most of her adult life. Many people have interpreted this as hypochondriacal, something of a melodrama of the Victorian times. Nightingale was rich and could take to her bed. Rumors have abounded among nursing students that she suffered from tertiary syphilis. She became ill during the Crimean War in May 1855 and was diagnosed with a severe case of Crimean fever. Today Crimean fever is recognized as Mediterranean fever and is categorized as brucellosis. She developed spondylitis, or inflammation of the spine. For the next 34 years, she managed to continue her writing and advocacy, often predicting her imminent death. Others have claimed that Nightingale suffered from bipolar disorder, causing her to experience long periods of depression alternating with remarkable bursts of productivity. Read about the various theories of her chronic disabling condition and reflect on your own conclusions about her mysterious illness. With supporting evidence, what are your conclusions about Nightingale's health condition?

Sources: Data from Dossey, B. (2000). *Florence Nightingale: Mystic, visionary, healer.* Philadelphia, PA: Lippincott Williams & Wilkins; Australian Nursing Federation. (2004). Nightingale suffered bipolar disorder. *Australian Nursing Journal, 12*(2), 33.

Classroom Activity 2

What would Florence Nightingale's résumé or curriculum vitae look like? Check out Nightingale's curriculum vitae at www.countryjoe.com/nightingale/cv.htm.

References

Abel, E. K. (1997). Take the cure to the poor: Patients' responses to New York City's tuberculosis program, 1894–1918. *American Journal of Public Health, 87*, 11.

American Nurses Association. (1965). *Educational preparation for nurse practitioners and assistants to nurses: A position paper.* New York, NY: Author.

American Nurses Association. (1991). *Nursing's agenda for health care reform: Executive summary.* Washington, DC: Author.

Andrews, G. (2003). Nightingale's geography. *Nursing Inquiry, 10*(4), 270–274.

Attewell, A. (1996). Florence Nightingale's health-at-home visitors. *Health Visitor, 6.9*(10), 406.

Australian Bureau of Statistics. (1985). Year book Australia, 1985. Retrieved from http://www.abs.gov.au/ausstats/abs@.nsf/featurearticlesbytitle/911B5AF72F818 795CA2569DE0024ED5A?OpenDocument

Australian Government. (2009). Women in action: Nurses and serving women. Retrieved from http://www.australia.gov.au/about-australia/australian-story /women-in-action

Australian Nursing and Midwifery Accreditation Council. (2014). About ANMAC: History. Retrieved from http://www.anmac.org.au/history

Australian Nursing and Midwifery Federation. (2015). About the ANMF. Retrieved from http://anmf.org.au/pages/about-the-anmf

Australian Nursing and Midwifery Federation (SA Branch). (2012). Our history. Retrieved from https://www.anmfsa.org.au/about-us/our-history/

Australian Nursing Federation. (2004). Nightingale suffered bipolar disorder. *Australian Nursing Journal, 12*(2), 33.

Barker, E. R. (1989). Care givers as casualties. *Western Journal of Nursing Research, 11*(5), 628–631.

Boorstin, D. J. (1985). *The discoverers: A history of man's search to know his world and himself.* New York, NY: Vintage.

Brainard, A. M. (1922). *The evolution of public health nursing.* Philadelphia, PA: Saunders.

Brockett, L. P., & Vaughan, M. C. (1867). *Women's work in the Civil War: A record of heroism: Patriotism and patience.* Philadelphia, PA: Seigler McCurdy.

Brooke, E. (1997). *Medicine women: A pictorial history of women healers.* Wheaton, IL: Quest Books.

Brown, E. L. (1936). *Nursing as a profession.* New York, NY: Russell Sage Foundation.

Brown, E. L. (1948). *Nursing for the future.* New York, NY: Russell Sage Foundation.

Brown, P. (1988). *Florence Nightingale.* Hats, UK: Exley Publications.

Brush, B. L., & Lynaugh, J. E. (1999). About this history. In B. L. Brush & J. E. Lynaugh (Eds.), *Nurses of all nations: A history of the International Council of Nurses, 1899–1999* (pp. xi–xvii). Philadelphia, PA: Lippincott Williams & Wilkins.

Buhler-Wilkerson, K. (1985). Public health nursing: In sickness or in health? *American Journal of Public Health, 75*, 1155–1156.

Bullough, V. L., & Bullough, B. (1978). *The care of the sick: The emergence of modern nursing.* New York, NY: Prodist.

Calabria, M. D. (1996). *Florence Nightingale in Egypt and Greece: Her diary and visions.* Albany, NY: State University of New York Press.

Canadian Association of Schools of Nursing. (n.d.). CASN/ACESI mission. Retrieved from http://www.casn.ca/about-casn/casnacesi-mission/

Canadian Museum of History. (n.d.). Canadian nursing history collection: A brief history of nursing in Canada from establishment of New France to present. Retrieved from http://www.historymuseum.ca/cmc/exhibitions/tresors/nursing/nchis01e.shtml

Canadian Nurses Association. (n.d.). History. Retrieved from http://www.cna-aiic.ca/en/about-cna/history

Canadian Nurses Foundation. (2014). Our history. Retrieved from http://cnf-fiic.ca/who-we-are/our-stories/our-history/#.VNwEqiifmmA

Carnegie, M. E. (1991). *The path we tread: Blades in nursing 1854–1990* (2nd ed.). New York, NY: National League for Nursing Press.

Cartwright, F. F. (1972). *Disease and history*. New York, NY: Dorset Press.

Christman, L. (1971). The nurse specialist as a professional activist. *Nursing Clinics of North America, 6*(2), 231–235.

Christy, T. E. (1975). The fateful decade: 1890–1900. *American Journal of Nursing, 75*(7), 1163–1165.

Cohen, M. N. (1989). *Health and the rise of civilization*. New Haven, CT: Yale University Press.

Cook, E. (1913). *The life of Florence Nightingale* (Vols. 1 and 2). London, England: Macmillan.

D'Antonio, P. (2002). Nurses in war. *Lancet, 360*(9350), 7–12.

Diamond, J. (1997). *Guns, germs, and steel: The fates of human societies*. New York, NY: W. W. Norton.

Dickens, C. (1844). *Martin Chuzzlewit*. New York, NY: Macmillan.

Dietz, D. D., & Lehozky, A. R. (1963). *History and modern nursing*. Philadelphia, PA: F. A. Davis.

Dock, L., & Stewart, I. (1931). *A short history of nursing from the earliest times to the present day* (3rd ed.). New York, NY: G. P. Putnam's Sons.

Donahue, M. P. (1985). *Nursing: The finest art*. St. Louis, MO: Mosby.

Dossey, B. (2000). *Florence Nightingale: Mystic, visionary, healer*. Philadelphia, PA: Lippincott Williams & Wilkins.

Ford, L. C. (1979). A nurse for all seasons: The nurse practitioner. *Nursing Outlook, 27*(8), 516–521.

Ford, L. C., & Silver, H. K. (1967). The expanded role of the nurse in child care. *Nursing Outlook, 15*(8), 43–45.

Frantz, A. K. (1998). Nursing pride: Clara Barton in the Spanish American War. *American Journal of Nursing, 98*(10), 39–41.

Goldmark, J. C. (1923). *Nursing and nursing education in the United States*. New York, NY: Macmillan.

Hamilton, D. (1988). Clinical excellence, but too high a cost: The Metropolitan Life Insurance Company Visiting Nurse Service (1909–1953). *Public Health Nursing, 5*, 235–240.

Hanlon, J. J., & Pickett, G. E. (1984). *Public health administration and practice* (8th ed.). St. Louis, MO: Mosby.

Heinrich, J. (1983). Historical perspectives on public health nursing. *Nursing Outlook, 32*(6), 317–320.

Howell, J. (1996). *Technology in the hospital*. Baltimore, MD: Johns Hopkins University Press.

Huch, M. (2001). Advanced practice nursing in the community. In K. S. Lundy & S. Janes (Eds.), *Community health nursing: Caring for the public's health* (pp. 968–980). Sudbury, MA: Jones and Bartlett.

Institute of Medicine. (1999). *To err is human: Building a safer health system*. Washington, DC: National Academy Press.

Institute of Medicine. (2001). *Crossing the quality chasm: A new health system for the 21st century*. Washington, DC: National Academy Press.

Institute of Medicine. (2003). *Health professions education: A bridge to quality*. Washington, DC: National Academy Press.

Institute of Medicine. (2011). *The future of nursing: Leading change, advancing health*. Washington, DC: National Academy Press.

International Council of Nurses. (n.d.). Who we are. Retrieved from http://www.icn.ch/who-we-are/who-we-are/

Judd, D. (2014). Nursing in the United States from the 1920s to the early 1940s: Education rather than training for nurses. In D. Judd & K. Stizman (Eds.), *A history of American nursing: Trends and eras* (2nd ed., pp. 148–180). Burlington, MA: Jones & Bartlett Learning.

Kalisch, P. A., & Kalisch, B. J. (1986). *The advance of American nursing* (2nd ed.). Boston, MA: Little, Brown.

Kalisch, P. A., & Kalisch, B. J. (2004). *American nursing: A history* (4th ed.). Philadelphia, PA: Lippincott Williams and Wilkins.

LeVasseur, J. (1998). Plato: Nightingale and contemporary nursing. *Image: Journal of Nursing Scholarship, 30*(3), 281–285.

Longfellow, H. W. (1857). Santa Filomena. *Atlantic Monthly, 1*, 22–23.

Lundy, K. S., Janes, S., & Hartman, S. (2001). Opening the door to health care in the community. In K. S. Lundy & S. Janes (Eds.), *Community health nursing: Caring for the public's health* (pp. 5–29). Sudbury, MA: Jones and Bartlett.

MacEachern, M. T. (1932). Which shall we choose: Graduate or student service? *Modern Hospital, 38*, 97–98, 102–104.

Mansell, D. J. (2004). *Forging the future: A history of nursing in Candada*. Ann Arbor, MI: Thomas Press.

Massachusetts Department of Higher Education. (2010). *Nurse of the future: Nursing core competencies*. Retrieved from http://www.mass.edu/currentinit/documents/NursingCoreCompetencies.pdf

McGann, S., Crowther, A., & Dougall, R. (2009). *A history of the Royal College of Nursing 1916–1990: A voice for nurses*. New York, NY: Manchester University Press.

Montag, M. L. (1959). *Community college education for nursing: An experiment in technical education for nursing*. New York, NY: McGraw-Hill.

Monteiro, L. A. (1985). Florence Nightingale on public health nursing. *American Journal of Public Health, 75*(2), 181–185.

Mosley, M. O. P. (1996). Satisfied to carry the bag: Three black community health nurses' contribution to health care reform, 1900–1937. *Nursing History Review, 4*, 65–82.

New South Wales Nurses and Midwives' Association. (2014). History. Retrieved from http://www.nswnma.asn.au/about-us/history/

Nightingale, F. (1860). *Notes on nursing: What it is and what it is not.* London, England: Harrison.

Nightingale, F. (1893). Sick-nursing and health-nursing. In B. Burdett-Coutts (Ed.), *Women's mission* (pp. 184–205). London, England: Sampson, Law, Marston and Co.

Nightingale, F. (1894). *Health teaching in towns and villages.* London, England: Spottiswoode & Co.

Nightingale, F. (1979). Cassandra. In M. Stark (Ed.), *Florence Nightingale's Cassandra.* Old Westbury, NY: Feminist Press.

Nursing and Midwifery Board of Australia. (n.d.). State and territory nursing and midwifery board members. Retrieved from http://www.nursingmidwiferyboard .gov.au/About/State-and-Territory-Nursing-and-Midwifery-Board-Members.aspx

Nutting, M. A., & Dock, L. L. (1907). *A history of nursing: The evolution of nursing systems from the earliest times to the foundation of the first English and American training schools for nurses.* New York, NY: G. P. Putnam's Sons.

The 100 people who made the millennium. (1997). *Life Magazine, 20*(10a).

Ontario Nurses' Association. (n.d.). Our history and milestones. Retrieved from http://www.ona.org/our_history.html

Palmer, I. S. (1977). Florence Nightingale: Reformer, reactionary, researcher. *Nursing Research, 26*(2), 13–18.

Palmer, I. S. (1982). *Through a glass darkly: From Nightingale to now.* Washington, DC: American Association of Colleges of Nursing.

Quality and Safety Education for Nurses. (2007). Quality and safety competencies. Retrieved from http://www.qsen.org/competencies.php

Rathbone, W. (1890). *A history of nursing in the homes of the poor.* Introduction by Florence Nightingale. London, England: Macmillan.

Registered Nurses' Association of Ontario. (n.d.). About RNAO. Retrieved from http://rnao.ca

Richardson, B. I. W. (1887). *The health of nations: A review of the works of Edwin Chadwick* (Vol. 2). London, England: Longmans, Green.

Roberts, M. (1954). *American nursing: History and interpretation.* New York, NY: Macmillan.

Robinson, V. (1946). *White caps: The story of nursing.* Philadelphia, PA: Lippincott.

Rosen, G. (1958). *A history of public health.* New York, NY: M.D. Publications.

Royal Australian Army Nursing Corps. (n.d.). Royal Australian Army Nursing Corps (RAANC). Retrieved from http://www.defence.gov.au/health/about/docs /RAANC.pdf

Royal British Nurses' Association. (n.d.). Registration of nurses. Retrieved from http://www.rbna.org.uk/registration.asp

Royal College of Nursing. (n.d.). Our history. Retrieved from http://www.rcn.org.uk /aboutus/our_history

Sabin, L. (1998). *Struggles and triumphs: The story of Mississippi nurses 1800–1950.* Jackson, MS: Mississippi Hospital Association Health, Research and Educational Foundation.

Sanger, M. (1928). *Motherhood in bondage.* New York, NY: Brentano's.

Seymer, L. (1954). *Selected writings of Florence Nightingale.* New York, NY: Macmillan.

Shryock, R. H. (1959). *The history of nursing: An interpretation of the social and medical factors involved.* Philadelphia, PA: Saunders.

Sitzman, K., & Judd, D. (2014a). Nursing in the American colonies from the 1600s to the 1700s: The influence of past ideas, traditions, and trends. In D. Judd & K. Sitzman (Eds.), *A history of American nursing: Trends and eras* (2nd ed., pp. 49–62). Burlington, MA: Jones & Bartlett Learning.

Sitzman, K., & Judd, D. (2014b). Nursing in the United States during the 1800s: Inspiration and insight lead to nursing reforms. In D. Judd & K. Sitzman (Eds.), *A history of American nursing: Trends and eras* (2nd ed., pp. 80–109). Burlington, MA: Jones & Bartlett Learning.

Smith, E. (1934). *Mississippi special public health nursing project made possible by federal funds*. Paper presented at the 1934 annual Mississippi Nurses Association meeting, Jackson, MS.

State board test pool examination. (1952). *American Journal of Nursing, 52,* 613.

Taylor, H. O. (1922). *Greek biology and medicine*. Boston, MA: Marshall Jones.

Tiffany, F. (1890). *The life of Dorothea Lynde Dix*. Boston, MA: Houghton Mifflin.

Tooley, S. A. (1910). *The life of Florence Nightingale*. London, England: Cassell and Co.

The University of Melbourne. (2015). The Australian nursing and midwifery history project: Military nursing. Retrieved from http://anmhp.unimelb.edu.au/history/military_nursing

Veterans Affairs Canada. (n.d.). The nursing sisters of Canada. Retrieved from http://www.veterans.gc.ca/eng/remembrance/those-who-served/women-and-war/nursing-sisters

Vicinus, M., & Nergaard, B. (1990). *Ever yours: Florence Nightingale: Selected letters*. Cambridge, MA: Harvard University Press.

Victorian Order of Nurses. (2009). History—a century of caring. Retrieved from http://www.von.ca/about/history.aspx

Wald, L. D. (1915). *The house on Henry Street*. New York, NY: Holt.

Wertz, R. W., & Wertz, D. C. (1977). *Lying-in: A history of childbirth in America*. New Haven, CT: Yale University Press.

Wheeler, W. (1999). Is Florence Nightingale holding us back? *Nursing 99, 29*(10), 22–23.

Williams, C. B. (1961). Stories from Scutari. *American Journal of Nursing, 61,* 88.

Winslow, C.-E. A. (1946). Florence Nightingale and public health nursing. *Public Health Nursing, 38,* 330–332.

Woodham-Smith, C. (1951). *Florence Nightingale*. New York, NY: McGraw-Hill.

Woodham-Smith, C. (1983). *Florence Nightingale*. New York, NY: Athenaeum.

Young, D. A. (1995). Florence Nightingale's fever. *British Medical Journal, 311,* 1697–1700.

Young, J. (2010). "Monthly" nurses, "sick" nurses, and midwives: Working-class caregivers in Toronto, 1830–91. In M. Rutherdale (Ed.), *Caregiving on the periphery: Historical perspectives on nursing and midwifery in Canada* (pp. 33–60). Montreal, Canada: McGill-Queen's University Press.

CHAPTER 2

Frameworks for Professional Nursing Practice

Kathleen Masters

Learning Objectives

After completing this chapter, the student should be able to:

1. Identify the four metaparadigm concepts of nursing.
2. Explain several theoretical works in nursing.
3. Discuss the Nurse of the Future concepts and core competencies.
4. Describe several non-nursing theories important to the discipline of nursing.
5. Begin the process of identifying theoretical frameworks of nursing that are consistent with a personal belief system.

Although the beginning of nursing theory development can be traced to Florence Nightingale, it was not until the second half of the 1900s that nursing theory caught the attention of nursing as a discipline. During the decades of the 1960s and 1970s, theory development was a major topic of discussion and publication. During the 1970s, much of the discussion was related to the development of one global theory for nursing. However, in the 1980s, attention turned from the development of a global theory for nursing as scholars began to recognize multiple approaches to theory development in nursing.

Because of the plurality in nursing theory, this information must be organized to be meaningful for practice, research, and further knowledge development. The goal of this chapter is to present an organized and practical overview of the major concepts, models, philosophies, and theories that are essential in professional nursing practice.

It can be helpful to define some terms that might be unfamiliar. A **concept** is a term or label that describes a phenomenon (Meleis, 2004). The phenomenon

Key Terms and Concepts

- » Concept
- » Conceptual model
- » Propositions
- » Assumptions
- » Theory
- » Metaparadigm
- » Person
- » Environment
- » Health
- » Nursing
- » Philosophies

Note: Excerpts adapted from Masters, K. (2015). *Nursing theories: A framework for professional practice* (2nd ed.). Burlington, MA: Jones & Bartlett Learning appear in this chapter.

described by a concept can be either empirical or abstract. An empirical concept is one that can be either observed or experienced through the senses. An abstract concept is one that is not observable, such as hope or caring (Hickman, 2002).

A **conceptual model** is defined as a set of concepts and statements that integrate the concepts into a meaningful configuration (Lippitt, 1973; as cited in Fawcett, 1994). **Propositions** are statements that describe relationships among events, situations, or actions (Meleis, 2004). **Assumptions** also describe concepts or connect two concepts and represent values, beliefs, or goals. When assumptions are challenged, they become propositions (Meleis, 2004). Conceptual models are composed of abstract and general concepts and propositions that provide a frame of reference for members of a discipline. This frame of reference determines how the world is viewed by members of a discipline and guides the members as they propose questions and make observations relevant to the discipline (Fawcett, 1994).

A **theory** "is an organized, coherent, and systematic articulation of a set of statements related to significant questions in a discipline that are communicated in a meaningful whole" (Meleis, 2007, p. 37). The primary distinction between a conceptual model and a theory is the level of abstraction and specificity. A conceptual model is a highly abstract system of global concepts and linking statements. A theory, in contrast, deals with one or more specific, concrete concepts and propositions (Fawcett, 1994).

A **metaparadigm** is the most global perspective of a discipline and "acts as an encapsulating unit, or framework, within which the more restricted ... structures develop" (Eckberg & Hill, 1979, p. 927). Each discipline singles out phenomena of interest that it will deal with in a unique manner. The concepts and propositions that identify and interrelate these phenomena are even more abstract than those in the conceptual models. These are the concepts that comprise the metaparadigm of the discipline (Fawcett, 1994).

The conceptual models and theories of nursing represent various paradigms derived from the metaparadigm of the discipline of nursing. Therefore, although each of the conceptual models might link and define the four metaparadigm concepts differently, the four metaparadigm concepts are present in each of the models.

The central concepts of the discipline of nursing are **person**, **environment**, **health**, and **nursing**. These four concepts of the metaparadigm of nursing are more specifically "The person receiving the nursing, the environment within which the person exits, the health–illness continuum within which the person falls at the time of the interaction with the nurse, and, finally, nursing actions themselves" (Flaskerud & Holloran, 1980, cited in Fawcett, 1994, p. 5).

Because concepts are so abstract at the metaparadigm level, many conceptual models have been developed from the metaparadigm of nursing. Subsequently, multiple theories have been derived from conceptual models in an effort to describe, explain, interpret, and predict the experiences, observations, and relationships observed in nursing practice.

Overview of Selected Nursing Theories

CRITICAL THINKING QUESTION *

What are the specific competencies for nurses in relation to theoretical knowledge? *

To apply nursing theory in practice, the nurse must have some knowledge of the theoretical works of the nursing profession. This chapter is not intended to provide an in-depth analysis of each of the theoretical works in nursing but rather provides an introductory overview of selected theoretical works to give you a launching point for further reflection and study as you begin your journey into professional nursing practice.

Theoretical works in nursing are generally categorized as either philosophies, conceptual models or grand theories, middle-range theories, or practice theories (also referred to as situation-specific theories) depending on the level of abstraction. We begin with the most abstract of these theoretical works, the philosophies of nursing.

Selected Philosophies of Nursing

Philosophies set forth the general meaning of nursing and nursing phenomena through reasoning and the logical presentation of ideas. Philosophies are broad and address general ideas about nursing. Because of their breadth, nursing philosophies contribute to the discipline by providing direction, clarifying values, and forming a foundation for theory development (Alligood, 2006).

Nightingale's Environmental Theory

Nightingale's philosophy includes the four metaparadigm concepts of nursing (**Table 2-1**), but the focus is primarily on the patient and the environment, with the nurse manipulating the environment to enhance patient recovery. Nursing interventions using Nightingale's philosophy are centered on the 13 canons, which follow (Nightingale, 1860/1969):

- *Ventilation and warming:* The interventions subsumed in this canon include keeping the patient and the patient's room warm and keeping the patient's room well ventilated and free of odors. Specific instructions

TABLE 2-1 Metaparadigm Concepts as Defined in Nightingale's Model	
Person	Recipient of nursing care.
Environment	External (temperature, bedding, ventilation) and internal (food, water, and medications).
Health	Health is "not only to be well, but to be able to use well every power we have to use" (Nightingale, 1969, p. 24).
Nursing	Alter or manage the environment to implement the natural laws of health.

included "keep the air within as pure as the air without" (Nightingale, 1860/1969, p. 10).

- *Health of houses:* This canon includes the five essentials of pure air, pure water, efficient drainage, cleanliness, and light.
- *Petty management:* Continuity of care for the patient when the nurse is absent is the essence of this canon.
- *Noise:* Instructions include the avoidance of sudden noises that startle or awaken patients and keeping noise in general to a minimum.
- *Variety:* This canon refers to an attempt at variety in the patient's room to avoid boredom and depression.
- *Taking food:* Interventions include the documentation of the amount of food and liquids that the patient ingests.
- *What food?* Instructions include trying to include patient food preferences.
- *Bed and bedding:* The interventions in this canon include comfort measures related to keeping the bed dry and wrinkle free.
- *Light:* The instructions contained in this canon relate to adequate light in the patient's room.
- *Cleanliness of rooms and walls:* This canon focuses on keeping the environment clean.
- *Personal cleanliness:* This canon includes measures such as keeping the patient clean and dry.
- *Chattering hopes and advices:* Instructions in this canon include the avoidance of talking without reason or giving advice that is without fact.
- *Observation of the sick:* This canon includes instructions related to making observations and documenting observations.

The 13 canons are central to Nightingale's theory but are not all inclusive. Nightingale believed that nursing was a calling and that the recipients of nursing care were holistic individuals with a spiritual dimension; thus, the nurse was expected to care for the spiritual needs of the patients in spiritual distress. Nightingale also believed that nurses should be involved in health promotion and health teaching with the sick and with those who were well (Bolton, 2006).

Although Nightingale's theory was developed long ago in response to a need for environmental reform, the nursing principles are still relevant today. Even as some of Nightingale's rationales have been modified or disproved by advances in medicine and science, many of the concepts in her theory have not only endured, but have been used to provide general guidelines for nurses for more than 150 years (Pfettscher, 2006).

Virginia Henderson: Definition of Nursing and 14 Components of Basic Nursing Care

Henderson made such significant contributions to the discipline of nursing during her more-than-60-year career as a nurse, teacher, author, and researcher that some refer to her as the Florence Nightingale of the 20th century (Tomey, 2006). She is perhaps best known for her definition of nursing, which was first published in 1955 (Harmer & Henderson, 1955) and then published in 1966 with minor revisions. According to Henderson (1996), the role of the nurse involves assisting the patient to perform activities that contribute to health, recovery, or a peaceful death, which the patient would perform without assistance if he or she possessed " the necessary strength, will, or knowledge" and to do so in a way that helps the patient gain independence rather than remain dependent on the nurse (p. 15). In her work, Henderson emphasized the art of nursing as well as empathetic understanding, stating that the nurse must "get inside the skin of each of her patients in order to know what he needs" (Henderson, 1964, p. 63). She believed that "the beauty of medicine and nursing is the combination of your heart, your head and your hands and where you separate them, you diminish them ..." (McBride, 1997, as cited by Gordon, 2001).

   Henderson identified 14 basic needs on which nursing care is based. These needs include the following:

- Breathe normally.
- Eat and drink adequately.
- Eliminate bodily wastes.
- Move and maintain desirable postures.
- Sleep and rest.
- Select suitable clothes; dress and undress.
- Maintain body temperature within normal range by adjusting clothing and modifying the environment.
- Keep the body clean and well groomed and protect the integument.
- Avoid dangers in the environment, and avoid injuring others.
- Communicate with others in expressing emotions, needs, fears, or opinions.
- Worship according to one's faith.
- Work in such a way that there is a sense of accomplishment.
- Play or participate in various forms of recreation.
- Learn, discover, or satisfy the curiosity that leads to normal development and health and use the available health facilities (Henderson, 1966, 1991).

Although Henderson did not consider her work a theory of nursing, and did not explicitly state assumptions or define each of the domains of nursing, her work includes the metaparadigm concepts of nursing (**Table 2-2**) (Furukawa & Howe, 2002).

Jean Watson: Philosophy and Science of Caring

According to Watson's theory (1996), the goal of nursing is to help persons attain a higher level of harmony within the mind–body–spirit. Attainment of that goal can potentiate healing and health (**Table 2-3**). This goal is pursued through transpersonal caring guided by carative factors and corresponding caritas processes.

TABLE 2-2	Metaparadigm Concepts as Defined in Henderson's Philosophy and Art of Nursing
Person	Recipient of nursing care who is composed of biological, psychological, sociological, and spiritual components.
Environment	External environment (temperature, dangers in environment); some discussion of impact of community on the individual and family.
Health	Based upon the patient's ability to function independently (as outlined in 14 components of basic nursing care).
Nursing	Assist the person, sick or well, in performance of activities (14 components of basic nursing care) and help the person gain independence as rapidly as possible (Henderson, 1966, p. 15).

Watson's theory for nursing practice is based on 10 carative factors (Watson, 1979). As Watson's work evolved, she renamed these carative factors into what she termed clinical caritas processes (Fawcett, 2005). *Caritas* means to cherish, to appreciate, and to give special attention. It conveys the concept of love (Watson, 2001). The 10 caritas processes are summarized here:

- Practice of loving kindness and equanimity for oneself and other
- Being authentically present and enabling and sustaining the deep belief system and subjective life world of self and the one being cared for
- Cultivating one's own spiritual practices; going beyond the ego self; deepening of self-awareness
- Developing and sustaining a helping–trusting, authentic caring relationship

TABLE 2-3	Metaparadigm Concepts as Defined in Watson's Philosophy and Science of Caring
Person (human)	A "unity of mind–body–spirit/nature" (Watson, 1996, p. 147); embodied spirit (Watson, 1989).
Healing space and environment	A nonphysical energetic environment; a vibrational field integral with the person where the nurse is not only in the environment but "the nurse IS the environment" (Watson, 2008, p. 26).
Health (healing)	Harmony, wholeness, and comfort.
Nursing	Reciprocal transpersonal relationship in caring moments guided by carative factors and caritas processes.

- Being present to, and supportive of, the expression of positive and negative feelings as a connection with a deeper spirit of oneself and the one being cared for
- Creatively using oneself and all ways of knowing as part of the caring process and engagement in artistry of caring–healing practices
- Engaging in a genuine teaching–learning experience within the context of a caring relationship, while attending to the whole person and subjective meaning; attempting to stay within the other's frame of reference
- Creating a healing environment at all levels, subtle environment of energy and consciousness whereby wholeness, beauty, comfort, dignity, and peace are potentiated
- Assisting with basic needs, with an intentional caring consciousness; administering human care essentials, which potentiate alignment of the mind–body–spirit, wholeness, and unity of being in all aspects of care; attending to both embodied spirit and evolving emergence
- Opening and attending to spiritual, mysterious, and unknown existential dimensions of life, death, suffering; "allowing for a miracle" (Watson, 2008)

Watson (2001) refers to the clinical caritas processes as the "core" of nursing, which is grounded in the philosophy, science, and the art of caring. She contrasts the core of nursing with what she terms the "trim," a term she uses to refer to the practice setting, procedures, functional tasks, clinical disease focus, technology, and techniques of nursing. The trim, Watson explains, is not expendable, but it cannot be the center of professional nursing practice (Watson, 1997, p. 50).

Regarding the value system that is blended with the 10 carative factors, Watson (1985) states:

> Human care requires high regard and reverence for a person and human life.... There is high value on the subjective–internal world of the experiencing person and how the person (both patient and nurse) is perceiving and experiencing health–illness conditions. An emphasis is placed upon helping a person gain more self-knowledge, self control, and readiness for self-healing. (pp. 34, 35)

The carative factors described by Watson provide guidelines for nurse–patient interactions; however, the theory does not furnish instructions about what to do to achieve authentic caring–healing relationships. Watson's theory is more about being than doing, but it provides a useful framework for the delivery of patient-centered nursing care (Neil & Tomey, 2006).

Patricia Benner's Clinical Wisdom in Nursing Practice

Benner's work has focused on the understanding of perceptual acuity, clinical judgment, skilled know-how, ethical comportment, and ongoing experiential learning (Brykczynski, 2010, p. 141). Also important in Benner's philosophy is an understanding of ethical comportment. According to Day and Benner (2002), good conduct is a product of an individual relationship with the patient that involves engagement in a situation combined with a sense of membership in a profession where professional conduct is socially embedded, lived, and embodied in the practices, ways of being, and responses to clinical situations and where clinical and ethical judgments are inseparable.

Benner's original domains and competencies of nursing practice were derived inductively from clinical situation interviews and observations of nurses in actual practice. From these interviews and observations, 31 competencies and 7 domains were identified and described. The 7 domains are the helping role, the teaching-coaching function, the diagnostic and patient monitoring function, effective management of rapidly changing situations, administering and monitoring therapeutic interventions and regimens, monitoring and ensuring the quality of healthcare practices, and organizational work role competencies (Benner, 1984/2001). Along with the identification of the competencies and domains of nursing, Benner identified five stages of skill acquisition based on the Dreyfus model of skill acquisition as applied to nursing along with characteristics of each stage. The stages identified included novice, advanced beginner, competent, proficient, and expert (Benner, 1984/2001).

Later, in an extension of her original work, Benner and her colleagues identified nine domains of critical care nursing. These domains are diagnosing and managing life-sustaining physiologic functions in unstable patients, using skilled know-how to manage a crisis, providing comfort measures for the critically ill, caring for patients' families, preventing hazards in a technological environment, facing death: end-of-life care and decision making, communicating and negotiating multiple perspectives, monitoring quality and managing breakdown, using the skilled know-how of clinical leadership and the coaching and mentoring of others (Benner, Hooper-Kyriakidis, & Stannard, 1999). In addition, the nine domains of critical care nursing practice are used as broad themes in data interpretation for the identification and description of six aspects of clinical judgment and skilled comportment. These six aspects are as follows:

- *Reasoning-in-transition:* Practical reasoning in an ongoing clinical situation
- *Skilled know-how:* Also known as embodied intelligent performance; knowing what to do, when to do it, and how to do it
- *Response-based practice:* Adapting interventions to meet the changing needs and expectations of patients
- *Agency:* One's sense of and ability to act on or influence a situation
- *Perceptual acuity and the skill of involvement:* The ability to tune into a situation and hone in on the salient issues by engaging with the problem and the person

TABLE 2-4 Metaparadigm Concepts as Defined in Benner's Philosophy	
Person	Embodied person living in the world who is a "self-interpreting being, that is, the person does not come into the world pre-defined but gets defined in the course of living a life" (Benner & Wrubel, 1989, p. 41).
Environment (situation)	A social environment with social definition and meaningfulness.
Health	The human experience of health or wholeness.
Nursing	A caring relationship that includes the care and study of the lived experience of health, illness, and disease.

- *Links between clinical and ethical reasoning:* The understanding that good clinical practice cannot be separated from ethical notions of good outcomes for patients and families (Benner et al., 1999)

Benner identifies and defines the four metaparadigm concepts of nursing in addition to the concepts previously discussed. The concepts of person, environment, health, and nursing as defined by Benner are summarized in **Table 2-4**.

Selected Conceptual Models and Grand Theories of Nursing

Conceptual models provide a comprehensive view and guide for nursing practice. They are organizing frameworks that guide the reasoning process in professional nursing practice (Alligood, 2006). At the level of the conceptual model, each metaparadigm concept is defined and described in a manner unique to the model, with the model providing an alternative way to view the concepts considered important to the discipline (Fawcett, 2005, pp. 17–18).

Martha Rogers's Science of Unitary Human Beings
According to Rogers (1994), nursing is a learned profession, both a science and an art. The art of nursing is the creative use of the science of nursing for human betterment.

Rogers's theory asserts that human beings are dynamic energy fields that are integrated with environmental energy fields so that the person and his or her environment form a single unit. Both human energy fields and environmental fields are open systems, pandimensional in nature and in a constant state of change. Pattern is the identifying characteristic of energy fields (**Table 2-5**).

Rogers identified the principles of helicy, resonancy, and integrality to describe the nature of change within human and environmental energy fields.

TABLE 2-5 Metaparadigm Concepts as Defined in Rogers's Theory	
Person	An irreducible, irreversible, pandimensional, negentropic energy field identified by pattern; a unitary human being develops through three principles: helicy, resonancy, and integrality (Rogers, 1992).
Environment	An irreducible, pandimensional, negentropic energy field, identified by pattern and manifesting characteristics different from those of the parts and encompassing all that is other than any given human field (Rogers, 1992).
Health	Health and illness as part of a continuum (Rogers, 1970).
Nursing	Seeks to promote symphonic interaction between human and environmental fields, to strengthen the integrity of the human field, and to direct and redirect patterning of the human and environmental fields for realization of maximum health potential (Rogers, 1970).

Together, these principles are known as the principle of homeodynamics. The helicy principle describes the unpredictable but continuous, nonlinear evolution of energy fields, as evidenced by a spiral development that is a continuous, nonrepeating, and innovative patterning that reflects the nature of change. Resonancy is depicted as a wave frequency and an energy field pattern evolution from lower to higher frequency wave patterns and is reflective of the continuous variability of the human energy field as it changes. The principle of integrality emphasizes the continuous mutual process of person and environment (Rogers, 1970, 1992).

Rogers used two widely recognized toys to illustrate her theory and constant interaction of the human–environment process. The Slinky illustrates the openness, rhythm, motion, balance, and expanding nature of the human life process, which is continuously evolving (Rogers, 1970). The kaleidoscope illustrates the changing patterns that appear to be infinitely different (Johnson & Webber, 2010, p. 142).

Rogers (1970) identified five assumptions that support and connect the concepts in her conceptual model:

- Man is a unified whole possessing his own integrity and manifesting characteristics more than and different from the sum of his parts (p. 47).
- Man and environment are continuously exchanging matter and energy with one another (p. 54).
- The life process evolves irreversibly and unidirectionally along the space–time continuum (p. 59).
- Pattern and organization identify man and reflect his innovative wholeness (p. 65).
- Man is characterized by the capacity for abstraction and imagery, language and thought, sensation, and emotion (p. 73).

Rogers's model is an abstract system of ideas but is applicable to practice, with nursing care focused on pattern appraisal and patterning activities. Pattern appraisal involves a comprehensive assessment of environmental field patterns and human field patterns of communication, exchange, rhythms, dissonance, and harmony through the use of cognitive input, sensory input, intuition, and language. Patterning activities can include interventions such as meditation, imagery, journaling, or modifying surroundings. Evaluation is ongoing and requires a repetition of the appraisal process (Gunther, 2006). This process of pattern appraisal continues as long as the nurse–patient relationship continues (Gunther, 2010).

Dorothea Orem's Self-Care Deficit Theory of Nursing

Orem describes her theory as a general theory that is made up of three related theories, the Theory of Self-Care, the Theory of Self-Care Deficit, and the Theory of Nursing Systems. The Theory of Self-Care describes why and how people care for themselves. The Theory of Self-Care Deficit describes and explains why people can be helped through nursing. The Theory of Nursing Systems describes and explains relationships that must exist and be maintained for nursing to occur. These three theories in relationship constitute Orem's general theory of nursing known as the Self-Care Deficit Theory of Nursing (Berbiglia, 2010; Orem, 1990; Taylor, 2006).

Theory of Self-Care

The Theory of Self-Care describes why and how people care for themselves and suggests that nursing is required in case of inability to perform self-care as a result of limitations. This theory includes the concepts of self-care agency, therapeutic self-care demand, and basic conditioning factors.

Self-care agency is an acquired ability of mature and maturing persons to know and meet their requirements for deliberate and purposive action to regulate their own human functioning and development (Orem, 2001, p. 492). The concept of self-care agency has three dimensions: development, operability, and adequacy. According to Orem (2001, p. 491), therapeutic self-care demand consists of the summation of care measures necessary to meet all of an individual's known self-care requisites. *Basic conditioning factors* refer to those factors that affect the value of the therapeutic self-care demand or self-care agency of an individual. Ten factors are identified: age, gender, developmental state, health state, pattern of living, healthcare system factors, family system factors, sociocultural factors, availability of resources, and external environmental factors (Orem, 2001).

Orem identifies three types of self-care requisites that are integrated into the theory of self-care and provide the basis for self-care. These include universal self-care requisites, developmental self-care requisites, and health deviation self-care requisites.

Universal self-care requisites are those found in all human beings and are associated with life processes. These requisites include the following needs:

- Maintenance of sufficient intake of air
- Maintenance of sufficient intake of water
- Maintenance of sufficient intake of food
- Provision of care associated with elimination processes and excrements
- Maintenance of a balance of activity and rest
- Maintenance of a balance between solitude and social interaction
- Prevention of hazards to human life, human functioning, and human well-being
- Promotion of human functioning and development within social groups in accordance with human potential, known limitations, and the human desire to be normal (Orem, 1985, pp. 90–91)

Developmental self-care requisites are related to different stages in the human life cycle and might include events such as attending college, marriage, and retirement. Broadly speaking, the development self-care requisites include the following needs:

- Bringing about and maintenance of living conditions that support life processes and promote the processes of development—that is, human progress toward higher levels of organization of human structures and toward maturation
- Provision of care either to prevent the occurrence of deleterious effects of conditions that can affect human development or to mitigate or overcome these effects from various conditions (Orem, 1985, p. 96)

Health-deviation self-care requisites are related to deviations in structure or function of a human being. There are six categories of health-deviation requisites:

- Seeking and securing appropriate medical assistance
- Being aware of and attending to the effects and results of illness states
- Effectively carrying out medically prescribed treatments
- Being aware of and attending to side effects of treatment
- Modifying self-concept in accepting oneself in a particular state of health
- Learning to live with the effects of illness and medical treatment (Orem, 1985, pp. 99–100)

Theory of Self-Care Deficit

The Theory of Self-Care Deficit explains that maturing or mature adults deliberately learn and perform actions to direct their survival, quality of life, and well-being; put more simply, it explains why people can be helped through nursing. According to Orem, nurses use five methods to help meet the self-care needs of patients:

- Acting for or doing for another
- Guiding and directing

- Providing physical or psychological support
- Providing and maintaining an environment that supports personal development
- Teaching (Johnson & Webber, 2010; Orem, 1995, 2001)

Theory of Nursing Systems

The Theory of Nursing Systems describes and explains relationships that must exist and be maintained for the product (nursing) to occur (Berbiglia, 2010; Taylor, 2006). Three systems can be used to meet the self-requisites of the patient: the wholly compensatory system, the partially compensatory system, and the supportive-educative system.

- In the *wholly compensatory system,* the patient is unable to perform any self-care activities and relies on the nurse to perform care.
- In the *partially compensatory system,* both the patient and the nurse participate in the patient's self-care activities, with the responsibility for care shifting from the nurse to the patient as the self-care demand changes.
- In the *supportive-educative system,* the patient has the ability for self-care but requires assistance from the nurse in decision making, knowledge, or skill acquisition. The nurse's role is to promote the patient as a self-care agent.

The system selected depends on the nurse's assessment of the patient's ability to perform self-care activities and self-care demands (Johnson & Webber, 2010; Orem, 1995, 2001).

There are eight general propositions for the Self-Care Deficit Theory of Nursing (although each of the three individual theories also has its own set of propositions) (Meleis, 2004):

- Human beings have capabilities to provide their own self-care or care for dependents to meet universal, developmental, and health-deviation self-care requisites. These capabilities are learned and recalled.
- Self-care abilities are influenced by age, developmental state, experiences, and sociocultural background.
- Self-care deficits should balance between self-care demands and self-care capabilities.
- Self-care or dependent care is mediated by age, developmental stage, life experience, sociocultural orientation, health, and resources.
- Therapeutic self-care includes actions of nurses, patients, and others that regulate self-care capabilities and meet self-care needs.
- Nurses assess the abilities of patients to meet their self-care needs and their potential of not performing their self-care.
- Nurses engage in selecting valid and reliable processes, technologies, or actions for meeting self-care needs.
- Components of therapeutic self-care are wholly compensatory, partly compensatory, and supportive-educative.

TABLE 2-6 Metaparadigm Concepts as Defined in Orem's Theory

Person (patient)	A person under the care of a nurse; a total being with universal, developmental needs, and capable of self-care.
Environment	Physical, chemical, biologic, and social contexts within which human beings exist; environmental components include environmental factors, environmental elements, environmental conditions, and developmental environment (Orem, 1985).
Health	"A state characterized by soundness or wholeness of developed human structures and of bodily and mental functioning" (Orem, 1995, p. 101).
Nursing	Therapeutic self-care designed to supplement self-care requisites. Nursing actions fall into one of three categories: wholly compensatory, partly compensatory, or supportive–educative system (Orem, 1985).

In addition to these other concepts, the four metaparadigm concepts of nursing are identified in Orem's theory (**Table 2-6**). Orem's theory clearly differentiates the focus of nursing and is one of the nursing theories that is most commonly used in practice.

Callista Roy's Adaptation Model

The Roy Adaptation Model presents the person as an adaptive system in constant interaction with the internal and the external environments. The main task of the human system is to maintain integrity in the face of environmental stimuli (Phillips, 2006). The goal of nursing is to foster successful adaptation (**Table 2-7**).

According to Roy and Andrews (1999), adaptation refers to "the process and outcome whereby thinking and feeling persons, as individuals or in groups,

TABLE 2-7 Metaparadigm Concepts as Defined in Roy's Model

Person	"An adaptive system with cognator and regulator subsystems acting to maintain adaptation in the four adaptive modes" (Roy, 2009, p. 12).
Environment	"All conditions, circumstances, and influences surrounding and affecting the development and behavior of persons and groups, with particular consideration of mutuality of person and earth resources" (Roy, 2009, p. 12).
Health	"A state and process of being and becoming an integrated and whole that reflects person and environment mutuality" (Roy, 2009, p. 12).
Nursing	The goal of nursing is "to promote adaptation for individuals and groups in the four adaptive modes, thus contributing to health, quality of life, and dying with dignity by assessing behavior and factors that influence adaptive abilities and to enhance environmental factors" (Roy, 2009, p. 12).

use conscious awareness and choice to create human and environmental integration" (p. 54). Adaptation leads to optimum health and well-being, to quality of life, and to death with dignity (Andrews & Roy, 1991). The adaptation level represents the condition of the life processes. Roy describes three levels: integrated, compensatory, and compromised life processes. An integrated life process can change to a compensatory process, which attempts to reestablish adaptation. If the compensatory processes are not adequate, compromised processes result (Roy, 2009, p. 33).

The processes for coping in the Roy Adaptation Model are categorized as "the regulator and cognator subsystems as they apply to individuals, and the stabilizer and innovator subsystems as applied to groups" (Roy, 2009, p. 33). A basic type of adaptive process, the regulator subsystem responds through neural, chemical, and endocrine coping channels. Stimuli from the internal and external environments act as inputs through the senses to the nervous system, thereby affecting the fluid, electrolyte, and acid–base balance, as well as the endocrine system. This information is all channeled automatically, with the body producing an automatic, unconscious response to it (p. 41).

The second adaptive process, the cognator subsystem, responds through four cognitive-emotional channels: perceptual and information processing, learning, judgment, and emotion. Perceptual and information processing includes activities of selective attention, coding, and memory. Learning involves imitation, reinforcement, and insight. Judgment includes problem solving and decision making. Defenses are used to seek relief from anxiety and make affective appraisal and attachments through the emotions (Roy, 2009, p. 41).

The cognator–regulator and stabilizer–innovator subsystems function to maintain integrated life processes. These life processes—whether integrated, compensatory, or compromised—are manifested in behaviors of the individual or group. Behavior is viewed as an output of the human system and takes the form of either adaptive responses or ineffective responses. These responses serve as feedback to the system, with the human system using this information to decide whether to increase or decrease its efforts to cope with the stimuli (Roy, 2009, p. 34).

Behaviors can be observed in four categories, or adaptive modes: physiologic-physical mode, self-concept–group identify mode, role function mode, and interdependence mode. Behavior in the *physiologic-physical mode* is the manifestation of the physiologic activities of all cells, tissues, organs, and systems making up the body. The *self-concept–group identity mode* includes the components of the physical self, including body sensation and body image, and the personal self, including self-consistency, self-ideal, and moral-ethical-spiritual self. The *role function mode* focuses on the roles of the person in society and the roles within a group, and the *interdependence mode* is a category of behavior related to interdependent relationships. This mode focuses on interactions related to the giving and receiving of love, respect, and value (Roy, 2009).

In the Roy Adaptation Model, three classes of stimuli form the environment: the focal stimulus (internal or external stimulus most immediately in the awareness of the individual or group), contextual stimuli (all other stimuli present in the situation that contribute to the effect of the focal stimulus), and residual stimuli (environmental factors within or outside human systems, the effects of which are unclear in the situation) (Roy, 2009, pp. 35–36).

The propositions of Roy's theory include the following:

- Nursing actions promote a person's adaptive responses.
- Nursing actions can decrease a person's ineffective adaptive responses.
- People interact with the changing environment in an attempt to achieve adaptation and health.
- Nursing actions enhance the interaction of persons with the environment.
- Enhanced interactions of persons with the environment promote adaptation (Meleis, 2004).

The Roy Adaptation Model is commonly used in nursing practice. To use the model in practice, the nurse follows Roy's six-step nursing process, which is as follows (Phillips, 2006):

- Assessing the behaviors manifested from the four adaptive modes (physiologic-physical mode, self-concept–group identity mode, role function mode, and interdependence mode)
- Assessing and categorizing the stimuli for those behaviors
- Making a nursing diagnosis based on the person's adaptive state
- Setting goals to promote adaptation
- Implementing interventions aimed at managing stimuli to promote adaptation
- Evaluating achievement of adaptive goals

Andrews and Roy (1986) point out that by manipulating the stimuli rather than the patient, the nurse enhances "the interaction of the person with their environment, thereby promoting health" (p. 51).

Betty Neuman's Systems Model

The Neuman Systems Model is a wellness model based on general systems theory in which the client system is exposed to stressors from within and without the system. The focus of the model is on the client system in relationship to stressors. The client system is a composite of interacting variables that include the physiologic variable, the psychological variable, the sociocultural variable, the developmental variable, and the spiritual variable (Neuman, 2002, pp. 16–17). Stressors are classified as intrapersonal, interpersonal, or extrapersonal depending on their relationship to the client system (p. 22).

The client system is represented structurally in the model as a series of concentric rings or circles surrounding a basic structure. These flexible concentric circles represent normal lines of defense and lines of resistance that function to preserve client system integrity by acting as protective mechanisms for the basic structure. The basic structure or central core consists of basic survival factors common to the species, innate or genetic features, and strengths and weaknesses of the system. The flexible line of defense forms the outer boundary of the defined client system; it protects the normal line of defense. The normal line of defense represents what the client has become or the usual wellness state. Adjustment of the five client system variables to environmental stressors determines its level of stability. The concentric broken circles surrounding the basic structure are known as lines of resistance. They become activated following invasion of the normal line of defense by environmental stressors (Neuman, 2002, pp. 16–18). The greater the quality of the client system's health, the greater protection is provided by the various lines of defense (Geib, 2006). In addition to these concepts, the four metaparadigm concepts of nursing are identified in Neuman's theory (**Table 2-8**).

Basic assumptions of the Neuman Systems Model include the following (Meleis, 2004; Neuman, 1995):

- Nursing clients have both unique and universal characteristics and are constantly exchanging energy with the environment.
- The relationships among client variables influence a client's protective mechanisms and determine the client's response.
- Clients present a normal range of responses to the environment that represent wellness and stability.
- Stressors attack flexible lines of defense and then normal lines of defense.
- Nurses' actions are focused on primary, secondary, and tertiary prevention.

TABLE 2-8 Metaparadigm Concepts as Defined In Neuman's Model	
Person (client system)	A composite of physiological, psychological, sociocultural, developmental, and spiritual variables in interaction with the internal and external environment; represented by central structure, lines of defense, and lines of resistance (Neuman, 2002).
Environment	All internal and external factors of influences surrounding the client system; three relevant environments identified are the internal environment, the external environment, and the created environment (Neuman, 2002, p. 18).
Health	A continuum of wellness to illness; equated with optimal system stability (Neuman, 2002, p. 23).
Nursing	Prevention as intervention; concerned with all potential stressors.

The Neuman Systems Model is health oriented, with an emphasis on prevention as intervention, and has been used in a wide variety of settings. Perhaps one of the greatest attractions to this model is the ease with which it can be used for families, groups, and communities as well as the individual client. The use of the model in practice requires only moderate adaptation of the nursing process with a focus on assessment of stressors and client system perceptions.

Imogene King's Interacting Systems Framework and Theory of Goal Attainment

King, in her Interacting Systems Framework, conceptualizes three levels of dynamic interacting systems that include personal systems (individuals), interpersonal systems (groups), and social systems (society). Individuals exist within personal systems, and concepts relevant to this system include body image, growth and development, perception, self, space, and time. Interpersonal systems are formed when two or more individuals interact. The concepts important to understanding this system include communication, interaction, role, stress, and transaction. Examples of social systems include religious systems, educational systems, and healthcare systems. Concepts important to understanding the social system include authority, decision making, organization, power, and status (King, 1981; Sieloff, 2006).

King's Theory of Goal Attainment was derived from her Interacting Systems Framework (Sieloff, 2006) and addresses nursing as a process of human interaction (Norris & Frey, 2006). The theory focuses on the interpersonal system interactions in the nurse–client relationship (**Table 2-9**). During the nursing process, the nurse and the client perceive one another, make judgments, and take action that results in reaction. Interaction results, and if

TABLE 2-9 Metaparadigm Concepts as Defined in King's Theory	
Person (human being)	A personal system that interacts with interpersonal and social systems.
Environment	Can be both external and internal. The external environment is the context "within which human beings grow, develop, and perform daily activities" (King, 1981, p. 18); the internal environment of human beings transforms energy to enable them to adjust to continuous external environmental changes (King, 1981, p. 5).
Health	"Dynamic life experiences of a human being, which implies continuous adjustment to stressors in the internal and external environment through optimum use of one's resources to achieve maximum potential for daily living" (King, 1981, p. 5).
Nursing	A process of human interaction, the goal of nursing is to help patients achieve their goals.

perceptual congruence exists, transactions occur (Sieloff, 2006). Outcomes are defined in terms of goals obtained. If the goals are related to patient behaviors, they become the criteria by which the effectiveness of nursing care can be measured (King, 1989, p. 156).

The propositions of King's Theory of Goal Attainment are as follows (King, 1981):

- If perceptual accuracy is present in nurse–client interactions, transactions will occur.
- If the nurse and client make transactions, goals will be attained.
- If goals are attained, satisfactions will occur.
- If goals are attained, effective nursing care will occur.
- If transactions are made in the nurse–client interactions, growth and development will be enhanced.
- If role expectations and role performance as perceived by the nurse and client are congruent, transactions will occur.
- If role conflict is experienced by nurse or client or both, stress in nurse–client interactions will occur.
- If nurses with special knowledge and skills communicate appropriate information to clients, mutual goal setting and goal attainment will occur.

King's theory can be implemented in practice using the nursing process where assessment focuses on the perceptions of the nurse and client, communication of the nurse and client, and interaction of the nurse and client. Planning involves deciding on goals and agreeing on how to attain goals. Implementation focuses on transactions made, and evaluation focuses on goals attained using King's theory (King, 1992).

Johnson's Behavioral System Model

Dorothy Johnson's model for nursing presents the client as a living open system that is a collection of behavioral subsystems that interrelate to form a behavioral system (**Table 2-10**). The seven subsystems of behavior proposed by Johnson include achievement, affiliative, aggressive, dependence, sexual, eliminative, and ingestive. Motivational drives direct the activities of the subsystems that are constantly changing because of maturation, experience, and learning (Johnson, 1980).

The achievement subsystem functions to control or master an aspect of self or environment to achieve a standard. This subsystem encompasses intellectual, physical, creative, mechanical, and social skills. The affiliative or attachment subsystem forms the basis for social organization. Its consequences are social inclusion, intimacy, and the formation and maintenance of strong social bonds. The aggressive or protective subsystem functions to protect and preserve the system. The dependency subsystem promotes helping or nurturing behaviors. The consequences include approval, recognition, and physical assistance.

TABLE 2-10	Metaparadigm Concepts as Defined in Johnson's Model
Person (human being)	A biopsychosocial being who is a behavioral system with seven subsystems of behavior.
Environment	Includes internal and external environment.
Health	Efficient and effective functioning of system; behavioral system balance and stability.
Nursing	An external regulatory force that acts to preserve the organization and integrity of the patient's behavior at an optimal level under those conditions in which the behavior constitutes a threat to physical or social health or in which illness is found (Johnson, 1980, p. 214).

The sexual subsystem has the function of procreation and gratification and includes development of gender role identity and gender role behaviors. The eliminative subsystem addresses "when, how, and under what conditions we eliminate," whereas the ingestive subsystem "has to do with when, how, what, how much, and under what conditions we eat" (Johnson, 1980, p. 213).

The nursing process for the behavioral system model is known as Johnson's nursing diagnostic and treatment process. The components of the process include the determination of the existence of a problem, diagnosis and classification of problems, management of problems, and evaluation of behavioral system balance and stability. When using Johnson's model in practice, the focus of the assessment process is obtaining information to evaluate current behavior in terms of past patterns, determining the impact of the current illness on behavioral patterns, and establishing the maximum level of health. The assessment is specifically related to gathering information related to the structure and function of the seven behavioral subsystems as well as the environmental factors that affect the behavioral subsystems (Holaday, 2006). The ultimate goals of nursing using the model are to maintain or restore behavioral system balance (Johnson, 1980).

Selected Theories and Middle-Range Theories of Nursing

Middle-range theory may be derived from a grand theory or a conceptual model, or may originate from practice perspectives. Middle-range theories are narrower in scope than grand theories and include concepts that are less abstract and therefore more amenable to testing in research and use in nursing practice.

Rosemarie Parse's Humanbecoming Theory

Parse's theory was originally called man-living-health (Parse, 1981). In 1992, Parse changed the name to *human becoming*, and then in 2007 again changed the name to *humanbecoming* (Mitchell & Bournes, 2010) to coincide with Parse's evolution of thought. The Humanbecoming Theory consists of three major themes: meaning, rhythmicity, and transcendence (Parse, 1998). Meaning is the linguistic and imagined content of something and the interpretation that one gives to something. Rhythmicity is the cadent, paradoxical patterning of the human–universe mutual process. Transcendence is defined as reaching beyond with possibles or the "hopes and dreams envisioned in multidimensional experiences powering the originating of transforming" (Parse, 1998, p. 29). The three major principles of the Humanbecoming Theory flow from these themes.

The first principle of the Humanbecoming Theory states, "Structuring meaning multidimensionally is cocreating reality through the languaging of valuing and imaging" (Parse, 1998, p. 35). This principle proposes that persons structure or choose the meaning of their realities and that the choosing occurs at levels that are not always known explicitly (Mitchell, 2006). This means that one person cannot decide the significance of something for another person and does not even understand the meaning of the event unless that person shares the meaning through the expression of his or her views, concerns, and dreams.

The second principle states, "Cocreating rhythmical patterns of relating is living the paradoxical unity of revealing—concealing and enabling—limiting while connecting—separating" (Parse, 1998, p. 42). This principle means that persons create patterns in life, and these patterns tell about personal meanings and values. The patterns of relating that persons create involve complex engagements and disengagements with other persons, ideas, and preferences (Mitchell, 2006). According to Parse (1998), persons change their patterns when they integrate new priorities, ideas, hopes, and dreams.

The third principle of the Humanbecoming Theory states, "Cotranscending with the possibles is powering unique ways of originating in the process of transforming" (Parse, 1998, p. 46). This principle means that persons are always engaging with and choosing from infinite possibilities. The choices reflect the person's ways of moving and changing in the process of becoming (Mitchell, 2006).

Three processes for practice have been developed from the concepts and principles in the Humanbecoming Theory, including the following (Parse, 1998, pp. 69, 70):

- Illuminating meaning is explicating what was, is, and will be. Explicating is making clear what is appearing now through language.
- Synchronizing rhythms is dwelling with the pitch, yaw, and roll of the human–universe process. Dwelling with is immersing with the flow of connecting–separating.
- Mobilizing transcendence is moving beyond the meaning moment with what is not yet. Moving beyond is propelling with envisioned possibles of transforming.

TABLE 2-11 Metaparadigm Concepts as Defined in Parse's Theory	
Person	An open being, more than and different than the sum of parts in mutual simultaneous interchange with the environment who chooses from options and bears responsibility for choices (Parse, 1987, p. 160).
Environment	Coexists in mutual process with the person.
Health	Continuously changing process of becoming.
Nursing	A learned discipline, the nurse uses true presence to facilitate the becoming of the participant.

In practice, nurses guided by the Humanbecoming Theory prepare to be truly present (**Table 2-11**) with others through focused attentiveness on the moment at hand through immersion (Parse, 1998).

Madeleine Leininger's Cultural Diversity and Universality Theory

Leininger (1995) defined transcultural nursing as both an area of study and an area of nursing practice. The main features of the Cultural Diversity and Universality Theory focus on "comparative cultural care (caring) values, beliefs, and practices" (p. 58) for either individuals or groups of people with similar or different cultures. The goal of transcultural nursing is the provision of nursing care that is culture specific in order to either promote health or to assist individuals face sickness or death "in culturally meaningful ways" (p. 58). Consistent with the focus of her theory, Leininger defined the metaparadigm concepts of nursing in a manner that causes the nurse to specifically consider culture in the delivery of competent nursing care (**Table 2-12**).

According to Leininger (2001), three modalities guide nursing judgments, decisions, and actions to provide culturally congruent care that is beneficial, satisfying, and meaningful to the persons the nurse serves. These three modes include cultural care preservation or maintenance, cultural care accommodation or negotiation, and cultural care repatterning or restructuring. Cultural care preservation or maintenance refers to those assistive, supportive, facilitative, or enabling professional actions and decisions that help people of a specific culture to maintain meaningful care values for their well-being, recover from illness, or deal with a handicap or dying. Cultural care accommodation or negotiation refers to those assistive, supportive, facilitative, or enabling professional actions and decisions that help people

TABLE 2-12	Metaparadigm Concepts as Defined in Leininger's Theory
Person	Human being, family, group, community, or institution.
Environment	Totality of an event, situation, or experience that gives meaning to human expressions, interpretations, and social interactions in physical, ecological, sociopolitical, and/or cultural settings (Leininger, 1991).
Health	A state of well-being that is culturally defined, valued, and practiced (Leininger, 1991, p. 46).
Nursing	Activities directed toward assisting, supporting, or enabling with needs in ways that are congruent with the cultural values, beliefs, and lifeways of the recipient of care (Leininger, 1995).

of a specific culture or subculture adapt to or negotiate with others for meaningful, beneficial, and congruent health outcomes. Cultural care repatterning or restructuring refers to the assistive, supportive, facilitative, or enabling professional actions and decisions that help patients reorder, change, or modify their lifeways for new, different, and beneficial health outcomes (Leininger & McFarland, 2006).

The nurse using Leininger's theory plans and makes decisions with clients with respect to these three modes of action. All three care modalities require coparticipation of the nurse and client working together to identify, plan, implement, and evaluate nursing care with respect to the cultural congruence of the care (Leininger, 2001).

Leininger developed the sunrise model, which she revised in 2004. She labeled this model as "an enabler," to clarify that although it depicts the essential components of the Cultural Diversity and Universality Theory, it is a visual guide for exploration of cultures.

Hildegard Peplau's Theory of Interpersonal Relations

In her theory, Peplau addresses all of nursing's metaparadigm concepts (Table 2-13), but she is primarily concerned with one aspect of nursing: how persons relate to one another. According to Peplau, the nurse–patient relationship is the center of nursing (Young, Taylor, & McLaughlin-Renpenning, 2001).

Peplau (1952) originally described four phases in nurse–patient relationships that overlap and occur over the time of the relationship: orientation, identification, exploitation, and resolution. In 1997, Peplau combined the phase of identification and exploitation, resulting in three phases: orientation, working, and termination. Nevertheless, most other theorists still consider the phases of identification and exploitation to be subphases of the working phase. During the orientation phase, a health problem has emerged that results in a "felt need," and professional assistance is sought (p. 18).

TABLE 2-13   Metaparadigm Concepts as Defined in Peplau's Theory

Person	Encompasses the patient (one who has problems for which expert nursing services are needed or sought) and the nurse (a professional with particular expertise) (Peplau, 1992, p. 14).
Environment	Forces outside the organism within the context of culture (Peplau, 1952, p. 163).
Health	"Implies forward movement of personality and other ongoing human processes in the direction of creative, constructive, productive, personal, and community living" (Peplau, 1992, p. 12).
Nursing	The therapeutic, interpersonal process between the nurse and the patient.

In the working phase, the patient identifies those who can help, and the nurse permits exploration of feelings by the patient. During this phase, the nurse can begin to focus the patient on the achievement of new goals. The resolution (termination) phase is the time when the patient gradually adopts new goals and frees himself or herself from identification with the nurse (Peplau, 1952, 1997).

Peplau (1952) also describes six nursing roles that emerge during the phases of the nurse–patient relationship: the role of the stranger, the role of the resource person, the teaching role, the leadership role, the surrogate role, and the counseling role. Over the course of Peplau's career, the nursing roles were refined to include teacher, resource, counselor, leader, technical expert, and surrogate. As a teacher, the nurse provides knowledge about a need or problem. In the role of resource, the nurse provides information to understand a problem. In the role of counselor, the nurse helps recognize, face, accept, and resolve problems. As a leader, the nurse initiates and maintains group goals through interaction. As a technical expert, the nurse provides physical care using clinical skills. And, as a surrogate, the nurse may take the place of another (Johnson & Webber, 2010, p. 125).

Peplau (1952) also described four psychobiological experiences: needs, frustration, conflict, and anxiety. According to Peplau, these experiences "all provide energy that is transformed into some form of action" (p. 71) and provide a basis for goal formation and nursing interventions (Howk, 2002).

Peplau, as one of the first theorists since Nightingale to present a theory for nursing, is considered a pioneer in the area of theory development in nursing. Prior to Peplau's work, nursing practice involved acting on, to, or for the patient such that the patient was considered an object of nursing actions. Peplau's work was the force behind the conceptualization of the patient as a partner in the nursing process (Howk, 2002, pp. 379–380). Although Peplau's book was first published in 1952, her model continues to be used extensively by clinicians and continues to provide direction to educators and researchers (Howk, 2002).

Nola Pender's Health Promotion Model

The Health Promotion Model is an attempt to portray the multidimensionality of persons interacting with their interpersonal and physical environments as they pursue health while integrating constructs from expectancy-value theory and social cognitive theory with a nursing perspective of holistic human functioning (Pender, 1996, p. 53). A summary of the metaparadigm concepts of nursing as defined by Pender is presented in **Table 2-14**.

There are three major categories to consider in Pender's health promotion model: (1) individual characteristics and experiences, (2) behavior-specific cognitions and affect, and (3) behavioral outcome. Personal factors include personal biological factors such as age, body mass index, pubertal status, menopausal status, aerobic capacity, strength, agility, or balance. Personal psychological factors include factors such as self-esteem, self-motivation, and perceived health status; personal sociocultural factors include factors such as race, ethnicity, acculturation, education, and socioeconomic status. Some personal factors are amenable to change, whereas others cannot be changed (Pender, Murdaugh, & Parsons, 2006, p. 52; 2011, pp. 45–46).

Behavior-specific cognitions and affect are behavior-specific variables within the Health Promotion Model. Such variables are considered to have motivational significance. In the Health Promotion Model, these variables are the target of nursing intervention because they are amenable to change. The behavior-specific cognitions and affect identified in the Health Promotion Model include (1) perceived benefits of action, (2) perceived barriers to action, (3) perceived self-efficacy, and (4) activity-related affect. Perceived benefits of action are the anticipated positive outcomes resulting from health behavior. Perceived barriers to action are the anticipated, imagined, or real blocks or personal costs of a behavior. Perceived self-efficacy refers to the judgment of personal capability to organize and execute a health-promoting behavior. It influences the perceived barriers to actions, such that higher efficacy results in lower perceptions of barriers. Activity-related affect refers to the subjective positive or negative feelings that occur before,

TABLE 2-14 Metaparadigm Concepts as Defined in Pender's Model	
Person	The individual, who is the primary focus of the model.
Environment	The physical, interpersonal, and economic circumstances in which persons live.
Health	A positive high-level state.
Nursing	The role of the nurse includes raising consciousness related to health-promoting behaviors, promoting self-efficacy, enhancing the benefits of change, controlling the environment to support behavior change, and managing barriers to change.

during, and following behavior based on the stimulus properties of the behavior. Activity-related affect influences perceived self-efficacy, such that the more positive the subjective feeling, the greater the perceived efficacy (Pender et al., 2006, pp. 52–54; 2011, pp. 46–48; Sakraida, 2010, p. 438; 2014, p. 399).

Commitment to a plan of action marks the beginning of a behavioral event. Interventions in the Health Promotion Model focus on raising consciousness related to health-promoting behaviors, promoting self-efficacy, enhancing the benefits of change, controlling the environment to support behavior change, and managing the barriers to change. Health-promoting behavior, which is ultimately directed toward attaining positive health outcomes, is the product of the Health Promotion Model (Pender et al., 2006, pp. 56–63; 2011, pp. 49–51).

Afaf Ibrahim Meleis's Transitions Theory

Transitions are a central concept of interest to nursing (Meleis, 2007, p. 467). Nurses interact with individuals experiencing transitions if those transitions relate to health, well-being, or self-care ability. Nurses also interact with individuals within environments that support or hamper personal, communal, familial, or population transitions (Meleis, 2010, p. 11).

Transition is a process triggered by a change that represents a passage from a fairly stable state to another fairly stable state (Meleis, 2010, p. 11). Transitions can be described in terms of types and patterns of transitions, properties of transition experiences, transition conditions, process indicators, outcome indicators, and nursing therapeutics (Meleis, Sawyer, Im, Hilfinger Messias, & Schumacher, 2000, p. 16).

Types of transitions include developmental, health and illness, situational, and organizational. Developmental transitions may include events such as the transition from childhood to adolescence, or from adulthood to old age. Health and illness transitions may include events such as diagnosis of chronic illness. Birth and death are examples of events that may lead to situational transitions. Patterns of transitions reflect the experience of multiple simultaneous transitions in the lives of individuals rather than single, sequential transition events (Meleis et al., 2000, p. 17).

Essential and interrelated properties of transition experiences have been identified that include awareness, engagement, change and difference, time span, and critical points and events (Meleis et al., 2000, p. 18). Awareness is related to perception, knowledge, and recognition of the transition experience; it is often reflected in the congruency between what is known about the process and responses and what the expected perceptions and responses of individuals in similar transitions are. Engagement is related to the involvement of the individual in the transition process, which may be manifested by activities such as seeking information. Change and difference are properties of transitions that are similar but not interchangeable. Either change may be the result of transition or the transition may result in change. All transitions involve change, but not all change is related to transition (Meleis et al., 2000, pp. 18–19). Confronting difference in the context of transitions refers to "unmet or divergent expectations, feeling different, being perceived as different, or seeing the work and others in different ways" (Meleis et al., 2000, p. 20). Time span refers to the flow and movement over time that occurs with all transitions. Individuals experiencing long-term transitions do not necessarily constantly experience a state of flux; however, such a state "may periodically surface, reactivating a latent transition experience" (Meleis et al., 2000, pp. 20–21). Thus, it is important to consider the possibility of variability over time and reassess outcomes (p. 21).

Most transitions include critical points or marker events such as birth, death, or diagnosis with an illness. Critical points are often associated with awareness of change or difference or increased engagement in the transition experience and may represent periods of heightened vulnerability. During the period of uncertainty, a number of critical points may occur depending on the nature of the transition. Final critical points are characterized by a sense of stabilization (Meleis et al., 2000, p. 21).

Transition conditions include facilitators and inhibitors, or the perceptions of and meanings attached to health and illness situations that facilitate or hinder progress toward achieving a healthy transition (Schumacher & Meleis, 1994). Perceptions and meanings are influenced by and in turn influence the conditions in which transitions occur. These facilitators and inhibitors include personal, community, or societal conditions. Personal conditions include meanings, cultural beliefs and attitudes, socioeconomic status, and preparation and knowledge. Community conditions may include community resources, support from family, and role models. Societal conditions may include stigmatization, marginalization, and cultural attitudes (Meleis et al., 2000, p. 21).

Patterns of response include process indicators and outcome indicators. Because transitions occur over time, process indicators that direct individuals toward health or toward vulnerability and risk may be identified through early assessment to promote health outcomes. Assessment of outcome indicators may be used to ascertain whether a transition process is healthy and may include efforts to determine whether the individual is feeling connected, interacting, being situated, and developing confidence and coping (Meleis et al., 2000, p. 24). Outcome indicators include mastery and development of identity. Mastery of new skills required to manage a transition and the development of a new fluid and integrative identity reflect a healthy outcome of the transition process (p. 26).

Nursing therapeutics are conceptualized as measures applicable to therapeutic intervention during transitions. The first nursing therapeutic is an assessment of readiness; it includes an assessment of each transition condition to determine readiness and allows clinicians to determine patterns of the transition experience. Preparation for transition is the second nursing therapeutic. It includes education to generate the best condition for transition. The third nursing therapeutic is role supplementation (Schumacher & Meleis, 1994), a deliberative process that is applied when role insufficiency or potential role insufficiency is identified. In this process, the conditions and strategies of role clarification and role taking are used to develop preventive or therapeutic measures to decrease, improve, or prevent role insufficiency (Meleis, 2010, p. 17). The metaparadigm concepts of nursing as defined by Meleis are summarized in **Table 2-15**.

Kristen Swanson's Theory of Caring

Swanson's Theory of Caring (1991, 1993, 1999a, 1999b) offers an explanation of what it means to practice nursing in a caring manner. In this theory, *caring* is defined as a "nurturing way of relating to a valued other toward whom one feels a personal sense of commitment and responsibility" (Swanson, 1991, p. 162). Swanson (1993) posits caring for a person's biopsychosocial and spiritual well-being is a fundamental and universal component of good nursing care.

Five additional concepts are integral to Swanson's Theory of Caring and represent the five basic processes of caring: maintaining belief, knowing, being with, doing for, and enabling.

- The concept of maintaining belief is sustaining faith in the other's capacity to get through an event or transition and face a future with meaning. This includes believing in the other's capacity and holding him or her in high esteem, maintaining a hope-filled attitude, offering realistic optimism, helping to find meaning, and standing by the one cared for, no matter what the situation (Swanson, 1991, p. 162).

TABLE 2-15 Metaparadigm Concepts as Defined in Meleis's Transitions Theory	
Person	Active beings who experience fundamental life patterns and who have perceptions of and attach meaning to transition experiences (Meleis et al., 2000, p. 21).
Environment	Environmental conditions expose persons to potential damage, problematic recovery, or delayed or unhealthy coping, contributing to vulnerability related to transitions.
Health	Consists of complex and multidimensional transitions that are characterized by flow and movement over time; healthy outcomes are defined in terms of the transition process.
Nursing	Being the primary caregiver for individuals and their families during the transition process and applying nursing therapeutics during transitions to promote healthy outcomes.

- The concept of knowing refers to striving to understand the meaning of an event in the life of the other, avoiding assumptions, focusing on the person cared for, seeking cues, assessing meticulously, and engaging both the one caring and the one cared for in the process of knowing (Swanson, 1991, p. 162).
- The concept of being with refers to being emotionally present to the other. It includes being present in person, conveying availability, and sharing feelings without burdening the one cared for (Swanson, 1991, p. 162).
- The concept of doing for refers to doing for others what one would do for oneself, including anticipating needs, comforting, performing skillfully and competently, and protecting the one cared for while preserving his or her dignity (Swanson, 1991, p. 162).
- The concept of enabling refers to facilitating the other's passage through life transitions and unfamiliar events by focusing on the event, informing, explaining, supporting, validating feelings, generating alternatives, thinking things through, and giving feedback (Swanson, 1991, p. 162).

These caring processes are sequential and overlapping. In fact, they might not exist separate from one another because each is an integral component of the overarching structure of caring (Wojnar, 2010, p. 746). According to Swanson (1999b), knowing, being with, doing for, enabling, and maintaining belief are essential components of the nurse–client relationship, regardless of the context. A summary of the metaparadigm concepts of nursing as defined by Swanson is included in **Table 2-16**.

Katharine Kolcaba's Theory of Comfort

Comfort, as described by Kolcaba (2004, p. 255) in the Theory of Comfort, is the immediate experience of being strengthened by having needs for relief, ease, and transcendence addressed in four contexts—physical, psychospiritual, sociocultural, and environmental; it is much more than simply the absence of pain or other physical discomfort. Physical comfort pertains to bodily

TABLE 2-16	Metaparadigm Concepts as Defined in Swanson's Theory of Caring
Person	"Unique beings who are in the midst of becoming and whose wholeness is made manifest in thoughts, feelings, and behaviors" (Swanson, 1993, p. 352).
Environment	"Any context that influences or is influenced by the designated client" (Swanson, 1993, p. 353).
Health	Health and well-being is "to live the subjective, meaning-filled experience of wholeness. Wholeness involves a sense of integration and becoming wherein all facets of being are free to be expressed" (Swanson, 1993, p. 353).
Nursing	Informed caring for the well-being of others (Swanson, 1991, 1993).

sensations and homeostatic mechanisms. Psychospiritual comfort pertains to the internal awareness of self, including esteem, sexuality, meaning in one's life, and one's relationship to a higher order or being. Sociocultural comfort pertains to interpersonal, family, societal relationships, and cultural traditions. Environmental comfort pertains to the external background of the human experience, which includes light, noise, color, temperature, ambience, and natural versus synthetic elements (Kolcaba, 2004, p. 258).

According to Kolcaba, comfort care encompasses three components: an appropriate and timely intervention to meet the comfort needs of patients, a mode of delivery that projects caring and empathy, and the intent to comfort. Comfort needs include patients' or families' desire for or deficit in relief, ease, or transcendence in the physical, psychospiritual, sociocultural, or environmental contexts of human experience. Comfort measures refer to interventions that are intentionally designed to enhance patients' or families' comfort (Kolcaba, 2004, p. 255).

The Theory of Comfort also addresses intervening variables—negative or positive factors over which nurses and institutions have little control but that affect the direction and success of comfort care plans. Examples of intervening variables are the presence or absence of social support, poverty, prognosis, concurrent medical or psychological conditions, and health habits (Kolcaba, 2004, p. 255).

An additional concept within the theory comprises the health-seeking behaviors of patients and families. Health-seeking behaviors are those behaviors that patients and families engage in either consciously or unconsciously while moving toward well-being. Health-seeking behaviors can be either internal or external and can include dying peacefully. It is posited that enhanced comfort results in engagement in health-seeking behaviors (Kolcaba, 2004, p. 255). The metaparadigm concepts of nursing as defined by Kolcaba are summarized in **Table 2-17**.

TABLE 2-17	Metaparadigm Concepts as Defined in Kolcaba's Theory of Comfort
Person	Recipients of care may be individuals, families, institutions, or communities in need of health care (Kolcaba, Tilton, & Drouin, 2006).
Environment	The environment includes any aspect of the patient, family, or institutional setting that can be manipulated by the nurse, a loved one, or the institution to enhance comfort (Dowd, 2010, p. 711).
Health	Health is considered optimal functioning of the patient, the family, the healthcare provider, or the community (Dowd, 2010, p. 711).
Nursing	Nursing is the intentional assessment of comfort needs, design of comfort interventions to address those needs, and reassessment of comfort levels after implementation compared to baseline (Dowd, 2010, p. 711).

Pamela Reed's Self-Transcendence Theory

Three major concepts are central to the Theory of Self-Transcendence: self-transcendence, well-being, and vulnerability. Self-transcendence is the capacity to expand self-boundaries intrapersonally, interpersonally, temporally, and transpersonally (Reed, 2008, p. 107; 2014, p. 111). The capacity to expand self-boundaries intrapersonally refers to a greater awareness of one's philosophy, values, and dreams. The capacity to expand interpersonally relates to others and one's environment. The capacity to expand temporally refers to integration of one's past and future in a way that has meaning for the present. Finally, the capacity to expand transpersonally refers to the capacity to connect with dimensions beyond the typically discernible world (p. 107). Self-transcendence is a characteristic of developmental maturity that is congruent with enhanced awareness of the environment and a broadened perspective on life. Self-transcendence is expressed through behaviors such as sharing wisdom with others, integrating physical changes of aging, accepting death as a part of life, and finding spiritual meaning in life (Reed, 2008, pp. 107–108).

Well-being is the second major concept of Reed's theory. Well-being is a sense of feeling whole and healthy, according to one's own criteria for wholeness and health. The definition of well-being depends on the individual or population. Indeed, indicators of well-being are as diverse as human perceptions of health and wellness. Examples of indicators of well-being are life satisfaction, positive self-concept, hopefulness, happiness, and having meaning in life. Well-being is viewed as a correlate and an outcome of self-transcendence (Reed, 2008; 2014, pp. 112–113).

The third major concept, vulnerability, is the awareness of personal mortality and the likelihood of experiencing difficult life situations. Self-transcendence emerges naturally in health experiences when a person is confronted with mortality and immortality. Life events such as illness, disability, aging, childbirth, or parenting—all of which heighten a person's sense of mortality, inadequacy, or vulnerability—can trigger developmental progress toward a renewed sense of identity and expanded self-boundaries (Reed, 2014, p. 113). According to Reed (2008, pp. 108–109), self-transcendence is evoked through life events and can enhance well-being by transforming losses and difficulties into healing experiences.

Additional concepts in Reed's theory include moderating-mediating factors and points of intervention. Moderating-mediating factors are personal and contextual variables such as age, gender, life experiences, and social environment that can influence the relationships between vulnerability and self-transcendence and between self-transcendence and well-being. Nursing activities that facilitate self-transcendence are referred to as points of intervention (Coward, 2010, p. 623). Two points of intervention are intertwined with the process of self-transcendence: Nursing actions can focus either directly on a person's inner resource for self-transcendence or indirectly on the personal

TABLE 2-18	Metaparadigm Concepts as Defined in Reed's Self-Transcendence Theory
Person	Persons are human beings who develop over the life span through interactions with other persons and within an environment (Coward, 2010, p. 622).
Environment	The environment is composed of family, social networks, physical surroundings, and community resources (Coward, 2010, p. 622).
Health	Well-being is a sense of feeling whole and healthy, according to one's own criteria for wholeness and health (Reed, 2008).
Nursing	The role of nursing activity is to assist persons through interpersonal processes and therapeutic management of their environment to promote health and well-being (Coward, 2010, p. 622).

and contextual factors that affect the relationship between vulnerability and self-transcendence and the relationship between self-transcendence and well-being (p. 621). The metaparadigm concepts of nursing as defined by Reed are summarized in **Table 2-18**.

Merle Mishel's Uncertainty in Illness Theory

The purpose of the Uncertainty in Illness Theory is to "describe and explain uncertainty as a basis for practice and research" (Mishel, 2014, p. 54). Uncertainty, the central concept of the theory, is defined as "the inability to determine the meaning of illness-related events inclusive of inability to assign definite value and/or to accurately predict outcomes" (p. 56). The second central concept in the theory, cognitive schema, is defined by Mishel as a "person's subjective interpretation of illness-related events" (p. 56).

The Uncertainty in Illness Theory is organized around three themes: antecedents of uncertainty, appraisal of uncertainty, and coping with uncertainty. Antecedents of uncertainty include the stimuli frame, cognitive capacities, and structure providers. According to the model, uncertainty is a result of these antecedents, with the major path to uncertainty being through the stimuli frame variables (Mishel, 2014, pp. 58–59). The stimuli frame encompasses the form, composition, and structure of the stimuli that the person perceives. It has three components: symptom pattern, event familiarity, and event congruence (pp. 56–57). The symptom pattern refers to the degree to which symptoms occur with enough consistency to be perceived as following a pattern. Event familiarity refers to the degree to which a situation is repetitive or contains recognized cues. Event congruence refers to the consistency between what is expected and what is experienced (Mishel, 1988). The stimuli frame is the foundation for cognitive schema or the person's interpretation of the events (Bailey & Stewart, 2014, p. 557). Cognitive capacities refer to the information-processing ability of the person, and structure providers refer to the resources such as education, social support, and credible authority available to assist the person as he or she interprets the stimuli frame. Thus, cognitive capacities and structure providers influence the components of the stimuli frame (Mishel, 2014, pp. 56–57).

The second theme, appraisal of uncertainty, refers to the process of placing a value on the uncertain event or situation. Appraisal of uncertainty has two components: inference and illusion. Inference refers to the evaluation of uncertainty by using examples; it is predicated on personality disposition, experience, knowledge, and contextual cues. Illusion comprises the construction of beliefs to create a positive outlook (Mishel, 2014, p. 57).

The third theme, coping with uncertainty, includes the concepts of danger, opportunity, coping, and adaptation. Danger refers to the possibility of a harmful outcome, whereas opportunity is the possibility of a positive outcome. Coping in the context of a danger appraisal encompasses activities directed toward reducing uncertainty and managing emotions; coping in the context of an opportunity appraisal comprises activities directed toward maintaining uncertainty (Mishel, 2014, pp. 57–58). Adaptation in the context of the uncertainty theory is defined as biopsychosocial behavior occurring within a person's range of usual behavior and is the outcome of coping (pp. 57–58).

The reconceptualized Uncertainty in Illness Theory presents the process of moving from uncertainty appraised as danger to uncertainty appraised as an opportunity and resource for a new view of life. The revised theory incorporates two new concepts: self-organization and probabilistic thinking. Self-organization refers to the reformulation of a new sense of order resulting from the integration of continuous uncertainty into self-structure, where uncertainty is accepted as the natural rhythm of life. Probabilistic thinking refers to the belief in a conditional world in which the expectation of certainty is abandoned (Bailey & Stewart, 2014, p. 558; Mishel, 2014, pp. 58–59).

The metaparadigm concepts of nursing as defined by Mishel are summarized in **Table 2-19**.

Cheryl Tatano Beck's Postpartum Depression Theory

Two major concepts are included in the Postpartum Depression Theory: postpartum mood disorders and loss of control. Postpartum mood disorders include postpartum depression, maternity blues, postpartum psychosis, postpartum obsessive–compulsive disorder, and postpartum-onset panic disorder (Beck, 2002). The second major concept in Beck's theory describes the experience of loss of control in all areas of women's lives. Loss of control is a basic psychosocial problem with which women attempt to cope through a four-stage process labeled by Beck as "teetering on the edge," referring to what women describe as walking a fine line between sanity and insanity.

TABLE 2-19	Metaparadigm Concepts as Defined in Mishel's Uncertainty in Illness Theory
Person	The concept of person is the central focus of the theory and may be an individual or the family of an ill individual (Mishel, 2014, p. 54); the individual is viewed as a biopsychosocial being who is an open system exchanging energy with the environment.
Environment	Not explicitly defined, but is acknowledged to exchange energy with the person system.
Health	Defined in terms of uncertainty in the context of the illness experience, with the concept of health or well-being being congruent with the formulation of a new life view and probabilistic thinking.
Nursing	Nurses are viewed as a part of the antecedent variable of structure providers (Mishel, 2014, p. 71).

The four stages of the coping process consist of (1) encountering terror in the form of symptoms such as anxiety attacks, fogginess, and obsessive thinking that hit unexpectedly and suddenly, (2) dying of self, as mothers who no longer know who they have become isolate themselves and contemplate and sometimes attempt self-destruction, (3) struggling to survive, as they battle the healthcare system and seek help from support groups and prayer, and (4) regaining control of their lives during transition and guarded recovery while mourning lost time with their infant (Beck, 1993).

Additional concepts in Beck's theory include predictors or risk factors for postpartum depression. These concepts include prenatal depression, childcare stress, life stress, social support, prenatal anxiety, marital satisfaction, history of depression, infant temperament, maternity blues, self-esteem, socioeconomic status, marital status, and unplanned or unwanted pregnancy (Beck, 2003, p. 397). Concepts that are used for screening in the Postpartum Depression Screening Scale include sleeping and eating disturbances, anxiety and insecurity, emotional lability, mental confusion, loss of self, guilt and shame, and suicidal thoughts (Beck & Gable, 2000). Modifications to the Postpartum Depression Theory have occurred as research reveals new information. In addition to these concepts, the four metaparadigm concepts of nursing are presented in the context of Beck's Postpartum Depression Theory. These concepts are summarized in **Table 2-20**.

The American Association of Critical-Care Nurses' Synergy Model for Patient Care

The Synergy Model is a conceptual framework for designing practice competencies to care for critically ill patients with a goal of optimizing outcomes for patients and families. Optimal outcomes are realized when the competencies of the nurse match the patient and family needs.

TABLE 2-20   Metaparadigm Concepts as Defined in Beck's Postpartum Depression Theory

Person	Described in terms of wholeness with biological, sociological, and psychological aspects, with personhood understood in the context of family and community (Maeve, 2014, p. 678).
Environment	Viewed broadly in terms of individual factors and external factors (Maeve, 2014, p. 678).
Health	Not defined explicitly; traditional ideas of physical and mental health are viewed as a consequence of women's responses to the contexts of their lives and environments (Maeve, 2014, p. 678).
Nursing	A caring profession with caring obligations; the nurse accomplishes the goals of health and wholeness through interpersonal interactions (Maeve, 2014, p. 678).

The Synergy Model for Patient Care is the result of the American Association of Critical-Care Nurses (AACN) envisioning a new paradigm for clinical practice. In 1993, the AACN Certification Corporation convened a think tank that included nationally recognized experts to develop a conceptual framework for certified practice. The initial work resulted in the description of 13 patient characteristics based on universal needs of patients and 9 characteristics required of nurses to meet patient needs. The patient characteristics identified were compensation, resiliency, margin of error, predictability, complexity, vulnerability, physiologic stability, risk of death, independence, self-determination, involvement in care decisions, engagement, and resource availability. The characteristics of nurses were engagement, skilled clinical practice, agency, caring practices, system management, teamwork, diversity responsiveness, experiential learning, and being an innovator–evaluator. The think tank suggested that the synergy emerging from the interaction between the patient needs and the nurse characteristics should result in optimal outcomes for the patient and that these characteristics of the nurse would determine competencies for certified practice (Hardin, 2005, pp. 3–4).

In 1995, the AACN Certification Corporation decided to refine this model, to conduct a study of practice and job analysis of critical care nurses, and to test the validity of the concepts in critical care nurses. The group refined the patient characteristics into eight concepts, merged the nurse characteristics into eight concepts, and delineated a continuum for the characteristics. The eight patient characteristics identified in the current model are resiliency, vulnerability, stability, complexity, resource availability, participation in care, participation in decision making, and predictability. The eight nurse characteristics are clinical judgment, advocacy, caring practices, collaboration, systems thinking, response to diversity, clinical inquiry, and facilitation of

TABLE 2-21 Metaparadigm Concepts as Defined in the Synergy Model for Patient Care	
Person	Persons are viewed in the context of patients who are biological, social, and spiritual entities who are present at a particular developmental stage.
Environment	The concept of environment is not explicitly defined; however, included in the assumptions is the idea that environment is created by the nurses for the care of the patient.
Health	The concept of health is not explicitly defined; an optimal level of wellness as defined by the patient is mentioned as a goal of nursing care.
Nursing	The purpose of nursing is to meet the needs of patients and families and to provide safe passage through the healthcare system during a time of crisis (Hardin, 2005, p. 8).

learning (Hardin, 2005, p. 4; 2013, p. 294). Each patient characteristic is placed on a scale from one to five, with the level of each patient characteristic being critical in terms of the competency required of the nurse (Hardin, 2005, pp. 4–7). The eight nurse characteristics can be considered essential competencies for providing care for critically ill patients. All eight competencies reflect an integration of knowledge, skills, and experience of the nurse. Each nurse characteristic can be understood on a continuum from one to five (Hardin, 2005, pp. 5–6).

The Synergy Model delineates three levels of outcomes: outcomes derived from the patient, outcomes derived from the nurse, and outcomes derived from the healthcare system. Outcomes data derived from the patient include functional changes, behavioral changes, trust, satisfaction, comfort, and quality of life. Outcomes data derived from nursing competencies include physiologic changes, the presence or absence of complications, and the extent to which treatment objectives are attained (Curley, 1998). Outcomes data derived from the healthcare system include readmission rates, length of stay, and cost utilization (Hardin, 2005, pp. 8–9). The metaparadigm concepts of nursing as defined in the Synergy Model for Patient Care are summarized in **Table 2-21**.

Nurse of the Future: Nursing Core Competencies

Although not a theory of nursing, the *Nurse of the Future: Nursing Core Competencies* (Massachusetts Department of Higher Education, 2010) document addresses the knowledge base and relationships among concepts important to the practice of nursing. In the context of nursing knowledge, the

TABLE 2-22	Metaparadigm Concepts as Defined in the *Nurse of the Future: Nursing Core Competencies*
Human being/patients	"The recipient of nursing care or services ... Patients may be individuals, families, groups, communities, or populations" (AACN, 1998, p. 2, as cited in Massachusetts Department of Higher Education, 2010, p. 7).
Environment	"The atmosphere, milieu, or conditions in which an individual lives, works or plays" (ANA, 2004, p. 47, as cited in Massachusetts Department of Higher Education, 2010, p. 7).
Health	"An experience that is often expressed in terms of wellness and illness, and may occur in the presence or absence of disease or injury" (ANA, 2004, p. 5, as cited in Massachusetts Department of Higher Education, 2010, p. 8).
Nursing	"....the protection, promotion, and optimization of health and abilities, prevention of illness and injury, alleviation of suffering through the diagnosis and treatment of human response, and advocacy in the care of individuals, families, groups, communities, and populations" (ANA, 2001, p. 5, as cited in Massachusetts Department of Higher Education, 2010, p. 8).

concepts of patient, environment, health, and nursing are defined and are presented in **Table 2-22**.

There arc 10 Nurse of the Future core competencies:

- *Patient-centered care:* "The Nurse of the Future will provide holistic care that recognizes an individual's preferences, values, and needs and respects the patient or designee as a full partner in providing compassionate, coordinated, age and culturally appropriate, safe and effective care" (Massachusetts Department of Higher Education, 2010, p. 9).
- *Professionalism:* "The Nurse of the Future will demonstrate accountability for the delivery of standard-based nursing care that is consistent with moral, altruistic, legal, ethical, regulatory, and humanistic principles" (Massachusetts Department of Higher Education, 2010, p. 13).
- *Leadership:* "The Nurse of the Future will influence the behavior of individuals or groups of individuals within their environment in a way that will facilitate the establishment and acquisition/achievement of shared goals" (Massachusetts Department of Higher Education, 2010, p. 17).
- *Systems-based practice:* "The Nurse of the Future will demonstrate an awareness of and responsiveness to the larger context of the health care system, and will demonstrate the ability to effectively call on micro-system resources to provide care that is of optimal quality and value" (Massachusetts Department of Higher Education, 2010, p. 19).

- *Informatics and technology:* "The Nurse of the Future will use information and technology to communicate, manage, knowledge, mitigate error, and support decision making" (Quality and Safety Education for Nurses [QSEN], 2007, as cited in Massachusetts Department of Higher Education, 2010, p. 22).
- *Communication:* "The Nurse of the Future will interact effectively with patients, families, and colleagues, fostering mutual respect and shared decision making to enhance patient satisfaction and health outcomes" (Massachusetts Department of Higher Education, 2010, p. 27).
- *Teamwork and collaboration:* "The Nurse of the Future will function effectively within nursing and interdisciplinary teams, fostering open communication, mutual respect, shared decision making, team learning, and development" (adapted from QSEN, 2007, as cited in Massachusetts Department of Higher Education, 2010, p. 31).
- *Safety:* "The Nurse of the Future will minimize risk of harm to patients and providers through both system effectiveness and individual performance" (QSEN, 2007, as cited in Massachusetts Department of Higher Education, 2010, p. 34).
- *Quality improvement:* "The Nurse of the Future uses data to monitor the outcomes of care processes, and uses improvement methods to design and test changes to continuously improve the quality and safety of health care systems" (QSEN, 2007, as cited in Massachusetts Department of Higher Education, 2010, p. 36).
- *Evidence-based practice:* "The Nurse of the Future will identify, evaluate, and use the best current evidence coupled with clinical expertise and consideration of patients' preferences, experience and values to make practice decisions" (adapted from QSEN, 2007, as cited in Massachusetts Department of Higher Education, 2010, p. 37).

The committee that designed the *Nurse of the Future: Nursing Core Competencies* also identified several assumptions and principles to serve as a framework. The assumptions include: (1) education and practice partnerships are key in developing an effective model, (2) it is imperative that leaders in nursing education and practice develop collaborative models to facilitate a minimum of a baccalaureate degree in nursing for all nurses, (3) a more effective education system must be created that will allow preparation of the nursing workforce to respond to the current and future healthcare needs of populations, (4) the nurse of the future will be proficient in a core set of competencies, and (5) nurse educators in education and practice settings will need to use different teaching strategies to integrate Nurse of the Future core competencies into the curriculum (Massachusetts Department of Higher Education, 2010, pp. 3–4).

The art and science of nursing are based on a framework of caring and respect for human dignity. A compassionate approach to patient care mandates that nurses provide care in a competent manner. The *Nurse of the Future: Nursing Core Competencies* provides a framework for the provision of competent nursing care (Massachusetts Department of Higher Education, 2010, p. 7).

Overview of Selected Non-Nursing Theories

Nursing as a discipline with a distinct body of theoretical knowledge has developed over time, but non-nursing theories have and still do influence nursing theory, research, and practice. Brief overviews of non-nursing theories that are commonly used in nursing follow.

General System Theory

Von Bertalanffy (1968) emphasized that systems are open to and interact with their environments, and that they can evolve as they acquire new properties. Rather than reducing an entity to the properties of its parts or elements, system theory focuses on the arrangement of and relations between the parts that connect them into a whole. This particular organization defines a system. Major concepts of general system theory include a system–environment boundary, input and output processes, and the organizational state of the system. General System Theory is founded on the premise that the world is composed of systems that are interconnected and influenced by one another. The two primary assumptions of the theory are that energy is needed to maintain an organizational state and that dysfunction in one system has an effect on other systems (Boulding, 1956). Roy's Adaptation Model, King's Interacting Systems Framework and Theory of Goal Attainment, and Neuman's System Model are all nursing theories that have foundations in general system theory.

Social Cognitive Theory

Social Cognitive Theory explains human behaviors in terms of dynamic reciprocal interactions among cognitive, behavioral, and environmental influences. According to Albert Bandura (1986), human behavior is learned observationally through modeling or observing others. Once a behavior is observed, the person forms an idea of how the new behavior is performed; on a later occasion, this coded information serves as a guide for action. Principles derived from Social Cognitive Theory are often used to promote behavior change.

Bandura incorporated the concept of self-efficacy into Social Learning Theory (now called Social Cognitive Theory) in 1977. The concept of self-efficacy refers to a person's confidence in his or her ability to take action and persist in that action to reach goals. The concept of self-efficacy can be important in influencing health behavior change (Bandura, 1997) and is frequently used by nurses engaged in health education and behavior modification. Nola Pender is a nurse theorist who identifies Social Learning Theory as central to her health promotion model, with the concept of self-efficacy being included as a central construct of the model (Sakraida, 2014, p. 398).

Stress and Coping Process Theory

Richard Lazarus suggested that stress might be an organizing concept for understanding a wide range of phenomena rather than a variable. Stress as conceptualized by Lazarus emphasizes the relationship of the person to the environment, with the judgment of whether a specific person–environment relationship is stressful dependent on cognitive appraisal (Lazarus & Folkman, 1984, p. 21). He identified three types of cognitive appraisal: primary, secondary, and reappraisal. Vulnerability is related to the concept of cognitive appraisal, because the vulnerable individual is one whose coping resources are deficient (Lazarus & Folkman, 1984, pp. 53–54). Patricia Benner credits Richard Lazarus with mentoring her in the area of stress and coping.

General Adaptation Syndrome

Hans Selye introduced the notion of a general adaptation syndrome in 1950 (Selye, 1950). In 1974, Selye defined stress as the nonspecific response of the body to any demand for change. General adaptation syndrome is based on physiologic and psychobiologic responses to stress. According to Selye, a stressor results in a three-stage response that includes alarm, resistance, and exhaustion, also known as coping with stress. The goals of coping with stress are adaptation and homeostasis (Selye, 1950, 1974).

Betty Neuman used Selye's definition of stress in her systems model (Lawson, 2014, p. 282). Sister Callista Roy also used concepts from Selye in the refinement of her adaptation model (Phillips & Harris, 2014, p. 304).

Relationship of Theory to Professional Nursing Practice

How will theory affect your nursing practice? Using a theoretical framework to guide your nursing practice assists you as you organize patient data, understand and analyze patient data, make decisions related to nursing interventions, plan patient care, predict outcomes of care, and evaluate patient outcomes (Alligood & Tomey, 2002). Why? The use of a theoretical framework provides a systematic and knowledgeable approach to nursing practice. The framework also becomes a tool that assists you to think critically as you plan and provide nursing care.

> **CRITICAL THINKING QUESTION** *
>
> Think about the definitions of the metaparadigm concepts and the assumptions or propositions of each of the theories presented. Which of the theories most closely matches your beliefs? *

How do you begin? Now that you know why nursing theory is important to your nursing practice, it is time to identify a theoretical framework that fits you and your practice. Alligood (2006) presented guidelines for selecting a framework for theory-based nursing practice. Following are the steps:

1. Consider the values and beliefs in nursing that you truly hold.
2. Write a philosophy of nursing that clarifies your beliefs related to person, environment, health, and nursing.
3. Survey definitions of person, environment, health, and nursing in nursing models.
4. Select two or three frameworks that best fit with your beliefs related to the concepts of person, environment, health, and nursing.
5. Review the assumptions of the frameworks that you have selected.
6. Apply those frameworks in a selected area of nursing practice.
7. Compare the frameworks on client focus, nursing action, and client outcome.
8. Review the nursing literature written by persons who have used the frameworks.
9. Select a framework and develop its use in your nursing practice.

Conclusion

As demonstrated by the descriptions of the philosophies, conceptual models, and theories presented in this chapter, there is a wide variety of perspectives and frameworks from which to practice nursing. There is no one right or wrong answer. Various nursing theories represent different realities and address different aspects of nursing (Meleis, 2007). For this reason, the multiplicity of nursing theories presented in this chapter should not be viewed as competing theories, but rather as complementary theories that can provide insight into different ways to describe, explain, and predict nursing concepts and/or prescribe nursing care. Curley (2007, p. 3) describes this understanding in an interesting way by comparing the multiplicity of nursing theories to a collection of maps of the same region. Each map might display a different characteristic of the region, such as rainfall, topography, or air currents. Although all of the maps are accurate, the best map for use depends on the information needed or the question being asked. This is precisely the case with the nurse's choice of nursing theories for practice.

So, begin with whichever theoretical framework seems to "fit," and then practice using it as you provide nursing care. "The full realization of nursing theory–guided practice is perhaps the greatest challenge that nursing as a scholarly discipline has ever faced" (Cody, 2006). So, be patient; developing your nursing practice guided by nursing theory takes time and practice. All nursing theories require in-depth study over time to master them fully (this chapter provides only a brief introduction), but the incorporation of theory into your practice can transform your nursing practice. The end result of this process will be seen in the excellent nursing care that you can provide to patients over the course of your professional nursing career.

CASE STUDY 2-1 ▪ MR. M.

Mr. M. is a 34-year-old Caucasian male who presents to the mental health clinic with depression and complaints of fatigue. An interview reveals that his wife and both of his children were killed in a traffic accident 6 months ago. The nurse knows that Mr. M. is vulnerable as a result of the loss of his family, but that self-transcendence is evoked through life events and that well-being can be enhanced by transforming losses and difficulties into healing experiences.

Case Study Questions

1. The nurse uses Reed's Self-Transcendence Theory to focus nursing activity for Mr. M. on facilitating self-transcendence. Based on the assessment, what intrapersonal strategies might be appropriate?

2. Which interpersonal strategies might be appropriate during follow-up visits to facilitate connecting to others?

Classroom Activity 1

Divide into small groups and give each group a copy of the same case study. Assign a different nursing theory to each group, and ask the groups to develop a plan of care using the assigned nursing theory as the basis for practice. Each group should share its plan of care with the class. Discuss the differences and similarities in the foci of care based on each of the selected theories.

Classroom Activity 2

Think about the metaparadigm concepts of nursing. Draw each of the concepts in relation to the other concepts to show your ideas of how each of the concepts interfaces with the others. Present your "conceptual model" to the class, and discuss your ideas about each of the concepts represented. This activity works best if you use colored pencils, crayons, or markers and a large piece of paper or newsprint. Actual student examples are presented in **Figure 2-1** and **Figure 2-2**.

Figure 2-1 Student conceptual model

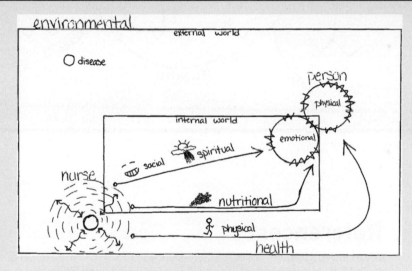

Source: Used with permission of Heather Grush.

Figure 2-2 Student conceptual model

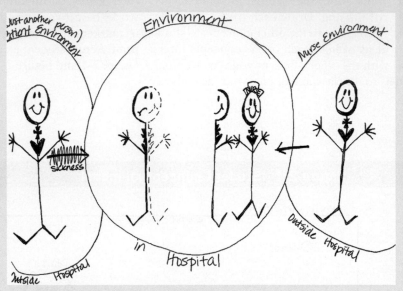

Source: Used with permission of Linzee McGinnis.

References

Alligood, M. R. (2006). Philosophies, models, and theories: Critical thinking structures. In M. R. Alligood & A. M. Tomey (Eds.), *Nursing theory: Utilization & application* (3rd ed., pp. 43–65). St. Louis, MO: Mosby.

Alligood, M. R., & Tomey, A. M. (2002). Significance of theory for nursing as a discipline and profession. In A. M. Tomey & M. R. Alligood (Eds.), *Nursing theorists and their work* (5th ed., pp. 14–31). St. Louis, MO: Mosby.

American Association of Colleges of Nursing. (1998). *The essentials of baccalaureate education for professional nursing practice*. Washington, DC: Author.

American Nurses Association. (2001). *Code of ethics for nurses with interpretive statements*. Silver Spring, MD: Author.

American Nurses Association. (2004). *Nursing: Scope and standards of practice*. Silver Spring, MD: Author.

Andrews, H. A., & Roy, C., Sr. (1986). *Essentials of the Roy adaptation model*. Norwalk, CT: Appleton-Century-Crofts.

Andrews, H. A., & Roy, C., Sr. (1991). *Essentials of the Roy adaptation model*. In C. Roy Sr. & H. A. Andrews (Eds.), *The Roy adaptation model: The definitive statement* (pp. 2–25). Norwalk, CT: Appleton & Lange.

Bailey, D. E., & Stewart, J. L. (2014). Merle H. Mishel: Uncertainty in illness theory. In M. R. Alligood (Ed.), *Nursing theorists and their work* (8th ed., pp. 555–573). Maryland Heights, MO: Mosby.

Bandura, A. (1977). Social learning theory: Toward a unifying theory of behavior change. *Psychological Review, 84*, 191–215.

Bandura, A. (1986). *Social foundations of thought and action: A social cognitive theory*. Englewood Cliffs, NJ: Prentice Hall.

Bandura, A. (1997). *Self-efficacy: The exercise of control*. New York, NY: W. H. Freeman.

Beck, C. (1993). Teetering on the edge: A substantive theory of postpartum depression. *Nursing Research, 42*(1), 42–48.

Beck, C. T. (2002). Postpartum depression: A metasynthesis. *Qualitative Health Research, 12*(4), 453–472.

Beck, C. T. (2003). Patient screening tool. Postpartum Depression Predictors Inventory—Revised. *Advances in Neonatal Care (Elsevier Science), 3*(1), 47–48.

Beck, C., & Gable, R. (2000). Postpartum Depression Screening Scale: Development and psychometric testing. *Nursing Research, 49*(5), 272–282.

Benner, P. (2001). *From novice to expert: Excellence and power in clinical nursing practice*. Upper Saddle River, NJ: Prentice Hall. (Original work published 1984)

Benner, P., Hooper-Kyriakidis, P., & Stannard, D. (1999). *Clinical wisdom and interventions in critical care: A thinking-in-action approach*. Philadelphia, PA: Saunders.

Benner, P., & Wrubel, J. (1989). *The primacy of caring: Stress and coping in health and illness*. Menlo Park, CA: Addison-Wesley.

Berbiglia, V. A. (2010). Orem's self-care deficit theory in nursing practice. In M. R. Alligood (Ed.), *Nursing theory: Utilization and application* (4th ed., pp. 261–286). Maryland Heights, MO: Mosby.

Bolton, K. (2006). Nightingale's philosophy in nursing practice. In M. R. Alligood & A. M. Tomey (Eds.), *Nursing theory: Utilization & application* (3rd ed., pp. 89–102). St. Louis, MO: Mosby.

Boulding, K. E. (1956). General systems theory: The skeleton of science. *Management Science, 2*(3), 197–208.

Brykczynski, K. A. (2010). Benner's philosophy in nursing practice. In M. R. Alligood (Ed.), *Nursing theory: Utilization and application* (4th ed., pp. 137–159). Maryland Heights, MO: Mosby.

Cody, W. K. (2006). Nursing theory–guided practice: What it is and what it is not. In W. K. Cody (Ed.), *Philosophical and theoretical perspectives for advanced nursing practice* (4th ed., pp. 119–121). Sudbury, MA: Jones and Bartlett.

Coward, D. D. (2010). Self-Transcendence Theory: Pamela G. Reed. In M. R. Alligood & A. M. Tomey (Eds.), *Nursing theorists and their work* (7th ed., pp. 618–637). Maryland Heights, MO: Mosby.

Curley, M. A. Q. (1998). Patient–nurse synergy: Optimizing patients' outcomes. *American Journal of Critical Care, 7*(1), 64–72.

Curley, M. A. Q. (2007). *Synergy: The unique relationship between nursing and patients*. Indianapolis, IN: Sigma Theta Tau International.

Day, L., & Benner, P. (2002). Ethics, ethical comportment, and etiquette. *American Journal of Critical Care, 11*(1), 76–79.

Dowd, T. (2010). Katharine Kolcaba: Theory of Comfort. In M. R. Alligood &A. M. Tomey (Eds.), *Nursing theorists and their work* (7th ed., pp. 706–721). Maryland Heights, MO: Mosby.

Eckberg, D. L., & Hill, L., Jr. (1979). The paradigm concept and sociology: A critical review. *American Sociological Review, 44,* 925–937.

Fawcett, J. (1994). *Analysis and evaluation of conceptual models of nursing.* Philadelphia, PA: F. A. Davis.

Fawcett, J. (2005). *Contemporary nursing knowledge: Analysis and evaluation of nursing models and theories* (2nd ed., pp. 553–585). Philadelphia, PA: F. A. Davis.

Flaskerud, J. H., & Holloran, E. J. (1980). Areas of agreement in nursing theory development. *Advances in Nursing Science, 3*(1), 1–7.

Furukawa, C. Y., & Howe, J. S. (2002). Definition and components of nursing: Virginia Henderson. In J. B. George (Ed.), *Nursing theories: The base for professional nursing practice* (5th ed., pp. 83–109). Upper Saddle River, NJ: Prentice Hall.

Geib, K. M. (2006). Neuman's systems model in nursing practice. In M. R. Alligood & A. M. Tomey (Eds.), *Nursing theory: Utilization & application* (3rd ed., pp. 229–254). St. Louis, MO: Mosby.

Gordon, S. C. (2001). Virginia Avenel Henderson: Definition of nursing. In M. Parker (Ed.), *Nursing theories and nursing practice*. Philadelphia, PA: F. A. Davis.

Gunther, M. (2006). Rogers' science of unitary human beings in nursing practice. In M. R. Alligood & A. M. Tomey (Eds.), *Nursing theory: Utilization & application* (3rd ed., pp. 283–306). St. Louis, MO: Mosby.

Gunther, M. (2010). Rogers' science of unitary human beings in nursing practice. In M. R. Alligood & A. M. Tomey (Eds.), *Nursing theory: Utilization & application* (4th ed., pp. 287–307). St. Louis, MO: Mosby.

Hardin, S. R. (2005). Introduction to the AACN Synergy Model for Patient Care. In S. R. Hardin & R. Kaplow (Eds.), *Synergy for clinical excellence: The AACN Synergy Model for Patient Care* (pp. 3–10). Sudbury, MA: Jones and Bartlett.

Hardin, S. R. (2013). The AACN Synergy Model. In S. J. Peterson & T. S. Bredow (Eds.), *Middle range theories: Application to nursing research* (3rd ed., pp. 294–305). Philadelphia, PA: Lippincott.

Harmer, B., & Henderson, V. (1955). *Textbook of the principles and practice of nursing.* New York, NY: Macmillan.

Henderson, V. (1964). The nature of nursing. *American Journal of Nursing, 64,* 62–68.

Henderson, V. (1966). *The nature of nursing: A definition and its implications for practice, research, and education.* New York, NY: Macmillan.

Henderson, V. (1991). *The nature of nursing: Reflections after 25 years.* New York, NY: National League for Nursing Press.

Hickman, J. S. (2002). An introduction to nursing theory. In J. B. George (Ed.), *Nursing theories: A base for professional nursing practice* (5th ed., pp. 1–20). Upper Saddle River, NJ: Prentice Hall.

Holaday, B. (2006). Johnson's behavioral system model in nursing practice. In M. R. Alligood & A. M. Tomey (Eds.), *Nursing theory: Utilization & application* (3rd ed., pp. 157–180). St. Louis, MO: Mosby.

Howk, C. (2002). Hildegard E. Peplau: Psychodynamic nursing. In A. M. Tomey & M. R. Alligood (Eds.), *Nursing theorists and their work* (5th ed., pp. 379–398). St. Louis, MO: Mosby.

Johnson, B. M., & Webber, P. B. (2010). *An introduction to theory and reasoning in nursing* (3rd ed.). Philadelphia, PA: Lippincott Williams & Wilkins.

Johnson, D. (1980). The behavioral systems model for nursing. In J. Riehl & C. Roy (Eds.), *Conceptual models for nursing practice* (2nd ed., pp. 207–216). New York, NY: Appleton-Century-Crofts.

King, I. M. (1981). *A theory of nursing: Systems, concepts, process.* New York, NY: Wiley.

King, I. M. (1989). King's general systems framework and theory. In J. P. Riehl-Sisca (Ed.), *Conceptual models for nursing practice* (3rd ed., pp. 149–158). Norwalk, CT: Appleton & Lange.

King, I. M. (1992). King's theory of goal attainment. *Nursing Science Quarterly, 5*(1), 19–26.

Kolcaba, K. (2004). Comfort. In S. J. Peterson & T. S. Bredow (Eds.), *Middle range theories: Application to nursing research* (pp. 255–273). Philadelphia, PA: Lippincott Williams & Wilkins.

Kolcaba, K., Tilton, C., & Drouin, C. (2006). Comfort theory: A unifying framework to enhance the practice environment. *Journal of Nursing Administration, 36*(11), 538–544.

Lawson, T. G. (2014). Betty Neuman: Systems model. In M. R. Alligood (Ed.), *Nursing theorists and their work* (8th ed., pp. 281–302). Maryland Heights, MO: Mosby.

Lazarus, R. S., & Folkman, S. (1984). *Stress, appraisal, and coping.* New York, NY: Springer.

Leininger, M. (1991). *Culture care diversity and universality: A theory of nursing.* New York: National League for Nursing Press.

Leininger, M. (1995). Transcultural nursing perspectives: Basic concepts, principles, and culture care incidents. In M. M. Leininger (Ed.), *Transcultural nursing: Concepts, theories, research, and practices* (2nd ed., pp. 57–92). New York, NY: McGraw-Hill.

Leininger, M. (2001). *Culture care diversity and universality: A theory of nursing.* Sudbury, MA: Jones and Bartlett.

Leininger, M. M., & McFarland, M. R. (2006). *Culture care diversity and universality: A worldwide theory of nursing* (2nd ed.). Sudbury, MA: Jones and Bartlett.

Lippitt, G. L. (1973). *Visualizing change: Model building and the change process.* Fairfax, VA: NTL Learning Resources.

Maeve, M. K. (2014). Cheryl Tatano Beck: Postpartum depression theory. In M. R. Alligood (Ed.), *Nursing theorists and their work* (8th ed., pp. 672–687). Maryland Heights, MO: Mosby.

Massachusetts Department of Higher Education. (2010). *Nurse of the future: Nursing core competencies.* Retrieved from http://www.mass.edu/currentinit/documents/NursingCoreCompetencies.pdf

McBride, A. B. (Narrator). (1997). *Celebrating Virginia Henderson* (Video). (Available from Center for Nursing Press, 550 West North Street, Indianapolis, IN 46202).

Meleis, A. I. (2004). *Theoretical nursing: Development & progress* (3rd ed.). Philadelphia, PA: Lippincott.

Meleis, A. I. (2007). *Theoretical nursing: Development & progress* (4th ed.). Philadelphia, PA: Lippincott.

Meleis, A. I. (2010). *Transitions theory: Middle-range and situation-specific theories in nursing research and practice.* New York, NY: Springer.

Meleis, A. I., Sawyer, L. M., Im, E. O., Hilfinger Messias, D. K., & Schumacher, K. (2000). Experiencing transitions: An emerging middle range theory. *Advances in Nursing Science, 23*(1), 12–28.

Mishel, M. H. (1988). Uncertainty in illness. *Image: The Journal of Nursing Scholarship, 20,* 225–231.

Mishel, M. H. (2014). Theories of uncertainty in illness. In M. J. Smith & P. R. Liehr (Eds.), *Middle range theory for nursing* (3rd ed., pp. 53–86). New York, NY: Springer.

Mitchell, G. J. (2006). Rosemarie Rizzo Parse: Human becoming. In A. M. Tomey & M. R. Alligood (Eds.), *Nursing theorists and their work* (6th ed., pp. 522–559). St. Louis, MO: Mosby.

Mitchell, G. J., & Bournes, D. A. (2010). Rosemarie Rizzo Parse: Humanbecoming. In M. R. Alligood & A. M. Tomey (Eds.), *Nursing theorists and their work* (7th ed., pp. 503–535). Maryland Heights, MO: Mosby.

Neil, R. M., & Tomey, A. M. (2006). Jean Watson: Philosophy and science of caring. In A. M. Tomey & M. R. Alligood (Eds.), *Nursing theorists and their work* (6th ed., pp. 91–115). St. Louis, MO: Mosby.

Neuman, B. (1995). *The Neuman systems model* (3rd ed.). Norwalk, CT: Appleton & Lange.

Neuman, B. (2002). The Neuman systems model. In B. Neuman & J. Fawcett (Eds.), *The Neuman systems model* (4th ed., pp. 3–34). Upper Saddle River, NJ: Prentice Hall.

Nightingale, F. (1969). *Notes on nursing: What it is and what it is not.* New York, NY: Dover. (Original work published 1860).

Norris, D., & Frey, M. A. (2006). King's system framework and theory in nursing practice. In M. R. Alligood & A. M. Tomey (Eds.), *Nursing theory: Utilization & application* (3rd ed., pp. 181–205). St. Louis, MO: Mosby.

Orem, D. (1985). *Nursing: Concepts of practice* (3rd ed.). New York, NY: McGraw-Hill.

Orem, D. (1990). A nursing practice theory in three parts, 1956–1989. In M. E. Parker (Ed.), *Nursing theories in practice* (pp. 47–60). New York, NY: National League for Nursing.

Orem, D. (1995). *Nursing: Concepts of practice* (5th ed.). St. Louis, MO: Mosby.

Orem, D. (2001). *Nursing: Concepts of practice* (6th ed.). St. Louis, MO: Mosby.

Parse, R. R. (1981). *Man–living–health: A theory of nursing.* New York, NY: Wiley.

Parse, R. R. (1987). *Nursing science: Major paradigms, theories, and critiques.* Philadelphia, PA: Saunders.

Parse, R. R. (1998). *The human becoming school of thought: A perspective for nurses and other health professionals.* Thousand Oaks, CA: Sage.

Pender, N. J. (1996). *Health promotion in nursing practice* (3rd ed.). Stamford, CT: Appleton & Lange.

Pender, N. J., Murdaugh, C. L., & Parsons, M. A. (2006). *Health promotion in nursing practice* (5th ed.). Upper Saddle River, NJ: Prentice Hall.

Pender, N. J., Murdaugh, C. L., & Parsons, M. A. (2011). *Health promotion in nursing practice* (6th ed.). Upper Saddle River, NJ: Prentice Hall.

Peplau, H. (1952). *Interpersonal relations in nursing.* New York, NY: G. P. Putnam's Sons.

Peplau, H. E. (1992). Interpersonal relations: A theoretical framework for application in nursing practice. *Nursing Science Quarterly, 5,* 13–18.

Peplau, H. E. (1997). Peplau's theory of interpersonal relations. *Nursing Science Quarterly, 10*(4), 162–167.

Pfettscher, S. A. (2006). Florence Nightingale: Modern nursing. In A. M. Tomey & M. R. Alligood (Eds.), *Nursing theorists and their work* (6th ed., pp. 71–90). St. Louis, MO: Mosby.

Phillips, K. D. (2006). Sister Callista Roy: Adaptation model. In A. M. Tomey & M. R. Alligood (Eds.), *Nursing theorists and their work* (6th ed., pp. 355–385). St. Louis, MO: Mosby.

Phillips, K. D., & Harris, R. (2014). Sister Callista Roy: Adaptation model. In M. R. Alligood (Ed.), *Nursing theorists and their work* (8th ed., pp. 303–331). Maryland Heights, MO: Mosby.

Quality and Safety Education for Nurses. (2007). Quality and safety competencies. Retrieved from http://www.qsen.org/competencies.php

Reed, P. G. (2008). Theory of self-transcendence. In M. J. Smith & P. R. Liehr (Eds.), *Middle range theory for nursing* (2nd ed., pp. 105–129). New York, NY: Springer.

Reed, P. G. (2014). Theory of self-transcendence. In M. J. Smith & P. R. Liehr (Eds.), *Middle range theory for nursing* (3rd ed., pp. 109–139). New York, NY: Springer.

Rogers, M. E. (1970). *An introduction to the theoretical basis of nursing*. Philadelphia, PA: F. A. Davis.

Rogers, M. E. (1992). Nursing science and the space age. *Nursing Science Quarterly, 5,* 27–34.

Rogers, M. E. (1994). The science of unitary human beings: Current perspectives. *Nursing Science Quarterly, 7,* 33–35.

Roy, C., Sr. (2009). *The Roy adaptation model* (3rd ed.). Upper Saddle River, NJ: Pearson.

Roy, C., Sr., & Andrews, H. A. (1999). *The Roy adaptation model* (2nd ed.). Stamford, CT: Appleton & Lange.

Sakraida, T. J. (2010). The health promotion model. In A. M. Tomey & M. R. Alligood (Eds.), *Nursing theorists and their work* (7th ed., pp. 434–453). St. Louis, MO: Mosby.

Sakraida, T. J. (2014). The health promotion model. In A. M. Tomey & M. R. Alligood (Eds.), *Nursing theorists and their work* (8th ed., pp. 396–416). St. Louis, MO: Mosby.

Schumacher, K. L., & Meleis, A. I. (1994). Transitions: A central concept in nursing. *Image: Journal of Nursing Scholarship, 26*(2), 119–127.

Selye, H. (1950). Stress and the general adaptation syndrome. *British Medical Journal, 4667,* 1383–1392.

Selye, H. (1974). *The stress of life*. New York, NY: McGraw-Hill.

Sieloff, C. L. (2006). Imogene King: Interacting systems framework and middle range theory of goal attainment. In A. M. Tomey & M. R. Alligood (Eds.), *Nursing theorists and their work* (6th ed., pp. 297–317). St. Louis, MO: Mosby.

Swanson, K. M. (1991). Empirical development of a middle range theory of caring. *Nursing Research, 40*(3), 161–166.

Swanson, K. M. (1993). Nursing as informed caring for the well-being of others. *Image: The Journal of Nursing Scholarship, 25*(4), 352–357.

Swanson, K. M. (1999a). The effects of caring, measurement, and time on miscarriage impact and women's well-being in the first year subsequent to loss. *Nursing Research, 48*(6), 288–298.

Swanson, K. M. (1999b). What's known about caring in nursing: A literary meta-analysis. In A. S. Hinshaw, J. Shaver, & S. Freetham (Eds.), *Handbook of clinical nursing research* (pp. 31–60). Thousand Oaks, CA: Sage.

Taylor, S. G. (2006). Self-care deficit theory of nursing. In A. M. Tomey & M. R. Alligood (Eds.), *Nursing theorists and their work* (6th ed., pp. 267–296). St. Louis, MO: Mosby.

Tomey, A. M. (2006). Nursing theorists of historical significance. In A. M. Tomey & M. R. Alligood (Eds.), *Nursing theorists and their work* (6th ed., pp. 54–67). St. Louis, MO: Mosby.

Von Bertalanffy, L. (1968). *General systems theory: Foundations, development, applications*. New York, NY: George Braziller.

Watson, J. (1979). Nursing: The philosophy and science of caring. Boston, MA: Little, Brown.

Watson, J. (1985). *Nursing: Human science and human care: A theory of nursing*. Sudbury, MA: Jones and Bartlett.

Watson, J. (1989). Watson's philosophy and theory of human caring in nursing. In J. P. Riehl-Sisca (Ed.), *Conceptual model for nursing practice* (3rd ed., pp. 219–236). Norwalk, CT: Appleton & Lange.

Watson, J. (1996). Watson's philosophy and theory of human caring in nursing. In J. P. Riehl-Sisca (Ed.), *Conceptual models for nursing practice* (pp. 219–235). Norwalk, CT: Appleton & Lange.

Watson, J. (1997). The theory of human caring: Retrospective and prospective. *Nursing Science Quarterly, 10,* 49–52.

Watson, J. (2001). Jean Watson: Theory of human caring. In M. E. Parker (Ed.), *Nursing theories and nursing practice* (pp. 343–354). Philadelphia, PA: F. A. Davis.

Watson, J. (2008). *Nursing: The philosophy and science of caring* (Rev. ed.). Boulder, CO: University Press of Colorado.

Wojnar, D. M. (2010). Kristin M. Swanson: Theory of caring. In M. R. Alligood & A. M. Tomey (Eds.), *Nursing theorists and their work* (7th ed., pp. 741–752). Maryland Heights, MO: Mosby.

Young, A., Taylor, S. G., & McLaughlin-Renpenning, K. (2001). *Connections: Nursing research, theory, and practice*. St. Louis, MO: Mosby.

CHAPTER 3

Philosophy of Nursing

Mary W. Stewart

Learning Objectives

After completing this chapter, the student should be able to:

1. Identify various philosophical views of truth.
2. Differentiate between values and beliefs.
3. Discuss the process of value clarification.
4. Explain the major components of nursing philosophy.
5. Articulate the purpose for having a personal philosophy of nursing.
6. Begin the development of a personal philosophy of nursing.

What is truth? Where do our ideas about truth originate? Why does truth matter?

The four principal domains of nursing—person, environment, health, and nursing—are the building blocks for all philosophies of nursing. As you are learning about these ideas, you are also learning that many nurses develop nursing theories or models. Think about it ... nurses creating theory! Yet, who better to describe our profession than professional nurses? All right, so maybe you are not that excited about this reality. Still, you have to admit that the ability to articulate nursing values and beliefs to guide us in our understanding of professional nursing is impressive. More than impressive, nursing theory is necessary.

In this chapter, we look more closely at nursing philosophy and its significance to professional nursing. We study the difference between beliefs and values and investigate the importance of values clarification. Finally, we examine guidelines for creating a personal philosophy of nursing.

Key Terms and Concepts

» Paradigm
» Realism
» Idealism
» Values
» Values clarification

Philosophy

Though no single definition of *philosophy* is uncontroversial, philosophy is defined in the following ways by the *American Heritage Dictionary of the English Language* (2000):

- Love and pursuit of wisdom by intellectual means and moral self-discipline
- Investigation of the nature, causes, or principles of reality, knowledge, or values, based on logical reasoning rather than empirical methods
- A system of thought based on or involving such inquiry; for example, the philosophy of Hume
- The critical analysis of fundamental assumptions or beliefs
- The disciplines presented in university curriculums of science and the liberal arts, except medicine, law, and theology
- The discipline comprising logic, ethics, aesthetics, metaphysics, and epistemology
- A set of ideas or beliefs relating to a particular field or activity; an underlying theory; for example, an original philosophy of advertising
- A system of values by which one lives; for example, has an unusual philosophy of life

Examples of philosophies can be found in university catalogs, clinical agency manuals, and nursing school handbooks—and they are prolific on the Internet. Needless to say, people have strong values and beliefs about many topics. A written statement of philosophy is a good way to communicate to others what you see as truth.

Some people are anxious to prescribe their own system of values to others by implying what "should be." However, each person or group of persons is responsible for delineating their particular philosophy. At the same time, how the insider's philosophy fits with the outsider's view is also important, particularly in situations such as nursing. Because nursing is inextricably linked to society, those of us within the profession must consider how society defines the values and beliefs within nursing.

So, how do we please everyone all the time? The answer is simple: We don't. We do, however, consider our own values and beliefs, which are interdependent of society, as we convey our professional philosophy of nursing. Does the philosophy ever change? Absolutely. As society and individuals change, our philosophy of nursing changes to be congruent with new and renewed understanding. How did we ever get started on this journey? A brief look at the beginnings of philosophy can help answer that question.

Early Philosophy

As society and individuals change, our philosophy of nursing changes to be congruent with new and renewed understanding. In the beginning, the Greeks moved from seeking supernatural to natural explanations. One assumption by the early Greek philosophers was that "something" had always existed. They did not question how something could come from nothing. Rather, they wanted to know what the "something" was. The pre-Socratics took the first step toward science in that they abandoned mythological thought and sought reason to answer their questions.

Heraclitus, a pre-Socratic philosopher, is well known for his thesis, Everything Is in Flux. He moved from simply looking at "being" to "becoming." A popular analogy he used was that of a river, saying, "You cannot step into the same river twice, for different and again different waters flow." More emphasis was placed on the senses versus reasoning.

On the other hand, Parmenides, who followed Heraclitus, said these two things: (1) Nothing can change, and (2) our sensory perceptions are unreliable. He is called the first metaphysician, a "hard-core philosopher." Metaphysics is the study of reality as a whole, including beyond the natural senses. What is the nature of reality? The universe? He starts with what it means and then moves to how the world must ultimately be. He does not go with his sense or experience. Parmenides thought that everything in the world had always been and that there was no such thing as change. He did, of course, sense that things changed, but his reason told him otherwise. He believed that our senses give us incorrect information and that we can rely only on our reason for acquiring knowledge about the world. This is called rationalism.

Probably a name more familiar to us is Socrates (469–399 B.C.), famous for the "know thyself" philosophy that focused on man, not nature. Plato wrote about his teacher, "Socrates ... believed in the immortal soul—all natural phenomena are merely shadows of the eternal forms or ideas. The soul, which existed before the body, longs to return to the world of ideas." Plato was a rationalist—we know with our reason.

Aristotle (384–322 B.C.) followed Socrates and Plato. His father was a physician, apparently framing his own interest in the natural world. He is known for his contribution to logic. Aristotle believed that the highest degree of reality is what we perceive with our senses. Unlike Plato, Aristotle did not believe in forms as separate from the real objects! When an object has both form and matter, it is called a substance. Aristotle said happiness was man's goal and came through balance of the following: life of pleasure and enjoyment, life as a free and responsible citizen, and life as a thinker and philosopher.

During the Neoplatonism age in the third century, philosophy became known as the soul's vehicle to return to its intelligible roots. There was an extrarational approach to reach union with the One. Thinking was that truth, and certainty was not found in this world. This was a revival of the "other worldliness" thinking of Plato.

The birth of Christianity and Western philosophy came at the death of classicism. Augustine of Hippo (A.D. 354–430) became a Christian and was attracted to Neoplatonism, where existence is divine. In that period, evil was defined as an absence or incompleteness. Saint Thomas Aquinas (A.D. 1225–1274) is credited with bringing theology and philosophy together.

Throughout the centuries, from the Greeks to the present day, people have debated the same questions: What is man? What is God? How do God and man relate? How does man relate to man? One can become dizzy thinking about the possibilities. Humans have been asking questions for a very long time, and thankfully, that practice is not about to change. People have searched for truth and will continue to do so. Therefore, we should not strive to find absolute answers; rather, we should endeavor to be comfortable with the questioning. **Table 3-1** provides an overview of the perspectives of truth through the ages. From the pre-Socratics to the poststructuralists and postmodern thinkers, ways of knowing and finding truth have changed.

TABLE 3-1   Overview of the Perspectives of Truth Through the Ages

School of Thought	Meaning of Truth (Philosophers)
Classical philosophers	Truth corresponds with reality, and reality is achieved through our perceptions of the world in which we live.
	Truth could be found in the natural world—through our sensory experiences. (Heraclitus, Aristotle)
	Truth can be found in the natural world—through our rational intellect. (Parmenides, Plato)
	Truth is found when one knows self. (Socrates)
	Truth is not of this world. (Plotinus)
Theocratics	Truth comes through an understanding of God.
	Truth can be found through both the senses and the intellect. (St. Thomas Aquinas)
Empiricists	Truth is based on experience and relating to our experiences. (Bacon, Locke, Hume, Mill)
Rationalists	All things are knowable by man's deductive reasoning. (Descartes, Spinoza)
Idealists	Truth exists only in the mind. (Berkeley, Hegel, Kant)

Positivists	Truth is science and the facts that science discovers. (Comte, Mill, Spencer)
Early existentialists	Truth is found through man's faith in his existence as it relates to God. (Kierkegaard)
Pragmatists	Truth is relative and practical—if it works, then it is truth. (James, Peirce, Dewey)
Relativists	Truth is always dependent on the knower and the knower's context. (Kuhn, Laudan)
Phenomenologists	Truth is in human consciousness. (Husserl, Heidegger)
Existentialists	If truth can be found, it can only be found through man's search for self. (Sartre, Merleau-Ponty, Gadamer)
Poststructuralists/ Postmodernists	Truth (if there is truth) is not singular and is always historical. Truth can be found in the deconstruction of language. (Derrida) Truth is (evolves from) the outcomes of events. (Foucault) Truth is created through dialogue with a purpose of emancipatory action. (Habermas, Freire) Truth is unique to gender. (Feminists)

Now, back to the real world: What is the purpose for this dialogue in a text on professional nursing? One of the critical theorists, Habermas, would say, "Communication is the way to truth." We have this discussion because it leads us to truth. In this case, the dialogue leads us to truth about nursing. What we hold as truth does not come through mere reading, studying, or debating. The truth comes through dialogue. Let's continue.

Paradigms

How do you see the world? Whether you know it or not, you have an established worldview or **paradigm**. A paradigm is the lens through which you see the world. Paradigms are also philosophical foundations that support our approaches to research (Weaver & Olson, 2006). The continuum of **realism** and **idealism** explains bipolar paradigms (**Box 3-1**). Most people today would agree that "somewhere in the middle" of these dichotomies lies truth.

Our philosophies are established from a lifelong process of learning and show us how we find truth. In other words, a philosophy is our method of knowing. The experiences we have with ourselves, others, and the environment provide structure to our thinking. Ultimately, our philosophies are

BOX 3-1	THE CONTINUUM OF REALISM AND IDEALISM

Realism
- The world is static.
- Seeing is believing.
- The social world is a given.
- Reality is physical and independent.
- Logical thinking is superior.

Idealism
- The world is evolving.
- There is more than meets the eye.
- The social world is created.
- Reality is a conception perceived in the mind.
- Thinking is dynamic and constructive.

demonstrated in the outcomes of our day-to-day living. Nurses' values and beliefs about the profession come from observation and experience (Buresh & Gordon, 2000).

Your worldview of nursing began long before you enrolled in nursing school. As far as you can remember, think back on your understanding of nursing. What did you think you would do as a nurse? Did you know a nurse? Did you have an experience with a nurse? What images of the nurse did you see on television or in the movies? Since that time, your worldview of nursing has changed. What experiences in school have changed your perspective of nursing? Undoubtedly, how you see nursing now will differ from your worldview in a few years—or even a few months.

Beliefs

A chief goal in this chapter is to provide a starting point for writing a personal philosophy of nursing. To do that, we must have a discussion of beliefs and values. *Beliefs* indicate what we value, and according to Steele (1979), beliefs have a faith component. Rokeach (1973) identifies three categories of beliefs: existential, evaluative, and prescriptive/proscriptive beliefs. Existential beliefs can be shown to be true or false. An example is the belief that the sun will come up each morning. Evaluative beliefs describe beliefs that make a judgment about whether something is good or bad. The belief that social drinking is immoral is an evaluative belief. Prescriptive and proscriptive beliefs refer to what people should (prescriptive) or should not (proscriptive) do. An example of a prescriptive or desirable belief is that everyone should vote. An example of an undesirable or proscriptive belief is that people should not be dishonest. Beliefs demonstrate a personal confidence in the validity of a person, object, or idea.

How would you define *person*? Look at the following attributes given to a person: (1) the ability to think and conceptualize, (2) the capacity to interact with others, (3) the need for boundaries, and (4) the use of language (Doheny, Cook, & Stopper, 1997). Would you agree? What about Maslow's description of humanness in terms of a hierarchy of needs with self-actualization at the top? Another possibility is that persons are the major focus of nursing. Do you see humans as good or evil?

CRITICAL THINKING QUESTION∗

Where do you see yourself and your understanding of truth on the continuum of realism and idealism? ∗

Consider the second concept in nursing: *environment*. How do you define the internal (within the person) and external (outside the person) environments? Is it important that nurses look beyond the individual toward the surroundings and structures that influence quality of human life? If yes, then how do you see the relationship between the internal and external environments? Is one dimension more important than the other? How do they interact with each other? Martha Rogers, a grand theorist in nursing, described the environment as continuous with the person, no boundaries, in constant exchange of energy. Would you agree?

Health is the third domain of nursing to ponder. Is health the same as the absence of illness? Is health perception? A person who is living and surviving may be described as "healthy." Would you support that as a comprehensive definition of health? Doheny et al. (1997) referred to health in the following way:

> Health is dynamic and ever changing, not a stagnant state. Health can be measured only in relative terms. No one is absolutely healthy or ill. In addition, health applies to the total person, including progression toward the realization and fulfillment of one's potential as well as maintaining physical, psychosocial health. (p. 19)

Maybe that definition is sufficient, but probably not. All definitions—including yours—have limitations. Definitions merely give us a way to express our beliefs and may, as our beliefs do, evolve over time.

Finally, consider common beliefs about *nursing*. Clarke (2006) posed that question in "So What Exactly Is a Nurse?"—an article addressing the problematic nature of defining nursing. The American Nurses Association (ANA) provided a much used definition of nursing in 1980: "Nursing is the diagnosis and treatment of human responses to actual and potential health problems" (p. 9). Fifteen years later, the ANA (1995, p. 6) expanded its basic definition of nursing to acknowledge four fundamental aspects. According to this definition, professional nursing includes attention to the full range of human experiences and responses to health and illness without restriction to a problem-focused orientation, integration of objective data with an understanding of the subjective experience of the patient, application of scientific knowledge to the processes of diagnosis and treatment, and provision of a caring relationship that facilitates health and healing. In 2003, the ANA added two essential features to this list that reflect nursing's commitment to meeting the needs of society

CRITICAL THINKING QUESTION⁎

What are your beliefs about the major concepts in nursing—person, environment, health, nursing?⁎

amid constant changes in the healthcare environment. These additional features are the advancement of nursing knowledge through scholarly inquiry and the influence on social and public policy for the promotion of social justice (p. 5).

The definition of nursing has been only slightly modified since the 2003 revision: "Nursing is the protection, promotion, and optimization of health and abilities, prevention of illness and injury, alleviation of suffering through the diagnosis and treatment of human response, and advocacy in the care of individuals, families, communities, and populations" (ANA, 2010, p. 10) with the newest revision (2015) specifically including the concept of facilitation of healing and adding groups to the list of recipients of nursing care. Four essential characteristics of nursing identified from the definition are "human responses or phenomena, theory application, nursing actions or interventions, and outcomes" (ANA, 2010, p. 10).

How would you define nursing? Understanding our beliefs and articulating them in definitions are beginning steps for developing a personal philosophy. Definitions tell us what things are. Our philosophy tells us how things are. One other piece must be addressed before we begin writing our personal philosophy: the topic of values.

Values

Values refer to what the normative standard should be, not necessarily to how things actually are. Values are the principles and ideals that give meaning and direction to our social, personal, and professional lives. Steele (1979) defines *value* as "an affective disposition towards a person, object, or idea" (p. 1). The values of nursing have been articulated by groups such as the ANA in the *Code of Ethics* (2001) and the American Association of Colleges of Nursing's (AACN) (2008) essentials for baccalaureate nursing education. The AACN essentials document calls for integration of professional nursing values in baccalaureate education; they are altruism, autonomy, human dignity, integrity, and social justice. Ways of teaching these values have been addressed in recent literature (Fahrenwald, 2003).

Nursing values have been identified as the fundamentals that guide our standards, influence practice decisions, and provide the framework used for evaluation (Kenny, 2002). Nevertheless, nursing has been criticized as not clearly articulating what our values are (Kenny, 2002). If nursing is to engage in the move to "interprofessional working," which is beyond uniprofessional and multiprofessional relationships, we have to define our values clearly. Interprofessional working validates what others provide in health care, and the relationships depend on mutual input and collaboration. Values in nursing need to be clearly articulated so that they can be discussed in the context of interprofessional partnership. We can then work together across traditional boundaries for the good of patients. Nursing offers something to health care that no one else does, but that *something* must first be clear to those of us in nursing. "It is not enough just to argue that caring is never value-free, and that values are a fundamental aspect of nursing. What is required is greater precision and clarity so that values can be identified by those within the profession and articulated beyond it" (Kenny, 2002, p. 66).

Statements such as those by the ANA and the AACN mentioned earlier are a step in the right direction. Others have identified nursing values using different language. Antrobus (1997) sees nursing values as humanistic and included (1) a nurturing response to someone in need, (2) a view of the whole individual, (3) an emphasis on the individual's perspective, (4) concentration on developing human potential, (5) an aim of well-being, and (6) maintenance of the nurse–patient relationship at the heart of the helping situation. Nursing values have also been listed as caregiving, accountability, integrity, trust, freedom, safety, and knowledge (Weis & Schank, 2000).

Rokeach (1973) makes the following assertions about values:

- Each person has a few.
- All humans possess the same values.
- People organize values into systems.
- Values are developed in response to culture, society, and personality.
- Behaviors are manifestations or consequences of values.

The process of valuing involves three steps: (1) choosing values, (2) prizing values, and (3) acting on values (Chitty, 2001). To choose a value is an intellectual stage in which a person selects a value from identified alternatives. Second, prizing values involves the emotional or affective dimension of valuing. When we "feel" a certain way about our values, it is because we have reached this second step. Finally, we have to act on our intellectual choice and emotion. This third step includes behavior or action that demonstrates our value. Ideally, a genuine value is evidenced by consistent behavior.

Steele (1979) distinguished between intrinsic and extrinsic values. An intrinsic value is required for living (e.g., food and water), whereas an extrinsic value is not required for living and is originated external to the person. According to Simon and Clark (1975), the following criteria must be met in acquiring values:

- Must be freely chosen
- Must be selected from a list of alternatives
- Must have thoughtful consideration of each of the outcomes of the alternatives
- Must be prized and cherished
- Must involve a willingness to make values known to others
- Must precipitate action
- Must be integrated into lifestyle

Value acquisition refers to when a new value is assumed, and *value abandonment* is when a value is relinquished. *Value redistribution* occurs when society changes views about a particular value. Values are more dynamic than attitude because values include motivation as well as cognitive, affective, and behavioral components. Therefore, people have fewer values than attitudes (feelings or dispositions toward a person, object, or idea). In the end, values determine our choices.

According to Steele (1979), values can compete with each other on our "hierarchy of values." We typically have values that we hold about education, politics, gender, society, occupations, culture, religion, and so on. The values that are higher in the hierarchy receive more time, energy, resources, and attention. For change to occur there must be conflict among the value system. For example, if a patient values both freedom from pain and long life but is diagnosed with bone cancer, a conflict in values will occur. If professional responsibilities and religious beliefs conflict, the solution is not as simple as "right versus wrong." Rather, it is the choice between two goods. For example, suppose you have strong religious views about abortion. During your rotation, you are assigned to care for someone who elects to have an abortion. As a nurse, you must balance the value of the patient's choice with your personal value about elective abortions. These decisions are not easy.

Dowds and Marcel (1998) conducted a study involving 40 female nursing students who were taking a psychology class. The students completed the World Hypothesis Scale, which provided 12 items, each with four possible explanations of an event. Each of the four explanations represented a distinct way of thinking. A list of definitions and descriptions of the different ways of thinking includes the following:

- *Contextualism*: Understanding is embedded in context; meaning is subjective and open to change and dependent on the moment in time and the person's perspective.
- *Formism*: Understanding events in relationship to their similarity to an ideal or objective standard comes from categorization (e.g., the classification of plants and animals in biology).
- *Mechanism*: Understanding is in terms of cause-and-effect relationships, the common approach used by modern medicine.
- *Organicism*: Understanding comes from patterns and relationships; must understand the whole to understand the parts (e.g., cannot look at a child's language development without looking at his or her overall development history).

The students ranked the explanations in terms of their preferences for understanding the event. Nursing students chose mechanistic thinking significantly more than all other ways of thinking and chose contextualistic thinking significantly less than the other worldviews. No other comparisons were significant among or between the four worldviews. In other words, the nursing students did not choose options that allowed for more than one right answer. They resisted the options that allowed for ambiguity. What this tells us in relationship to values is that we can say that we value human response and the whole individual, but do we really? Human situations are dynamic, fluid, and open for multiple options. Nursing claims to respond to these contextual needs, but do we?

Values Clarification

Clarifying our values is an eye-opening experience. The process of **values clarification** can occur in a group or individually and helps us understand who we are and what is most important to us. The outcome of values clarification is positive because the outcome is growth. If the process occurs in a group, there must be trust within the group. No one should be embarrassed or intimidated. Everyone is respected.

Values clarification exercises help people discern their individual values. A simple approach to begin the process is considering your responses to statements such as "Patients have a right to know everything that is in the medical record." What is your immediate reaction? How do you feel about the options available in this situation? Have you acted on these beliefs in the past? Another statement to consider is this: "Everyone should have equal access to health care—regardless of income." Ask yourself the same questions. Other exercises involve real or hypothetical clinical situations. For example, a 19-year-old male with human immunodeficiency virus is totally dependent. His parents remain at his bedside but do not say a word. Another example is a single mom who has recently been diagnosed with multiple sclerosis. What about a 70-year-old man who loses his wife of 42 years, only to remarry a woman who is soon diagnosed with dementia? Reflect. What questions do you have? Why are these people in these situations? Does that matter? What in the patient's life choices conflicts with your choices? Share this with your peers, your friends, and your teachers. In values clarification, one should consider the steps identified earlier as necessary for value acquisition: (1) choosing freely from among alternatives, (2) experiencing an emotional connection, and (3) demonstrating actions consistent with a stated value.

We act on values as the climax of the values clarification process. We are more aware, more empathetic to others, and have greater insight to ourselves and those around us for having gone through this process. Our words and actions are not so different, and we become more content with the individuals we are (i.e., self-actualization). Values clarification also allows us to be more open to accepting others' choice of values.

We must keep in mind that values vary from person to person. Returning to the concept of health, if we asked several people "What is health?" we would get different responses because it means different things to different people. Most likely, we would find that others do not place health as high in their hierarchy of values as we do. This helps explain why some people go to the physician for every little ailment, whereas others wait until the situation is critical. Maintaining a nonjudgmental attitude about the values of others is crucial to the nurse–patient relationship.

Do you believe there is more than one right answer to situations? How do you value the whole individual? What barriers prevent us from responding to the contextual needs of our patients?*

In health care, we need to clarify values for both the consumer and provider in society. Referring once again to health, we recognize that although the majority of our society states that health is a right, not a privilege, not everyone has health care. Is health positioned at the top of society's hierarchy of values? We also have to assess the individual's values for congruency with the societal values. As research gives us new options to consider, continual reassessment of values is essential. A questioning attitude is healthy and necessary.

As a profession, nursing is responsible for clarifying our values on a regular basis. Just as society places a value on health, society also determines the value of nursing in the provision of health. Additionally, nurses need to be involved in all levels where decisions based on values are made, particularly with ethical decisions. The values that nursing supports need to be communicated clearly to those making the policies that affect the health of our society.

Values clarification is done for the purpose of understanding self—to discover what is important and meaningful (Steele, 1979). Throughout life, the process continues as it gives direction to life. As you work through the course of values clarification, keep in mind that personal and professional values are not necessarily the same.

KEY COMPETENCY 3-1

Examples of Applicable *Nurse of the Future: Nursing Core Competencies*

Professionalism:

Knowledge (K7) Understands ethical principles, values, concepts, and decision making that apply to nursing and patient care

Skills (S7c) Identifies and responds to ethical concerns, issues, and dilemmas that affect nursing practice

Attitudes/Behaviors (A7c) Clarifies personal and professional values and recognizes their impact on decision making and professional behavior

Source: Massachusetts Department of Higher Education. (2010). *Nurse of the future: Nursing core competencies* (p. 14). Retrieved from http://www.mass.edu/currentinit /documents/ NursingCoreCompetencies.pdf

Developing a Personal Philosophy of Nursing

Before we begin writing our individual nursing philosophies, consider the following comments about philosophy. According to Doheny et al. (1997), philosophy is defined as "beliefs of a person or group of persons" and "reveals underlying values and attitudes regarding an area" (p. 259). In this concise definition, these authors mentioned the building blocks of philosophy that we have discussed thus far: attitudes, beliefs, and values. Another definition that is not as concise reads, "Nursing philosophy is a statement of foundational and universal assumptions, beliefs, and principles about the nature of knowledge and truth (epistemology) and about the nature of the entities—nursing practice and human healing processes—represented in the metaparadigm (ontology)" (Reed, 1999, p. 483). Finally, philosophy "looks at the nature of things and aims to provide the meaning of nursing phenomena" (Blais, Hayes, Kozier, & Erb, 2002, p. 90).

In *Nursing's Agenda for the Future*, the ANA (2002) identified the need for nurses to "believe, articulate, and demonstrate the value of nursing" (p. 15). To do that, each professional nurse is responsible for clearly articulating a personal philosophy of nursing. Suggestions for developing personal professional philosophies have been presented in the literature (Brown & Gillis, 1999).

The overall purpose of personal philosophy is to define how one finds truth. Because there are different ways of knowing, each person has a unique way of finding truth, in other words, identifying our individual philosophy. Therefore, your philosophy of nursing will be unique.

How do you start writing? A suggested guide for writing your personal philosophy of nursing is in **Box 3-2**. When defining nursing, you may refer to definitions by professional individuals or groups. You may also choose to write an original definition, which is certainly acceptable. A final challenge would be this: Once you have used words to describe your personal philosophy, try drawing it. This exercise can enlighten you to gaps in your understanding and further clarify the picture for you.

Writing a philosophy does not have to be a difficult exercise. In fact, you have one already—you just need to practice putting it on paper. Keep in mind that your philosophy will change over time. In addition, composing a nursing philosophy will help you see yourself as an active participant in the profession.

Consider the scene if no one in nursing had a philosophy. What would happen? Unfortunately, we would find ourselves doing tasks without considering

CRITICAL THINKING QUESTIONS ✳

Do I believe in health care for everyone? Does health care for everyone have value to me as a person? Does it have value to me as a nurse? What value does universal health care have to my patients? ✳

BOX 3-2 GUIDE FOR WRITING A PERSONAL PHILOSOPHY OF NURSING

1. Introduction
   a. Who are you?
   b. Where do you practice nursing?
2. Define nursing.
   a. What is nursing?
   b. Why does nursing exist?
   c. Why do you practice nursing?
3. What are your assumptions or underlying beliefs about:
   a. Nurses?
   b. Patients?
   c. Other healthcare providers?
   d. Communities?
4. Define the major domains of nursing and provide examples:
   a. Person
   b. Health
   c. Environment
5. Summary
   a. How are the domains connected?
   b. What is your vision of nursing for the future?
   c. What are the challenges that you will face as a nurse?
   d. What are your goals for professional development?

How does my personal philosophy fit with the context of nursing? Does it fit? What areas, if any, need assessing? ✳

the rationale and performing routines in the absence of purpose. Most likely, we would find ourselves devalued by our patients and fellow care providers.

Although our individual philosophies vary, there are similarities that link us in our universal philosophy as a profession. As a whole, we are kept on track by continually evaluating our attitudes, beliefs, and values. We can evaluate our efforts by reflecting on our philosophies. In the process of personal and professional reflection, we are challenged to reach global relevancy and to begin the development of a global nursing philosophy (Henry, 1998).

KEY COMPETENCY 3-2

Examples of Applicable *Nurse of the Future: Nursing Core Competencies*

Professionalism:

Knowledge (K8A) Understands responsibilities inherent in being a member of the nursing profession

Skills (S8a) Understands the history and philosophy of the nursing profession

Attitudes/Behaviors (A8b) Values and upholds altruistic and humanistic principles

Source: Massachusetts Department of Higher Education. (2010). *Nurse of the future: Nursing core competencies.* (p. 15). Retrieved from http://www.mass.edu/currentinit /documents/ NursingCoreCompetencies.pdf

Conclusion

In this chapter, we have discussed one of the most ambiguous concepts in professional disciplines—nursing philosophy. The history of philosophy helps us to see that asking questions about humans, environment, health, and nursing is a continual process that leads to a better understanding of truth in our profession. Our own values and beliefs must be clarified so that we can authentically respond to the healthcare needs of our patients and to society as a whole. All along the way, our philosophies are changing. Therefore, we must constantly question the values of our profession, our society, and ourselves—aiming to better the health of all people worldwide.

Hegel, an early philosopher, said, "History is the spirit seeking freedom." On this path of searching for truth, we ask the same question, but in different contexts and with distinct experiences. The answers for one person do not provide the same satisfaction for another person. Through our individual and collective searching, we become *truth knowers*. Habermas, the supporter of dialogue, would suggest that the journey does not end with communication and questioning alone. When truth is revealed, oppressive forces are acknowledged, and the truth knowers are then responsible to move to action. Through that action comes a change in the social structure and the hope of rightness in the world.

Classroom Activity 1

Take about 15 minutes after the discussion related to developing a philosophy of nursing to begin answering the questions in Box 3-2. Jot down answers to the questions in Box 3-2. Ask questions as necessary while still in the classroom. This simple activity will make it easier when writing a personal philosophy of nursing.

Classroom Activity 2

After thinking about your answers to the questions in Box 3-2 related to the metaparadigm concepts (person, health, environment, and nursing), draw each of these concepts as you define them on a separate piece of paper. Save your drawings, and think about them and refine them as you develop your philosophy of nursing. This activity works best if you use colored pencils, crayons, or markers. An example is presented in **Figure 3-1**.

Figure 3-1   Drawing of the concept of person

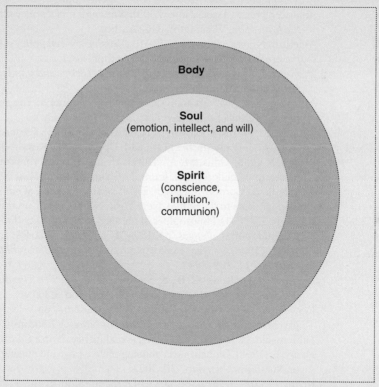

Body

Soul
(emotion, intellect, and will)

Spirit
(conscience,
intuition,
communion)

Source: Masters, K. (2006). *Drawing of concept of person*. Unpublished classroom exercise, as adapted from Nee, W. (1968). *The spiritual man*. New York, NY: Christian Fellowship Publishers.

References

American Association of Colleges of Nursing. (2008). *The essentials of baccalaureate education for professional nursing practice.* Washington, DC: Author.

American Heritage dictionary of the English language (4th ed.). (2000). Boston, MA: Houghton Mifflin.

American Nurses Association. (1980). *Nursing: A social policy statement.* Washington, DC: Author.

American Nurses Association. (1995). *Nursing's social policy statement.* Washington, DC: Author.

American Nurses Association. (2001). *Code of ethics for nurses with interpretive statements.* Washington, DC: Author.

American Nurses Association. (2002, April). *Nursing's agenda for the future: A call to the nation.* Retrieved from http://infoassist.panpha.org/docushare/dsweb/Get/Document-1884/PP-2002-APR-Nsgagenda.pdf

American Nurses Association. (2003). *Nursing's social policy statement: The essence of the profession.* Washington, DC: Author.

American Nurses Association. (2010). *Nursing's social policy statement: The essence of the profession.* Silver Spring, MD: Author.

American Nurses Association. (2015). *Nursing: Scope and standards of practice* (3rd ed.). Silver Spring, MD: Author.

Antrobus, S. (1997). An analysis of nursing in context: The effects of current health policy. *Journal of Advanced Nursing, 45,* 447–453.

Blais, K. K., Hayes, J. S., Kozier, B., & Erb, G. (2002). *Professional nursing practice: Concepts and perspectives* (4th ed.). Upper Saddle River, NJ: Prentice Hall.

Brown, S. C., & Gillis, M. A. (1999). Using reflective thinking to develop personal professional philosophies. *Journal of Nursing Education, 38,* 171–176.

Buresh, B., & Gordon, S. (2000). *From silence to voice: What nurses know and must communicate to the public.* New York, NY: Cornell University Press.

Chitty, K. K. (2001). Philosophies of nursing. In K. K. Chitty (Ed.), *Professional nursing: Concepts and challenges* (pp. 199–217). Philadelphia, PA: Saunders.

Clarke, L. (2006). So what exactly is a nurse? *Journal of Psychiatric and Mental Health Nursing, 13,* 388–394.

Doheny, M. O., Cook, C. B., & Stopper, M. C. (1997). *The discipline of nursing: An introduction* (4th ed.). Stamford, CT: Appleton & Lange.

Dowds, B. N., & Marcel, B. B. (1998). Students' philosophical assumptions and psychology in the classroom. *Journal of Nursing Education, 37,* 219–222.

Fahrenwald, N. L. (2003). Teaching social justice. *Nurse Educator, 28,* 222–226.

Henry, B. (1998). Globalization, nursing philosophy, and nursing science. *Image: Journal of Nursing Scholarship, 30,* 302.

Kenny, G. (2002). The importance of nursing values in interprofessional collaboration. *British Journal of Nursing, 11*(1), 65–68.

Massachusetts Department of Higher Education. (2010). *Nurse of the future: Nursing core competencies.* Retrieved from http://www.mass.edu/currentinit/documents/NursingCoreCompetencies.pdf

Masters, K. (2006). *Drawing of concept of person.* Unpublished classroom exercise.

Nee, W. (1968). *The spiritual man.* New York, NY: Christian Fellowship Publishers.

Reed, P. G. (1999). A treatise on nursing knowledge development for the 21st century: Beyond postmodernism. In E. C. Polifroni & M. Welch (Eds.), *Perspectives on philosophy of science in nursing* (pp. 478–490). Philadelphia, PA: Lippincott.

Rokeach, M. (1973). *The nature of human values.* New York, NY: Free Press.

Simon, S. B., & Clark, J. (1975). *Beginning values clarification: A guidebook for the use of values clarification in the classroom.* San Diego, CA: Pennant Press.

Steele, S. (1979). *Values clarification in nursing.* New York, NY: Appleton-Century-Crofts.

Weaver, K., & Olson, J. K. (2006). Understanding paradigms used for nursing research. *Journal of Advanced Nursing, 53*, 459–469.

Weis, D., & Schank, M. J. (2000). An instrument to measure professional nursing values. *Journal of Nursing Scholarship, 32*, 201–204.

CHAPTER 4

Foundations of Ethical Nursing Practice

Janie B. Butts and Karen L. Rich

Learning Objectives

After completing this chapter, the student should be able to:

1. Discuss the meaning of key terms associated with ethical nursing practice.
2. Compare and contrast ethical theories and approaches that might be used in nursing practice.
3. Discuss each of the popular bioethical principles as they relate to nursing practice: autonomy, beneficence, nonmaleficence, and justice.
4. Justify the importance of the *Code of Ethics for Nurses with Interpretive Statements* for professional nursing practice.
5. Explain how nurses can identify and analyze dilemmas in nursing practice.

Scientific and technological advances, economic realities, pluralistic worldviews, and global communication make it impossible for nurses to ignore important ethical issues in the world community, their individual lives, and their work. As controversial and sensitive ethical issues continue to challenge nurses and other healthcare professionals, many professionals have begun to develop an appreciation for personal philosophies of ethics and the diverse viewpoints of others.

Often ethical directives are not clearly evident, which leads some people to argue that ethics can be based merely on personal opinions. However, if nurses are to enter into the global dialogue about ethics, they must do more than practice ethics based simply on their personal opinions, their intuition, or the unexamined beliefs proposed by other people. It is important for nurses to have a basic understanding of the various concepts, theories, approaches, and principles used in ethics throughout history and to identify and analyze ethical issues and dilemmas relevant to nurses in this century. Mature ethical sensitivities are critical to professional nursing practice.

Key Terms and Concepts

- » Ethics
- » Morals
- » Bioethics
- » Nursing ethics
- » Moral reasoning
- » Values
- » Wholeness of character
- » Integrity
- » Basic dignity
- » Personal dignity
- » Virtues
- » Deontology
- » Utilitarianism
- » Ethic of care
- » Ethical principlism
- » Autonomy

Note: Fourth edition chapter revised by Janie B. Butts.

Ethics

Ethics, a branch of philosophy, means different things to different people. When the term is narrowly defined according to its original use, ethics is the study of ideal human behavior and ideal ways of being. The approaches to ethics and the meanings of ethically related concepts have varied over time among philosophers and ethicists. As a philosophical discipline of study, ethics is a systematic approach to understanding, analyzing, and distinguishing matters of right and wrong, good and bad, and admirable and deplorable as they exist along a continuum and as they relate to the well-being of and the relationships among sentient beings. Ethical determinations are applied through the use of formal theories, approaches, and codes of conduct.

As contrasted with the term *ethics,* **morals** are specific beliefs, behaviors, and ways of being based on personal judgments derived from one's ethics. One's morals are judged to be good or bad through systematic ethical analysis. Because the word *ethics* is used when one might literally be referring to a situation of morals, the process-related conception of ethics is sometimes overlooked today. People often use the word *ethics* when referring to a collection of actual beliefs and behaviors, thereby using the terms *ethics* and *morals* in essentially synonymous ways.

Bioethics

The terms *bioethics* and *healthcare ethics* are sometimes used interchangeably in the literature. **Bioethics** is a specific domain of ethics focused on moral issues in the field of health care. Callahan (1995) calls it "the intersection of ethics and the life sciences—but also an academic discipline" (p. 248). Bioethics evolved into a discipline all its own as a result of life-and-death moral dilemmas encountered by physicians, nurses, other healthcare professionals, patients, and families.

In his book *The Birth of Bioethics,* Albert Jonsen (1998) designated a span of 40 years, from 1947 to 1987, as the era when bioethics was evolving as a discipline. This era began with the Nuremberg Tribunal in 1947, when Nazi physicians were charged and convicted for the murderous and tortuous war crimes that these physicians had labeled as scientific experiments during the early 1940s. The 10 judgments in the final court ruling of the Nazi trial provided the basis for the worldwide Nuremberg Code of 1947. This code became a document to protect human subjects during research and experimentation.

The 1950s and 1960s were preliminary years before the actual birth of bioethics. A transformation was occurring during these years as technology advanced. In this era, a new ethic was emerging about life and extension of life through technology. The development of the polio vaccine, organ transplantation, life support, and many other advances occurred. Scientists and physicians were forced to ask the questions: "Who should live?" "Who should die?"

"Who should decide?" (Jonsen, 1998, p. 11). Many conferences and workshops during the 1960s and 1970s addressed issues surrounding life and death.

By 1970, the public, physicians, and researchers were referring to these phenomena as bioethics (Johnstone, 1999). Today, bioethics is a vast interdisciplinary venture that has engrossed the public's interest from the time of its conception. The aim of bioethicists today is to continue to search for answers to deep philosophical questions about life, death, and the significance of human beings and to help guide and control public policy.

Nursing Ethics

"It is the real-life, flesh-and-blood cases that raise fundamental ethical questions" (Fry & Veatch, 2000, p. 1) in nursing. **Nursing ethics** sometimes is viewed as a subcategory of the broader domain of bioethics, just as medical ethics is a subcategory of bioethics. However, controversy continues about whether nursing has unique moral problems in professional practice. Nursing ethics, similar to all healthcare ethics, usually begins with cases or problems in practice.

Some nursing ethicists distinguish issues of nursing ethics from broader bioethical issues in nursing practice and actually view nursing ethics as a separate field because of unique ethical problems in relationships between nurses and patients, families, physicians, and other professionals. The key criteria for distinguishing issues of nursing ethics from bioethics are that nurses are the primary agents in the scenario, and ethical issues are viewed from a nursing rather than a medical perspective.

Moral Reasoning

In general, reasoning involves using abstract thought processes to solve problems and to formulate plans (Angeles, 1992). More specifically, **moral reasoning** pertains to making decisions about how humans ought to be and act. Deliberations about moral reasoning go back to the days of the ancient Greeks when Aristotle, in *Nicomachean Ethics*, discussed the intellectual virtue of wisdom as being necessary for deliberation about what is good and advantageous in terms of moving toward worthy ends (Broadie, 2002).

Moral reasoning can be described by what Aristotle (Broadie, 2002) called the intellectual virtue of wisdom (*phronêsis*), also known as prudence. Virtue is an excellence of intellect or character. The virtue of wisdom is focused on the good achieved from being wise, that is, knowing how to act in a particular situation, practicing good deliberation, and having a disposition consistent with excellence of character (Broadie, 2002). Therefore, prudence involves more than having good intentions or meaning well. It includes knowing "what is what" but also transforming that knowledge into well-reasoned decisions.

Deliberation, judgment, and decision are the steps in transforming knowledge into action. Prudence becomes truth in action (Pieper, 1966).

More recently, in 1981, Lawrence Kohlberg reported his landmark research about moral reasoning based on 84 boys he had followed for more than 20 years. Kohlberg defined six stages ranging from immature to mature moral development. Kohlberg did not include any women in his research but expected that his six-stage scale could be used to measure moral development in both males and females. When the scale was applied to women, they seemed to score only at the third stage of the sequence, a stage in which Kohlberg described morality in terms of interpersonal relationships and helping others. Kohlberg viewed this third stage of development as deficient in terms of mature moral reasoning.

In light of Kohlberg's exclusion of females in his research and the negative implications of women being placed within the third stage of moral reasoning, Carol Gilligan raised the concern of gender bias. Gilligan, in turn, published an influential book in 1982, *In a Different Voice*, in which she argued that women's moral reasoning is different but is not deficient (Gilligan, 1993; Grimshaw, 1993; Thomas, 1993). The distinction usually made between the ethics of Kohlberg and Gilligan is that Kohlberg's is a male-oriented ethic of justice and Gilligan's is a more feminine ethic of care. The Kohlberg–Gilligan justice–care debate is relevant in feminist ethics.

Often the work of nurses does not involve independent moral reasoning and decision making with regard to the well-publicized issues in bioethics, such as withdrawing life support. Independent moral reasoning and decision making for nurses usually occurs more in the day-to-day care and relationships between nurses and their patients and between nurses and their coworkers. Nurses' moral reasoning, similar to the findings of Gilligan, often is based on caring and the needs of good interpersonal relationships. However, this does not negate what nurses can learn from studying Aristotle and his virtue of *phronêsis*. Nurses' moral reasoning needs to be deliberate and practically wise to facilitate patients' well-being.

Values in Nursing

In the *Code of Ethics for Nurses with Interpretive Statements*, the American Nurses Association (ANA, 2015a) emphasizes values as integral to moral reasoning in professional nursing. **Values** refer to a group's or individual's evaluative judgment about what is good or what makes something desirable. Values in nursing encompass appreciating what is important for both the profession and nurses personally, as well as what is important for patients.

In the code (discussed in more detail later in this chapter), the ANA (2015a) includes statements about **wholeness of character**, which pertains to knowing the values of the nursing profession and one's own authentic moral values, integrating these two belief systems, and expressing them appropriately.

Integrity is an important feature of wholeness of character. According to the code, maintaining integrity involves acting consistently with personal values and the values of the profession. In a healthcare system often burdened with constraints and self-serving groups and organizations, threats to integrity can be a serious pitfall for nurses. When nurses feel pressured to do things that conflict with their values, such as to falsify records, deceive patients, or accept verbal abuse from others, emotional and moral suffering can occur. A nurse's values must guide moral reasoning and actions, even when other people challenge those beliefs. When compromise is necessary, the compromise must not be such that it compromises personal or professional values.

Recognizing the dignity of oneself and each patient is another essential nursing value that should be given priority in moral reasoning. Pullman (1999) described two conceptions of dignity. One type, called **basic dignity**, is intrinsic, or inherent, and dwells within all humans, with all humans being ascribed this moral worth. The other type, called **personal dignity**, often mistakenly equated with autonomy, is an evaluative type. Judging others and describing behaviors as dignified or undignified are of an evaluative nature. Personal dignity is a socially constructed concept that fluctuates in value from community to community, as well as globally. Most often than not, personal dignity is highly valued.

Ethical Theories and Approaches

Within each ethical theory or approach, a normative framework serves as the foundational statements. Individuals who apply a particular theory or approach know what beliefs and values are right and wrong and what is and is not acceptable according to the particular ethical system. Normative ethical theories function as moral guides in answering the question: "What ought I do or not do?" Theory helps to provide guidance in moral thinking and justification for moral actions. Optimally, ethical theories and approaches should help people to discern commonplace morality and strengthen moral judgments "in the face of moral dilemmas" (Mappes & DeGrazia, 2001, p. 5).

Virtue Ethics

Since the time of Aristotle (384–322 B.C.), **virtues**, *arête* in Greek, have referred to excellences of intellect or character. Aristotle, the Greek philosopher, was a prominent thinker and writer of virtue ethics. Virtue ethics pertains to questions of "What sort of person must I be to achieve my life's purpose?" and "What makes one a good or excellent person?" rather than "What is right or good to do based on my duty or to achieve good consequences?" Virtues are intellectual and character traits or habits developed throughout one's life. The idea behind virtue ethics is when people are faced with complex moral dilemmas or situations, they will choose the right course of action because doing the right thing comes from a virtuous person's basic character. Aristotle believed moral character, personal effort, training, and practice must occur if a person is to develop. Examples of virtues include benevolence, compassion, courage, justice, generosity, truthfulness, wisdom, and patience.

Natural Law Theory

Saint Thomas Aquinas (1225–1274), who had a great influence on natural law theory as disseminated by Roman Catholic writers of that century, was himself influenced by Aristotle's work. Most versions of natural law theory today have their basis in Aquinas's basic philosophy. According to natural law theory, the rightness of actions is self-evident from the laws of nature, which in most cases is orchestrated by a lawgiver God. Morality is determined not by customs and human preferences but is commanded by the law of reason, which is implanted in nature and human intellect. Natural law ethicists believe behavior that is contrary to their views of the laws of nature is immoral. One example includes an artificial means of birth control.

Deontology

Deontology refers to actions that are duty based, not based on their rewards, happiness, or consequences. One of the most influential philosophers for the deontologic way of thinking was Immanuel Kant, an 18th-century German philosopher. In his classic work, *Groundwork of the Metaphysics of Morals*, Kant (1785/2003) defined a person as a rational human being with freedom, moral worth, and ideally having a good will, which means a person should act from a sense of duty. Because of their rationality, Kant believed, humans have the freedom to make moral judgments. Therefore, Kant argued that people ought to follow a universal framework of moral maxims, or rules, to guide right actions because it is only through performing dutiful actions that people have moral worth. Even when individuals do not want to act from duty, they are required to do so if they want to be ethical. Maxims apply to everyone universally and become the laws for guiding conduct. Moral actions should be ends in themselves, not the means to ends (Kant, 1785/2003). In fact, when people use others as a means to an end, such as deliberately using another person to reach one's personal goals, they are not treating other people with the dignity they deserve.

Kant distinguished between two types of duties: hypothetical imperatives and categorical imperatives. Hypothetical imperatives are duties or rules people ought to observe if certain ends are to be achieved. Hypothetical imperatives are sometimes called "if–then" imperatives, which are conditional: for instance, "If I want to pass my nursing course, then I should be diligent in my studies."

However, Kant believed moral actions must be based on unconditional reasoning. Where moral actions are concerned, duties and laws are absolute and universal. Kant called these moral maxims, or duties, categorical imperatives. When acting according to a categorical imperative, one should ask this question: "If I perform this action, would I will that it become a universal law?" No action can ever be judged as right if the action cannot have the potential to become a binding law for all people. For example, Kant's ethics would impose the categorical imperative that one can never tell a lie for any reason because if a person lies in any instance, the person cannot rationally wish permission to lie should universally become a law for everyone.

Utilitarianism

Contrasted with deontology, the ethical approach of **utilitarianism** is to promote the greatest good that is possible in situations (i.e., the greatest good for the greatest number). Jeremy Bentham (1789/1988) in his book *The Principles of Morals and Legislation*, promoted the theory of utilitarianism. Bentham believed each form of happiness is equal and each situation or action should be evaluated according to its production of happiness, good, or pleasure. John Stuart Mill (1863/2002) challenged Bentham's view in his book, *Utilitarianism*, and pointed out that experiences of pleasure and happiness do have different qualities and are not equal. For example, intellectual pleasures of humans have more value than physical pleasures of nonhuman animals.

Utilitarians place great emphasis on what is best for groups, not individual people. In doing so, the focus is on moral acts that produce the most good in terms of the most happiness, with the least amount of harm. By aiming for the most happiness, this theory focuses on good consequences, utility (usefulness), or good ends. Although happiness is the goal, utilitarianism is not based merely on subjective preferences or judgments of happiness. Commonsense ethical directives agreed upon by groups of people are usually applied.

Ethic of Care

The **ethic of care** has a history in feminist ethics, which has a focus in the moral experiences of women. In the ethic of care approach, personal relationships and relationship responsibilities are emphasized. Important concepts in this approach are compassion, empathy, sympathy, concern for others, and caring for others. Carol Gilligan with her study on gender differences in moral development (see the Moral Reasoning section earlier in this chapter) had a significant influence on the ethic of care approach.

People who uphold the ethic of care think in terms of particular situations and individual contexts, not in terms of impersonal universal rules

Think about the ethical theories and approaches in this section and the moral conflicts you have experienced in the past. Have you used one of these approaches to resolve a conflict? Which theory or approach have you used? ✳

and principles. In resolving moral conflicts and understanding a complex situation, a person must use critical thinking to inquire about relationships, circumstances, and the problem at hand. The situation must be brought to light with "caring, consideration, understanding, generosity, sympathy, helpfulness, and a willingness to assume responsibility" (Munson, 2004, p. 788).

Ethical Principlism

Ethical principlism, a popular approach to ethics in health care, involves using a set of ethical principles drawn from the common or widely shared conception of morality. The four most common principles used in bioethics are autonomy, beneficence, nonmaleficence, and justice. In 1979, Tom Beauchamp and James Childress published the first edition of *Principles of Biomedical Ethics*, which featured these four principles. Currently, the book is in its seventh edition, and the four principles have become an essential foundation for analyzing and resolving bioethical problems.

These principles, which are closely associated with rule-based ethics, provide a framework to support moral behavior and decision-making. However, the principles do not form a theory and do not provide a well-defined decision-making model. The framework of principlism provides a prima facie model. As a prima facie model, principles are applied based on rules and justifications for moral behavior. Often, more than one principle is relevant in ethical situations, and no conflict occurs. When relevant principles conflict in any situation, judgment must be used in weighing which principle should take precedence in guiding actions.

Autonomy

The word *autonomy* is a derivative of "the Greek *autos* ('self') and *nomos* ('rule, governance, or law')" (Beauchamp & Childress, 2009, p. 99). **Autonomy,** then, involves one's ability to self-rule and to generate personal decisions independently. Some people argue that autonomy has a top priority among the four principles, but there is no general consensus about this issue. Many people argue for a different principle, such as beneficence, to take priority. Ideally, when using a framework of principlism, no one principle should automatically be assumed to rule supreme.

The principle of autonomy sometimes refers to respect for autonomy (Beauchamp & Childress, 2012). In the domain of health care, respect for a patient's autonomy includes situations such as (1) obtaining informed consent for treatment, (2) facilitating patient choice regarding treatment options, (3) accepting patients' refusal of treatment, (4) disclosing medical information, diagnoses, and treatment options to patients, and (5) maintaining confidentiality. It is important to note that a patient's right to respect for autonomy is not unqualified. In cases of endangering or harming others, for example, through communicable diseases or acts of violence, people lose their basic rights to self-determination.

Beneficence

The principle of **beneficence** consists of deeds of "mercy, kindness, and charity" (Beauchamp & Childress, 2001, p. 166). Beneficence in nursing implies nurses' actions should benefit patients and facilitate their well-being. Beneficent nursing actions include obvious interventions such as lifting side rails on the patient's bed to prevent falls. More subtle actions also might be considered to be beneficent and kind actions, such as taking time to make phone calls for a frail, older patient who is unable to do so herself.

Occasionally, nurses can experience ethical conflicts when confronted with having to make a choice between respecting a patient's right to self-determination (autonomy) and the principle of beneficence. Nurses might decide to act in ways they believe are for a patient's "own good" rather than allowing patients to exercise their autonomy. The deliberate overriding of a patient's autonomy in this way is called **paternalism**. An example of a paternalistic action is for a nurse to decide a patient must try to ambulate in the hall, even though the patient moans and complains of being too tired from his morning whirlpool treatment. In that case, the nurse is aware that the patient wants to wait until a later time but insists otherwise. Nurses must weigh carefully the value of paternalistic actions and determine whether they are truly in the patient's best interest. Justified paternalism often involves matters of patient safety.

Nonmaleficence

Nonmaleficence, the injunction to "do no harm," is often paired with beneficence, but a difference exists between the two principles. Beneficence requires taking action to benefit others, whereas nonmaleficence involves refraining from actions that might harm others. Nonmaleficence has a wide scope of implications in health care, which includes most notably avoiding negligent care, as well as making decisions regarding withholding or withdrawing treatment and regarding the provision of extraordinary or heroic treatment.

Justice

The fourth major principle, **justice**, is a principle in healthcare ethics, a virtue, and the foundation of a duty-based ethical framework of moral reasoning. In other words, the concept of justice is quite broad in the field of ethics. Justice refers to the fair distribution of benefits and burdens. The justice bioethical principle most often refers to the allocation of scarce healthcare resources. Most of the time, difficult resource allocation decisions derive from attempts to answer questions regarding who has a right to health care, who will pay for healthcare costs, and what is fair.

KEY COMPETENCY 4-1

Examples of Applicable *Nurse of the Future: Nursing Core Competencies*

Professionalism:

Attitudes/Behaviors (A7a) Values the application of ethical principles in daily practice

Source: Massachusetts Department of Higher Education. (2010). *Nurse of the future: Nursing core competencies* (p. 14). Retrieved from http://www.mass.edu/currentinit /documents/NursingCoreCompetencies.pdf

Professional Ethics and Codes

Professional nursing education began in the 1800s in England at Florence Nightingale's school with a focus on profession-shaping ethical precepts and values. By the end of the 1800s, modern nursing had been established, and ethics was becoming a discussion topic in nursing. The Nightingale Pledge of 1893 was written under the leadership of a Detroit nursing school principal, Lystra Gretter, to establish nursing as an art and a science. Six years later, in 1899, the International Council of Nurses (ICN) established its own organization and was later a pioneer in developing a code of ethics for nurses.

At the turn of the 20th century, Isabel Hampton Robb, an American nurse leader, wrote the first book on nursing ethics, titled *Nursing Ethics: For Hospital and Private Use* (1900/1916). In Robb's book, the titles of the chapters were descriptive of the times and moral milieu, such as the chapters titled "The Probationer," "Uniform," "Night-Duty," and "The Care of the Patient," which addressed nurse–physician, nurse–nurse, and nurse–public relationships. The emphasis in the code was initially on physicians because male physicians usually trained nurses in the Nightingale era. Nurses' technical training and obedience to physicians remained at the forefront of nursing responsibilities into the 1960s. For example, the ICN's *Code of Ethics for Nurses* reflected technical training and obedience to physicians as late as 1965. By 1973, the ICN code shifted from a focus on obedience to physicians to a focus on patient needs, where it remains to this day.

Although the code is a nonnegotiable guide for nurses, no code can provide absolute or complete rules free of conflict and ambiguity. Because codes are unable to provide exact directives for ethical decision-making and action in all situations, some ethicists believe virtue ethics provides a better approach to ethics because the emphasis is on an agent's character rather than on rules, principles, and laws (Beauchamp & Childress, 2009). Proponents of virtue ethics consider that if a nurse's character is not virtuous, the nurse cannot be depended on to act in good or moral ways, even with a professional code as a guide. Professional codes do serve a useful purpose in providing direction to healthcare professionals. Ultimately, one must remember that codes do not eliminate moral dilemmas and are of no use without professionals' motivation to act morally.

ANA's *Code of Ethics for Nurses*

In 1926, the *American Journal of Nursing* (*AJN*) published "A Suggested Code" by the ANA, but the code was never adopted. In 1940, *AJN* published "A Tentative Code," but again it was never adopted (Davis, Fowler, & Aroskar, 2010). The ANA adopted its first official code in 1950. Three more code revisions occurred before the creation of the interpretive statements in 1976. The ANA added the word *ethics* to the publication title of the

KEY COMPETENCY 4-2

Examples of Applicable *Nurse of the Future: Nursing Core Competencies*

Professionalism:

Skills (S7a) Incorporates American Nurses Association's *Code of Ethics* into daily practice; (S7f) Applies a professional nursing code of ethics and professional guidelines to clinical practice

Attitudes/Behaviors (A7b) Values acting in accordance with codes of ethics and accepted standards of practice

Source: Massachusetts Department of Higher Education. (2010). *Nurse of the future: Nursing core competencies* (p. 14). Retrieved from http://www.mass.edu/currentinit /documents/NursingCoreCompetencies.pdf

2001 code. The seventh edition, published in 2015, is the latest revision. (See Appendix B for the provisions of the ANA code.)

Standards of professional performance require registered nurses to practice ethically and use the *Code of Ethics for Nurses with Interpretive Statements* (2015a) to guide practice (ANA, 2010, p. 47; 2015c). The ANA (2015a) outlined nine nonnegotiable provisions, each with interpretive statements for an illustration of detailed narratives for ethical decision making in clinical practice, education, research, administration, and self-development. Deontology and normative ethics largely serve as the basis for the code. Although they are detailed enough to guide decision making on a wide range of topics, the interpretive statements are not inclusive enough to predict every single ethical decision or action in the process of nurses carrying out their roles. A clear patient focus in the code obliges nurses to remain attentive and loyal to all patients in their care, but nurses must also be watchful for ethical issues and conflicts of interest that could lead to potentially negative decisions in care and relationships with patients. Politics in institutions and cost-cutting strategic plans are among other negative forces in today's environment.

The ANA (2015a) explores a variety of topics in the code (**Box 4-1**). The interpretive statements illustrate many moral situations. For example, Provision 6 illustrates wisdom, honesty, and courage as essential virtues to produce an image of a morally good nurse. When these virtues are habitually practiced, they promote the values of human dignity, well-being, respect, health, and independence. These values reflect what is important for the nurse personally and for patients.

BOX 4-1 **EXAMPLES OF SOME THEMES IN THE *CODE OF ETHICS FOR NURSES WITH INTERPRETIVE STATEMENTS***

- Respect for autonomy
- Relationships
- Patients' interests
- Collaboration
- Privacy
- Competent practice
- Accountability and delegation
- Self-preservation
- Environment and moral obligation
- Contributions to the nursing profession
- Human rights
- Articulation of professional codes by organizations

Source: Modified from the American Nurses Association. (2015a). *Code of ethics for nurses with interpretive statements.* Silver Spring, MD: Author.

Notably, the ANA (2015a) devoted Provision 5.1 to the subject of respect and duty to self and others, as accentuated in the first two sentences of that section: "Moral respect accords moral worth and dignity to all human beings regardless of their personal attributes or life situation. Such respect extends to oneself as well: the same duties that we owe to others we owe to ourselves" (p. 19). Another feature of the code is the emphasis on wholeness of character and preservation of self-integrity. Wholeness of character relates to nurses' professional relationships with patients and recognition of the values within the nursing profession, one's own authentic moral values, integration of these belief systems, and expressing them appropriately. Personal integrity involves nurses extending attention and care to their own requisite needs. Many times nurses who do not regard themselves as worthy of care cannot give comprehensive care to others. Recognizing the dignity of oneself and of each patient is essential to providing a morally enhanced level of care.

The ICN Code of Ethics for Nurses

The ICN adopted its first *Code of Ethics for Nurses* in 1953. The most recent revision of the ICN code occurred in 2012. Similar to the ANA code, the elements in the ICN code form a deontological, normative ethics framework for nurses to internalize before using it as a guide for nurses in practice, education, research, and leadership. The fundamental responsibilities of promoting health, preventing illness, restoring health, and alleviating suffering emanates from the role of nursing. The four principal elements contained within the ICN code involve standards related to nurses and people, practice, the profession, and coworkers. The ICN code (2012) is available in Appendix C of this title.

A Common Theme of the ANA and ICN Codes

A theme common to the ANA (2015a) and ICN (2012) codes is a focus on the importance of nurses delivering compassionate patient care aimed at alleviating suffering. The codes reflect this topic throughout both documents and with the patient as the central focus of nurses' work. The codes, which apply to all nurses in all settings and roles, are nonnegotiable ethical nursing standards with a focus on social values, people, relationships, and professional ideals. They share values such as respect, privacy, equality, and advocacy. Nurses should protect the moral space in which patients receive care and uphold the agreement with patients on an individual and collective basis. Protecting the moral space of patients necessitates nurses providing compassionate care and supporting the bioethical principles of autonomy, beneficence, nonmaleficence, and justice. Nursing care includes important responsibilities of promoting health and preventing illness, but the heart of nursing care has always involved caring for patients who are experiencing varying degrees of physical, psychological, and spiritual suffering.

Both codes illustrate the idea of nurses' moral self-respect. The ANA code's (2015a) self-respect language similarly is reflected in the ICN code (2012): "The nurse maintains a standard of personal health such that the ability to provide care is not compromised" (p. 3). Self-respect compares to one's personal regard. Personal regard involves nurses extending attention and care to their own requisite needs. Nurses who do not regard themselves as worthy of care usually cannot fully care for others.

Ethical Analysis and Decision Making in Nursing

Ethical issues and dilemmas are ever present in healthcare settings. Many times, ethical issues are so prevalent in practice that nurses do not even realize they are making minute-by-minute ethical decisions (Chambliss, 1996; Kelly, 2000). Whether or not nurses are cognizant of the ethical matters at the time when they make decisions, they use their critical thinking skills to respond to many of these everyday decisions. Answers to the questions "What is the right thing to do for my patient?" and "What sort of nurse do I want to be?" are important to professional nursing practice. All ethical decisions must derive from considered judgments based on the following variables:

- Personal values
- Professional values and competencies
- The ethical principles of autonomy, beneficence, nonmaleficence, and justice
- The justification for the decision based on the theory of deonotology, utilitarianism, or social justice, or an approach such as virtue ethics, ethic of care, or human rights

Ethical Dilemmas and Conflicts

An **ethical dilemma** is a situation in which an individual is compelled to make a choice between two actions that will affect the well-being of a sentient being, and both actions can be reasonably justified as being good, neither action is readily justifiable as good, or the goodness of the actions is uncertain. One action must be chosen, thereby generating a quandary for the person or group who must make the choice.

In addition to general, situational ethical dilemmas, dilemmas can arise from conflicts between nurses, other healthcare professionals, the healthcare organization, and the patient and family. A dilemma might involve nurses making a choice between staying to work an extra shift during a situation of inadequate staffing and going home to rest after a very tiring 8 hours of work. Nurses in this situation might believe that patients will not receive safe or good care if they do not stay to work the extra shift, but these nurses also might not provide safe care if they stay at the hospital because of already being tired from a particularly hard day of work.

Moral Suffering

Many times nurses experience disquieting feelings of anguish or uneasiness consistent with the term **moral suffering**, which nurses experience as they attempt to sort out their emotions and subsequently find themselves in situations that are morally unsatisfactory or when forces beyond their control prevent them from influencing or changing these perceived unsatisfactory moral situations. Suffering can occur because nurses believe that situations must be changed to bring well-being to themselves and others or to alleviate the suffering of themselves and others.

Moral suffering can arise, for example, from disagreements with institutional policy, such as a mandatory overtime or on-call policy that nurses believe does not allow adequate time for their psychological well-being. Nurses also might disagree with physicians' orders that the nurses believe are not in patients' best interest, or they might disagree with the way a family treats a patient or makes patient care decisions. These are but a few examples of the many types of nursing encounters that lead to moral suffering.

Another important, but often unacknowledged, source of moral suffering involves nurses freely choosing to act in ways that they, themselves, know is not morally commendable. An example of a difficult situation is when a nurse covers up a patient care error made by a valued nurse best friend. On the other hand, nurses might experience moral suffering when they act courageously by doing what they believe is morally right, despite anticipated disturbing consequences. Sometimes, doing the right thing or acting as a virtuous person would act is a difficult feat.

Some people view suffering as something to accept and to transform, if possible. Others react to situations with fear, bitterness, and anxiety. It is important to remember that wisdom and inner strength are often most increased during times of greatest difficulty.

Using a Team Approach

When patients are weakened by any debilitating illness or disease, whether end-of-life, acute, or chronic, families will react to the pain and suffering of their loved one. Decisions regarding treatment can become sensitive and challenging for everyone concerned. Members of the healthcare team might question the decision-making capacity of the patient or family. The patient's or family's decision might conflict with the doctor and healthcare team's opinions regarding treatment. Nurses who care for patients and interact with families sometimes find themselves caught in the middle of these conflicts.

When trying to navigate ethically laden situations, patients and families can experience extreme anguish and suffering. An end-of-life patient scenario is one example that particularly brings out unprocessed and visceral emotions in patients and families (**Box 4-2**).

Most problematic ethical decisions in health care are not unilateral decisions—not by physicians, nurses, or any other single person. Even so, nurses are an integral part of the larger team of decision makers. Although nurses often make ethical decisions independently, many ethical dilemmas require nurses to participate interdependently with others in the decision-making

---

BOX 4-2 TEAM APPROACH TO END-OF-LIFE SCENARIO

A patient, who is the mother, and her children have received disturbing news of the mother's diagnosis of metastatic breast cancer and its grave prognosis of only a short time left to live. While explaining the disease process to the patient and children, Dr. Lang and Nurse Ali together might increase the depth of information on the prognosis so the family can come to an informed agreement.

What if the doctor informed the patient or family members that, based on his experience and past evidence, the continuance of medical treatment would be nonbeneficial and medically futile?

Did you know....?

- The foremost ethical obligation of any doctor is to make every effort to discuss the meaning of the grave prognosis and medical futility intervention with the family and end-of-life patient and the anticipated events to come. See the chapter *Ethical Issues in Professional Nursing Practice* for the definition of medical futility.
- If a doctor believes treatment is medically futile, the American Medical Association's latest opinions of end-of-life care specify:
  - The doctor should not feel ethically obligated to provide treatment to prolong life if it is determined that medical treatment would not be beneficial; if this is the case, then
  - The focus of care should shift from one of treatment to interventions to promote comfort and closure (AMA, 1994, 1997).
- A discussion between the patient, her children, and the doctor and nurse team should take place to negotiate a joint satisfactory resolution.

What do you think?

What is your role as the nurse for the patient? How would you interact if the children confront you alone and insist on continuing some degree of treatment, but the doctor(s) had already agreed and documented that medical treatment, if continued, would be futile? Before you answer the questions, search the interpretive statements of Provisions 1.4 and 1.5 in ANA *Code of Ethics for Nurses with Interpretive Statements* (2015b).

process. In analyzing healthcare ethics and decision making, nurses participate in extensive dialogue with others through committees, clinical team conferences, and other channels. Nurses play a significant role in the ethical analysis and discussions of a larger team, usually an ethics consultation team or ethics committee.

The ethics committee usually consists of physicians, nurses who represent their patients, an on-staff chaplain, nurses who regularly participate on the consultative team, a social worker, administrative personnel, possibly a legal representative, a representative for the patient in question or surrogate decision maker, and others drafted by the team. The number and membership of the ethics team vary among organizations and specific cases. When ethical disputes arise among any members of a patient's healthcare team, including disputes with patients and families, nurses often are the ones who seek an ethics consultation. It is within the purview and ethical duty of nurses to seek help and advice from the ethics team if they encounter moral dilemmas or experience moral suffering because of the issues.

In healthcare settings, moral reasoning to resolve an ethical dilemma is often a case-based, or bottom-up, inductive, casuistry approach. This approach begins with relevant facts about a particular case and moves toward a resolution through a structured analysis. A practical case-based ethical analysis approach that is used commonly by nurses and other healthcare professionals is the Four Topics Method or, often called in jargon, the 4-Box Approach (Jonsen, Siegler, & Winslade, 2010, p. 8). The Four Topics Method, developed by Albert Jonsen, Mark Siegler, and William Winslade, was first published in 1982 in their book *Clinical Ethics: A Practical Approach to Ethical Decisions in Clinical Medicine*, which is in its seventh edition (2010).

This case-based approach facilitates critical thinking about the issues and problems of a particular situation and facilitates construction of the case through information gathering in a structured format. Each problematic ethical case undergoes analysis according to four major topics: medical indications, patient preferences, quality of life, and contextual features (Jonsen et al., 2010). Nurses and other healthcare professionals on the team gather information in an attempt to answer the questions in each of the four "boxes" or topical categories.

In the medical indications topical category, questions are addressed in the context of the principles of beneficence and nonmaleficence. The questions include:

- What is the patient's medical problem? history? diagnosis? prognosis?
- Is the problem acute? chronic? critical? emergent? reversible?
- What are the goals of treatment?
- What are the probabilities of success?
- What are the plans in case of therapeutic failure?
- In sum, how can this patient be benefited by medical and nursing care, and how can harm be avoided? (Jonsen et al., 2010, p. 8)

In the quality of life topical category, questions are addressed in the context of the principles of beneficence, nonmaleficence, and respect for autonomy. The questions include:

- What are the prospects, with or without treatment, for a return to normal life?
- What physical, mental, and social deficits is the patient likely to experience if treatment succeeds?
- Are there biases that might prejudice the provider's evaluation of the patient's quality of life?
- Is the patient's present or future condition such that his or her continued life might be judged undesirable?
- Is there any plan and rationale to forgo treatment?
- Are there plans for comfort and palliative care? (Jonsen et al., 2010, p. 8)

In the patient preferences topical category, questions are addressed in the context of respect for autonomy. The questions include:

- Is the patient mentally capable and legally competent? Is there evidence of incapacity?
- If competent, what is the patient stating about preferences for treatment?
- Has the patient been informed of benefits and risks, understood this information, and given consent?
- If incapacitated, who is the appropriate surrogate? Is the surrogate using appropriate standards for decision making?
- Has the patient expressed prior preferences, e.g., advance directives?
- Is the patient unwilling or unable to cooperate with medical treatment? If so, why?
- In sum, is the patient's right to choose being respected to the extent possible in ethics and law? (Jonsen et al., 2010, p. 8)

In the contextual features topical category, questions are addressed in the context of the principles of loyalty and fairness. The questions include:

- Are there family issues that might influence treatment decisions?
- Are there provider issues that might influence treatment decisions?
- Are there financial and economic factors?
- Are there religious and cultural factors?
- Are there limits on confidentiality?
- Are there problems of allocations of resources?
- How does the law affect treatment decisions?
- Is clinical research or teaching involved?
- Is there any conflict of interest on the part of the providers or the institution? (Jonsen et al., 2010, p. 8)

The Four Topics Method promotes a dialogue among the patient, family, and members of the healthcare ethics team. Each patient's case is unique and needs consideration as such, but the subject matter concerning the dilemma

KEY COMPETENCY 4-4

Examples of Applicable
*Nurse of the Future: Nursing
Core Competencies*

Professionalism:

Knowledge (K7) Understands
ethical principles, values,
concepts, and decision
making that apply to nursing
and patient care

Skills (S7b) Utilizes an
ethical decision-making
framework in clinical
situations

Source: Massachusetts Department of
Higher Education. (2010). *Nurse of the
future: Nursing core competencies* (p. 14).
Retrieved from http://www.mass.edu
/currentinit/documents/NursingCore
Competencies.pdf

involves common threads among cases, such as withdrawing or withholding treatment and right to life. Applicability of the four fundamental bioethical principles—autonomy, beneficence, nonmaleficence, and justice—needs consideration along with data generated by using the Four Topics Method in analyzing a patient's case. Each topic includes principles appropriate for each of the four topics. The additional principles of fairness and loyalty are included in the contextual features section.

Intense emotional conflicts between healthcare professionals and the patient and family can occur and hurt feelings can result. Nurses need to be sensitive and open to the needs of patients and families, particularly during these times. As information is transferred back and forth between the healthcare professionals and the patients and families, an attitude of respect is indispensable in keeping the lines of communication open. Nurses play an essential role in the decision-making process in bioethical cases because of their traditional roles as patient advocate, caregiver, and educator. Nurses must attempt to maximize the values and needs of patients and families. A key component in preserving patient autonomy, respect, and dignity is for the nurse to have all of the essential information necessary for wise and skillful decisions.

Conclusion

With any type of ethical matters in health care, a nurse must ask "What is good in terms of how one wants to be?" and "What is good in terms of what one ought to do?" Becoming ethically savvy does not just happen in nursing. Nurses must consciously cultivate ethical habits and use theoretical knowledge about how to navigate ethical dilemmas. Moral suffering cannot be eliminated from nursing practice, but the cultivation of wisdom and skill in decision making can help to alleviate some of its effects.

CASE STUDY 4-1 ▪ MS. CRANFORD

You are the student nurse caring for Ms. Cranford. She is a mentally competent woman, age 87, who has lived alone since her husband died 10 years ago. She presented to the ER with chest pain, feeling faint, a pulse of 48, and a blood pressure of 98/56. The doctor and the nurse team stabilized Ms. Cranford with medications and intravenous fluids and admitted her to the intensive care unit. The intensive care unit doctor and nurse later informed Ms. Cranford and her only son that she would need a heart pacemaker to regulate her heartbeat. After the doctor explained the procedure and risks involved, Ms. Cranford pondered the situation for a long while before discussing it with her son and doctor. Her medical history includes long-term adult-onset diabetes, chronic renal failure, and arterial insufficiency. She felt very tired and decided that she did not want the pacemaker. Once Ms. Cranford told her son her wishes, he was quite upset and apprehensive about her decision. The son met with the doctor to discuss the options. Together, they approached Ms. Cranford in an attempt to persuade her to change her mind, but she continued to refuse the recommended treatment. Ms. Cranford and her son argued. The doctor tried to explain to Ms. Cranford that the pacemaker was in her "best interest," and would involve minimal risks to her. She felt as if they were "ganging up" on her. Once the registered nurse became aware of the problem, you and the nurse decide to visit with Ms. Cranford and her son to assess and evaluate the ethical issues involved with her case.

Case Study Questions

Imagine that you are a nurse on the ethics committee consulted about Ms. Cranford's case. Answer the following questions:

1. What are the central ethical issues and questions in this case?

2. Which principles are in conflict in this case?

3. What did the physician mean by "best interest" for Ms. Cranford?

4. Use the Four Topics Method to discuss issues, to identify additional needed information, and to analyze this case. What are your recommendations on behalf of the ethics committee?

5. What is the role of the nurses caring for Ms. Cranford in resolving this situation with the ethics team, her other healthcare providers, Ms. Cranford, and her son?

References

American Medical Association. (1994, June). Opinion 2.035 - futile care. Retrieved from http://www.ama-assn.org/ama/pub/physician-resources/medical-ethics/code-medical-ethics/opinion2035.page

American Medical Association. (1997, June). Opinion 2.037 - medical futility in end-of-life care. Retrieved from http://www.ama-assn.org/ama/pub/physician-resources/medical-ethics/code-medical-ethics/opinion2037.page

American Nurses Association. (2010). *Nursing: Scope and standards of practice* (2nd ed.). Silver Spring, MD: Author.

American Nurses Association. (2015a). *Code of ethics for nurses with interpretive statements*. Silver Spring, MD: Author.

American Nurses Association. (2015b). *Code of ethics for nurses with interpretive statements*. Silver Spring, MD: Author. Read-only digital copy. Retrieved from http://www.nursingworld.org/MainMenuCategories/EthicsStandards/CodeofEthicsforNurses/Code-of-Ethics-For-Nurses.html

American Nurses Association. (2015c). *Nursing: Scope and standards of practice* (3rd ed.). Silver Spring, MD: Author.

Angeles, P. A. (1992). *The Harper Collins dictionary of philosophy* (2nd ed.). New York, NY: Harper Perennial.

Beauchamp, T. L., & Childress, J. F. (1979). *Principles of biomedical ethics*. New York, NY: Oxford University Press.

Beauchamp, T. L., & Childress, J. F. (2001). *Principles of biomedical ethics* (5th ed.). New York, NY: Oxford University Press.

Beauchamp, T. L., & Childress, J. F. (2009). *Principles of biomedical ethics* (6th ed.). New York, NY: Oxford University Press.

Beauchamp, T. L., & Childress, J. F. (2012). *Principles of biomedical ethics* (7th ed.). New York, NY: Oxford University Press.

Bentham, J. (1988). *The principles of morals and legislation*. Loughton, Essex, England: Prometheus. (Original work published 1789)

Broadie, S. (2002). Philosophical introduction. In S. Broadie & C. Rowe (Eds., C. Rowe Trans.), *Aristotle nicomachean ethics* (pp. 9–90). New York, NY: Oxford University Press.

Callahan, D. (1995). Bioethics. In W. T. Reich (Ed.), *Encyclopedia of bioethics:* Revised edition (Vol. 1, pp. 247–256). New York, NY: Simon & Schuster Macmillan.

Chambliss, D. F. (1996). *Beyond caring: Hospitals, nurses, and the social organization of ethics*. Chicago, IL: University of Chicago Press.

Davis, A. J., Fowler, M. D., & Aroskar, M. A. (2010). Ethical dilemmas and nursing practice (5th ed.). Boston, MA: Pearson.

Fry, S., & Veatch, R. M. (2000). *Case studies in nursing ethics* (2nd ed.). Sudbury, MA: Jones and Bartlett.

Gilligan, C. (1993). *In a different voice: Psychological theory and women's development*. Cambridge, MA: Harvard University Press.

Grimshaw, J. (1993). The idea of a female ethic. In P. Singer (Ed.), *A companion to ethics* (pp. 491–499). Oxford, England: Blackwell.

International Council of Nurses. (2012). *The ICN code of ethics for nurses*. Geneva, Switzerland: Author. Retrieved from http://www.icn.ch/images/stories/documents/about/icncode_english.pdf

Johnstone, M. J. (1999). *Bioethics: A nursing perspective* (3rd ed.). Sydney, Australia: Harcourt Saunders.

Jonsen, A. (1998). *The birth of bioethics*. New York, NY: Oxford University Press.

Jonsen, A. R., Siegler, M., & Winslade, W. J. (2010). *Clinical ethics: A practical approach to ethical decisions in clinical medicine* (7th ed.). New York, NY: McGraw-Hill.

Kant, I. (2003). *Groundwork of the metaphysics of morals*. New York, NY: Oxford University Press. (Original work published 1785)

Kelly, C. (2000). *Nurses' moral practice: Investing and discounting self*. Indianapolis, IN: Sigma Theta Tau International.

Kohlberg, L. (1981). *Essays on moral development: The philosophy of moral development* (Vol. 1). San Francisco, CA: Harper Row.

Mappes, T. A., & DeGrazia, D. (2001). *Biomedical ethics* (5th ed.). Boston, MA: McGraw-Hill.

Massachusetts Department of Higher Education. (2010). *Nurse of the future: Nursing core competencies*. Retrieved from http://www.mass.edu/currentinit/documents/NursingCoreCompetencies.pdf

Mill, J. S. (2002). *Utilitarianism*. (G. Sher, Trans.). Indianapolis, IN: Hackett Publishing. (Original work published 1863)

Munson, R. (2004). *Intervention and reflection: Basic issues in medical ethics* (7th ed.). Victoria, Australia: Thomson Wadsworth.

Pieper, J. (1966). *The four cardinal virtues*. Notre Dame, IN: University of Notre Dame Press.

Pullman, D. (1999). The ethics of autonomy and dignity in long-term care. *Canadian Journal on Aging, 18*(1), 26–46.

Robb, I. H. (1916). *Nursing ethics: For hospital and private use*. Cleveland, OH: E. C. Koeckert. (Original work published 1900)

Thomas, L. (1993). Morality and psychological development. In P. Singer (Ed.), *A companion to ethics* (pp. 464–475). Oxford, England: Blackwell.

CHAPTER 5

Social Context of Professional Nursing

Mary W. Stewart, Katherine Elizabeth Nugent, Rowena W. Elliott, and Kathleen Masters

Learning Objectives

After completing this chapter, the student should be able to:

1. Describe the social context of professional nursing.
2. Identify factors that influence the public's image of professional nursing.
3. Identify ways that nurses can promote an accurate image of professional nursing.
4. Discuss the gender gap in nursing.
5. Recognize connections between changing demographics and cultural competence.
6. Evaluate current barriers to health care in our society.
7. Discuss present trends in society that influence professional nursing.
8. Identify present trends associated with the profession of nursing.

When you hear the word *nurse*, what images, thoughts, perceptions, and assumptions come to mind? Ask yourself, "Why did I have those perceptions and assumptions about nurses?" The answer to your question reveals much about the social context of nursing or how society views nurses and the nursing profession. For many, the image that first comes into view is one of a white female who is dressed in a meticulously ironed white uniform with white hose, white shoes, and wearing a stiff white cap. For those of us in nursing, we recognize that this traditional American view of nursing is rarely seen in the real world of professional nursing. So, how do we communicate the true image of nursing in the 21st century?

In this chapter, we explore the social context of professional nursing and identify major influences that affect nursing in today's society. This quest for a deeper understanding of nursing challenges us to identify our

Key Terms and Concepts

» Stereotypes
» Cultural competence
» Access to care
» Incivility
» Violence
» Global aging
» Consumerism
» Complementary and alternative medicine
» Disaster preparedness
» Nursing shortage
» Nursing faculty shortage

individual responsibilities in educating our patients and the public about professional nursing as well as meeting our professional obligations to the public. The end result is not necessarily an immediate change in the picture that comes to mind when one says "nursing"; however, we might begin to see nursing and those of us committed to nursing in new, more accurate ways.

Nursing's Social Contract with Society

A mutually beneficial relationship exists between nursing and society. The profession of nursing grew out of a need within society and continues to evolve based on the needs of society. Because nursing has a responsibility to society, the interest of the profession must be perceived as serving the interests of society. Society provides the nursing profession with the authority to practice, grants the profession authority over functions, and grants autonomy over professional affairs. The profession is expected to regulate itself and act responsibly. This relationship is the essence of nursing's social contract with society (American Nurses Association [ANA], 2010, pp. 3, 5).

Foundational to nursing's social contract with society are some basic values. In brief, these values include that humans manifest an essential unity of mind, body, and spirit; human experience is contextually and culturally defined; health and illness are human experiences; and the relationship between the nurse and the patient occurs within the context of the values and beliefs of the patient and the nurse. In addition, public policy and the healthcare delivery system influence the health and well-being of society and professional nursing, and individual responsibility and interprofessional involvement are essential (ANA, 2010, pp. 6–7).

According to *Nursing's Social Policy Statement* (ANA, 2010, pp. 4–5), nursing is particularly active in relation to six key areas of health care that include the organization, delivery, and financing of quality health care; provision for the public's health though health promotion, disease prevention, and environmental measures; and expansion of nursing and healthcare knowledge (through research and evidence in practice) and application of technology. Also included are expansion of healthcare resources and health policy to enhance capacity for self-care; definitive planning for health policy and regulation; and duties under extreme conditions, which means that nurses weigh their duty to provide care with obligations to their own health during extreme emergencies.

Public Image of Nursing

The public values nursing. According to a Gallup poll in 2014, nurses received the top ranking for honesty and ethical standards (Riffkin, 2014). The honor of being the most trusted profession has been bestowed on the profession of nursing every year but one since 1999, when nursing was first added to the Gallup poll. The only year when nurses did not rank number one was in 2001 when firefighters took the top spot after the September 11th terrorist attacks. When asked to defend this nationwide trust of nurses, people often respond with anecdotal stories of personal experiences with nurses. Popular stories include those of relatives or friends who are nurses and positive experiences with nurses in a clinical setting. The fact that nurses serve society seems to have an automatically positive impact on society's value of nursing.

Although the trust is evident, there remains a gap between the public's perception of the nursing profession and the reality of nursing. For example, the general public might think that it requires only 2 years to become a registered nurse (RN), with the "training" consisting primarily of learning to administer medications, providing personal care, and sitting at the bedside. However, reality provides a stark revelation that nurses are educated at the baccalaureate, master's degree, and doctoral levels and work in areas of education, research, and independent clinical practice.

Nurses are aware of the gaps in society's knowledge of nursing. Hence, nurses should take the lead in making sure the public has an accurate picture of the vast knowledge and expertise that are present in the 3 million RNs in the United States (U.S. Department of Health and Human Services [USDHHS], 2010). So, where do we start? We must first begin with the realization that not all nurses are the same. As previously stated, many well-educated persons do not understand the various educational programs available to become an RN. Likewise, knowledge about the differences in preparation and responsibility of licensed practical nurses, RNs, and advanced practice nurses is lacking.

As you are preparing to be a professional nurse, ask yourself, "How do I clarify and communicate the significance of professional nursing?" First, become familiar with the scope of practice of professional nurses and understand the multifaceted roles for which you are being educated. Second, be able to identify the unique place that professional nurses have in the healthcare system. This comes by acquiring knowledge of the nursing profession and being aware of the roles, responsibilities, and contributions of other healthcare professionals. Most important, it is imperative you share your story of nursing. Although the public holds nurses in high regard, they know very little about what nurses actually do (Buresh & Gordon, 2000). Without articulating more clearly and loudly on our profession's behalf, we might be at a loss when trying to defend our place in the current healthcare system.

Suzanne Gordon, an award-winning journalist, has dedicated much of her career to telling the stories of nursing. Not a nurse herself, Gordon writes to empower nurses to find their voice and be heard. Gordon is committed to obtaining a first-hand account from nurses as they face the real challenges of being a nurse that include (1) inconvenient problems of improving patient safety (Gordon, Buchanan, & Bretherton, 2008), (2) the challenges of standing up for themselves, their patients, and the nursing profession (Gordon, 2010), and (3) the effect of cutting healthcare costs on patient care (Gordon, 2005), to name a few. If a journalist can commit to sharing "our" stories, that should provide a spark of motivation in us to share our experiences, triumphs, and defeats.

When nurses are asked about the nurse's reluctance to promote nursing effectively, the responses are riddled with excuses such as a lack of time, resources, and support from colleagues. Professional nurses work in very demanding, stressful, and taxing jobs. Frequently, we are so consumed with the responsibilities of our work that we fail to notice what we are actually getting accomplished. Additionally, we rarely take time to become fully aware of and celebrate what our nursing colleagues are doing within the profession. Professional nursing organizations exist to communicate and support these achievements. However, only a small percentage of RNs are actually members of their professional nursing associations.

Better insight into professional nursing must start with nurses at all levels of practice and education. Once we have obtained the necessary insight, we can provide a clear picture of the nursing profession to society. When these two actions are taken, the public image of nursing will be directly reflective of the reality of nursing. We want to maintain the positive impression the public now holds of nursing and sustain the earned trust, but nursing and the public deserve a great deal more than that. All of us should be convinced of the expertise that professional nursing offers: mastery of complicated technological skills; appreciation for the whole person; commitment to public health for all people; a keen knowledge of anatomy, physiology, pathophysiology, biochemistry, pharmacology, and other disciplines; the ability to think critically and connect the dots in today's ever-changing healthcare system; and proficiency in communication. The list continues.

Media's Influence

It is obvious that the media (television, radio, Internet) play a major role in how society views professional nursing. Historically, the nurse has been portrayed in the media in a variety of ways. First, the nurse appears as a young, seductive female whose principal qualification is the length of her slender legs and the amount of cleavage showing through her uniform. Needless to say, this nurse is usually depicted as one who is not educated and lacks common sense and intelligence. Another popular view of the nurse as portrayed by the media is an unattractive, overweight, and mean female. Her intelligence is not

---

KEY COMPETENCY 5-1

Examples of Applicable *Nurse of the Future: Nursing Core Competencies*

Professionalism:

Knowledge (K5b) Understands the culture of nursing and the health care system

Skills (S5b) Promotes and maintains a positive image of nursing

Source: Massachusetts Department of Higher Education. (2010). *Nurse of the future: Nursing core competencies* (p. 14). Retrieved from http://www.mass.edu/currentinit/documents/NursingCoreCompetencies.pdf

questioned, but her compassion for others is highly debatable. This nurse is shown as threatening and uncaring. Neither of these views is accurate, and probably no one would argue with this. At the same time, we continue to be perplexed when asked to define or describe the professional nurse.

In their book *From Silence to Voice: What Nurses Know and Must Communicate to the Public*, Buresh and Gordon (2006) state that "a profession's public status and credibility are enhanced by having its expertise acknowledged in the journalistic media" (p. 1). Buresh and Gordon also cite the study "Who Counts in News Coverage of Health Care," where the data show that many professional groups had a greater voice on health issues compared to nurses. Physicians were quoted the most in media, followed by government, business, education, public relations, and so forth. This is significant and shocking because nurses are the largest group of healthcare professionals, yet we are the most silent group. As nurses, we have been complacent about refuting the negative stereotypes portrayed in the media. Furthermore, we have been lax in articulating our expertise to the media.

Buresh and Gordon (2006) describe three communication challenges faced by the nursing profession that need to be addressed:

1. Not enough nurses are willing to talk about their work.
2. When nurses and nursing organizations do talk about their work, too often they intentionally project an inaccurate picture of nursing by using a "virtue" instead of a "knowledge" script.
3. When nursing groups give voice to nursing, they sometimes bypass, downplay, or even devalue the basic nursing work that occurs in direct care of the sick while elevating an image of "elite" nurses in advanced practice, administration, and academia. (p. 4)

Nurses should face the **stereotypes** present in our society and erase the lines that define us. To do this, we must first recognize our value to society and ourselves. When introducing ourselves in the professional role, we should do so with confidence and clarity. For example, we can say, "Good morning, Mr. Smith. I'm Susan Jones, your registered nurse." Such day-to-day engagement is important. We must tell the world what we do.

In *From Silence to Voice*, the authors identify the following actions to promote the real image of nursing:

- Educate the public in daily life.
- Describe the nurse's work.
- Make known the agency—independent thinker—of the RN.
- Deal with the fear of angering the physician.
- Accept thanks from others.
- Be ready to take advantage of openings to promote nursing.

CRITICAL THINKING QUESTION ✳

How can you, as a student nurse, tell members of society what professional nurses do? ✳

- Respond to queries with real-life stories from nursing.
- Tell the details.
- Avoid using nursing jargon.
- Be prepared ahead of time to tell your story.
- Do not suppress your enthusiasm.
- Reflect the nurse's clinical judgment and competency.
- Connect your work to pressing contemporary issues.
- Respect patient confidentiality.
- Deal with and confront the fear of failure.

In an effort to address the challenges faced by nursing, Buresh and Gordon (2006) provide a history and understanding of modern media and provide examples of how to interconnect with them. Knowing how news media work, how to write a letter to the editor, how to present oneself on television or radio, and how to converse with community groups are among the guidelines provided. Being proactive is essential, especially at a time when healthcare costs and cuts demand that only the fundamental players are left standing. Society needs to know that nurses are fundamental players.

Sigma Theta Tau International commissioned the 1997 Woodhull Study on Nursing and the Media, which reported the lack of representation that nurses have in the media (Sigma Theta Tau International, 1998). In approximately 20,000 articles from 16 major news publications, nurses were cited only 3% of the time. Among the healthcare industry publications, only 1% of the references were nurses. Although nurses are highly relevant participants in patients' stories, they were neglected in almost every case. Key recommendations from the Woodhull Study include the following:

- Nurses and media should be proactive in establishing ongoing dialogue.
- If the aim is to provide comprehensive coverage of health care, the media should include information by and about nurses.
- Training should be provided to nurses on how to speak about business, management, and policy issues.
- *Health care* needs to be clearly identified as the umbrella term for specific disciplines, such as medicine and nursing.
- Nurses with doctoral degrees should be identified correctly as doctors, and those with medical doctorate (MD) degrees should be identified as physicians.
- Language needs to reflect the diverse options for health care by avoiding phrases such as "Consult your doctor." Rather, media need to state, "Consult your primary healthcare provider."

In recent years, we have seen more accurate portrayals of nurses supported in the media. Instead of portraying sexual prowess or disrespect and anger, nurses have been presented as intelligent, competent, and essential to patient care. Johnson & Johnson continues the Campaign for Nursing's Future to raise public awareness of professional nursing. This positive promotion has supported student and faculty recruitment into the profession. Johnson & Johnson has taken additional steps to recognize the courageous efforts of many nurses, including those who were intensely engaged in responding during national crises such as Hurricane Katrina. Nurses must continually evaluate the portrayal of nurses in the media. After all, if the image is inaccurate, we have a responsibility to correct it.

The Gender Gap
Women in Nursing

In Western culture, women have traditionally been socialized as the more passive of the genders—to avoid conflict and yield to authority. The implications of this conventional thought are still evident in nursing practice today. Many nurses lack confidence in dealing with conflict and communicating with those in authority. For some, it is a matter of short supply of energy and too many other commitments. Others perceive assertiveness as clashing with people's expectations. We should ask ourselves, "Isn't the reward of knowing we do a good job enough?" For female nurses who assume multiple personal and professional roles, career is often not at the top of our priorities. This can be attributed to the fact that the role of women in past society was primarily geared toward family responsibility, not career. Many women who chose nursing did so without the expectation of a long-term commitment to the profession. Rather, nursing was a "good job" when and if a woman needed to work. This centeredness on service continues in nursing today, albeit with less intensity than in the past.

The women's movement in the 1960s empowered intelligent career-seeking women to enter professions other than the traditional ones of teaching and nursing. After some years of competing for students, nursing saw a return of interest in the 1980s and 1990s. At this point, more women chose nursing as a career because nursing provided a natural complement to their gifts, not because it was one of only a few options available to them (Chitty & Campbell, 2001). As the message of varied opportunities for women and men in nursing is shared, the social status of all nurses is elevated.

Another facet of women in nursing is the changing demographic of women entering the nursing profession. In the United States, a larger number of women from underrepresented groups are becoming nurses. According to the USDHHS (2010), approximately 170,235 RNs living in the United States obtained their initial nursing education in another country or U.S. territory. There was an increase from 3.7% in 2004 to 5.6% in 2008.

About 50% of the internationally educated RNs living in the United States in 2008 were from the Philippines, 11.5% were from Canada, and 9.3% were from India.

Men in Nursing

At the start of the new millennium, men represented approximately 5.4% of the RN population in the United States (Trossman, 2003). By 2004, men comprised 5.8% of the RN population, and then 6.6% in 2008 (USDHHS, 2010). This steady increase can be attributed to recruitment campaigns focused on attracting men into nursing. For example, the Oregon Center for Nursing (2002) created a poster of men in nursing with the slogan "Are you man enough to be a nurse?" The Mississippi Hospital Association published an all-male calendar with monthly features of men in nursing, ranging from men who were nursing students to practicing professionals in a variety of roles. The calendar was used as a recruiting tool to help encourage men, young and old, to consider career opportunities in nursing (Health Careers Center, 2012). These strategies help diminish the stigma associated with men in nursing.

The ANA inducted the first man into its Hall of Fame in 2004 (ANA, 2007). Dr. Luther Christman was recognized for his 65-year career and contributions to the profession, including the founding of the American Assembly for Men in Nursing. In 2007, the ANA established the Luther Christman Award to recognize the contributions of men in nursing. Current literature also helps to keep the discussion of men in nursing at the forefront. In 2006, *Men in Nursing* journal was launched as the first professional journal dedicated to addressing the issues and topics facing the growing number of men who work in the nursing field.

Although a seemingly recent topic, men have served in nursing roles throughout history. In the 13th century, men played a vital role in providing nursing care to vulnerable individuals. John Ciudad (1495–1550) opened a hospital in Grenada, Spain, so that he (along with friends) could provide care to the mentally ill, the homeless, and abandoned children (Blais, Hayes, Kozier, & Erb, 2001). Saint Camillus de Lellis (1550–1614) was the founder of the Nursing Order of Ministers of the sick. Men in this order were charged with providing care to alcoholics and those affected by the plague (Blais et al., 2001). In the United States, in the 1700s James Derham was an African American man who worked as a nurse in New Orleans and was subsequently able to buy his freedom and become the first African American physician in the United States.

Despite her many contributions to the nursing profession, Florence Nightingale did not encourage the participation of men in nursing. She believed that traits such as nurturance, gentleness, empathy, and compassion were needed to provide care and that these traits existed primarily in women.

Nightingale opposed men being nurses and stated that their "hard and horny" hands were not fit to "touch, bathe, and dress wounded limbs, however gentle their hearts may be" (Chung, 2000, p. 38). Thus, nursing became a predominately female discipline in the late 1800s.

Even with negative societal perceptions and stereotypes, men are now more open to pursuing nursing as a career choice (Berlin, Stennett, & Bednash, 2004). In the fall of 2003, the percentage of men enrolled in undergraduate schools of nursing was 8.4%. In 2014, the percentage of male students enrolled in baccalaureate nursing programs increased to 11.7%. Male students enrolled in master's degree nursing programs represented 10.8% of that group of students. Male students represented 9.6% of the students enrolled in research-focused doctoral programs and 11.7% of students enrolled in practice-focused doctoral programs (American Association of Colleges of Nursing [AACN], 2015a). These increases are largely the result of diminishing misconceptions and increased recruiting efforts. Men tend to prefer distinct practice areas, including high-technology, fast-paced, and intense environments. Emergency departments, intensive care units, operating rooms, and nurse anesthesiology are examples of areas to which men are often attracted (American Society of Registered Nurses, 2008; Gibbs & Waugaman, 2004). Some speculate that men make these choices to avoid potential role strain if they were to choose other areas, such as obstetrics and pediatrics, and because they prefer areas that require more technical expertise (American Society of Registered Nurses, 2008).

There is some debate that men in nursing have an advantage over their female peers. It is not unusual for patients to assume that a male nurse is a physician or a medical student. On the other hand, men in nursing have been mistaken for orderlies. However, the percentage of men in leadership roles in nursing is much higher than the percentage of men in nursing overall. This is partly because male nurses are more oriented and motivated to upgrade their professional status (American Society of Registered Nurses, 2008). As a result, women in nursing are challenged to learn how to promote themselves within the profession.

What issues and challenges do men face in nursing? According to research conducted by Armstrong (2002) and Keogh and O'Lynn (2007), male nurses are unfairly stereotyped in the profession as homosexuals, low achievers, and feminine. These false assumptions and perceptions deter other men from entering the profession, create gender-based barriers in nursing schools, and decrease retention rates of male nurses once they are licensed. Also, because most nursing faculty are female, most nursing textbooks are written by females, and most leaders in nursing are female, men might have to learn new ways of thinking and understanding to find a comfortable place of belonging in the nursing profession. For example, it is reported that a male nursing student was having difficulty answering questions on a nursing examination. When the student shared a sample question with his wife (who was not a nurse), she answered the question correctly (Brady & Sherrod, 2003).

What advantages do women have in nursing? What advantages do men have in the profession? What are the risks of being gender exclusive? ✳

As a consequence of gender bias, some patients might refuse or feel reluctant to allow men in the nursing role to care for them (American Society of Registered Nurses, 2008; Cardillo, 2001). During labor and delivery, patients and their partners might request a female nurse to be at the bedside. Overall, the presence of a male nurse alone in the room with a patient is out of the ordinary. On the other hand, male nurses are assumed to be physically stronger and willing to do the heavier tasks of nursing care, such as lifting and moving patients (Cardillo, 2001). Still, many men and women are learning to appreciate and enjoy the emerging culture in the profession (Meyers, 2003). The old biases continue to disappear as patients and providers become more educated about the need for gender diversity in nursing.

Changing Demographics and Cultural Competence

Despite national trends of increasing diversity, with ethnic and racial minorities reaching almost one-third of the U.S. population, minorities overall are underrepresented in the healthcare profession. The 2010 U.S. Census reports that 63.7% of the population is white and non-Hispanic. In contrast, the RN population remains predominantly female (94.2%) and 83.2% white, non-Hispanic (Health Resources and Services Administration [HRSA], 2010). The Sullivan Commission (2004) highlights the diversity gap in its hallmark report *Missing Persons: Minorities in the Health Professions*. Together, African Americans, Hispanic Americans, and American Indians make up more than 25% of the U.S. population but only 9% of the nation's nurses, 6% of its physicians, and 5% of dentists. Similar disparities show up in the faculties of health professional schools. For example, minorities make up less than 10% of baccalaureate nursing faculties, 8.6% of dental school faculties, and only 4.2% of medical school faculties. If the trends continue, the health workforce of the future will resemble the population even less than it does today. If these data are viewed in the context of the prediction that no racial or ethnic group will compose a majority by the year 2050, such a decline in a diverse workforce could be catastrophic.

In 2003, the Institute of Medicine (IOM) warned of the "unequal treatment" minorities face when encountering the healthcare system. Cultural differences, a lack of access to health care, high rates of poverty, and unemployment contribute to the substantial ethnic and racial disparities in health status and health outcomes (IOM, 2003b). Health services research shows that minority health professionals are more likely to serve minority and medically underserved populations. Increasing the number of underrepresented minorities in the health professions as well as improving the cultural competency of providers are key strategies for reducing health disparities (Betancourt, Green, Carrillo, & Ananeh-Firempong, 2003; IOM, 2003b).

Cultural competence in multicultural societies continues as a major initiative for health care and specifically for nursing. The mass media, healthcare policymakers, the Office of Minority Health and other governmental organizations, professional organizations, the workplace, and health insurance payers are addressing the need for individuals to understand and become culturally competent as one strategy to improve quality and eliminate racial, ethnic, and gender disparities in health care (Purnell & Paulanka, 2008).

Culturally competent healthcare providers reduce patient care error and increase access to and satisfaction with health care. The beginning of cultural competence is self-awareness. Culture has a powerful unconscious impact on health professionals and the care they provide. Purnell and Paulanka (2008) believe that self-knowledge and understanding promote strong professional perceptions that free healthcare providers from prejudice and facilitate culturally competent care.

Nursing has a long history of incorporating culture into nursing practice (DeSantis & Lipson, 2007). In 2008, the AACN released a publication identifying cultural competency in baccalaureate nursing education (AACN, 2008). Yet some maintain that no matter how culturally competent the nurse might be, the patient's experience remains structured in the nurse's culture (Dean, 2005). Despite nurses' best efforts to understand the culture of the patient, nurses often fail to understand that the patient might be experiencing health care for the first time, not in his or her own culture, but in the nurse's culture of healthcare delivery. The understanding of this concept associated with cultural competence increases the reality of the urgency of increasing the diversity in the nursing workforce.

The National Advisory Council on Nurse Education and Practice (NACNEP) was established to advise the secretary of the USDHHS and Congress on policy issues related to Title VIII programs administered by HRSA. NACNEP identified as an issue the need to increase the racial and ethnic diversity of the RN workforce. In its third report, NACNEP recommended that the country "expand the resources available to develop models that will effectively recruit and graduate sufficient numbers of racial/ethnic students to reflect the nation's diverse population" (NACNEP, 2003).

Currently, most RNs are white women, but more minority students are enrolling in nursing programs now than in past decades. In 2014, 30.1% of students enrolled in baccalaureate programs were minorities, as were 31.9% of nurses enrolled in masters programs, 28.7% of nurses enrolled in practice-focused doctoral programs, and 29.7% of nurses enrolled in research-focused doctoral programs. These numbers have increased substantially since 2005,

KEY COMPETENCY 5-2

Examples of Applicable
*Nurse of the Future: Nursing
Core Competencies*

Patient-Centered Care:

Knowledge (K4) Describes
how diverse cultural, ethnic,
spiritual and socioeconomic
backgrounds function as
sources of patient, family,
and community values

Skills (S4b) Implements
nursing care to meet
holistic needs of patient on
socioeconomic, cultural,
ethnic, and spiritual values
and beliefs influencing
health care and nursing
practice

Attitudes/Behaviors (A4b)
Recognizes impact of
personal attitudes, values,
and beliefs regarding
delivery of care to diverse
clients

Source: Massachusetts Department of Higher
Education. (2010). *Nurse of the future:
Nursing core competencies* (p. 10). Retrieved
from http://www.mass.edu/currentinit
/documents/NursingCoreCompetencies.pdf

when only 24.1% of students enrolled in baccalaureate programs, 22% of nurses enrolled in masters programs, and 18.4% of nurses enrolled in research-focused doctoral programs were minorities (AACN, 2015a).

The Joint Commission and the National Committee for Quality Assurance also identified the need for healthcare professionals to recognize and respect cultural differences, including dialects, regional differences, and slang (Levine, 2012). In an effort to respond to this national message, many hospitals and healthcare agencies have initiated the use of interactive patient-engagement technology as part of their education programs. These services are provided in several languages, including Russian, Spanish, and Mandarin. Nurses know that illness and associated stress, pain, and fear can hinder patients' comprehension when learning about their condition and treatment plan. Language barriers compound the problem, resulting in major obstacles to learning and subsequent issues with adhering to the treatment plan. As nursing focuses more on cultural behaviors, norms, and practices, healthcare outcomes can move in a positive direction (Levine, 2012).

As the general population of healthcare consumers becomes increasingly diverse, there is a greater need for culturally competent care (Jacob & Carnegie, 2002). To provide such nursing care, we must strive for a nursing population that more accurately represents the communities we serve. As the population continues to become more diverse, culturally competent care will be the basis for quality care, access to care, and alleviation of health disparities, thus promoting healthier population outcomes. Being culturally competent, that is, having the ability to interact appropriately with others through cultural understanding, is an expectation for people entering the nursing profession (Grant & Letzring, 2003), keeping in mind that there is a difference between *learning of* another culture and *learning from* another culture.

Access to Health Care

Many Americans have health insurance coverage and access to some of the best healthcare professionals in the nation. However, a large number of individuals experience disparities in our healthcare system. These disparities, or unfair differences in access, can result in poor quality and quantity of health care. According to the Agency for Healthcare Research and Quality (AHRQ, 2010), individuals who are at greatest risk for experiencing healthcare disparities are racial and ethnic minorities and those with a low socioeconomic status. Lack of health insurance is the most significant contributing factor to a decrease in disease prevention and thus is one of the foci of the Patient Protection and Affordable Care Act. Although lack of health insurance has a major effect on access to health care, other factors, such as continuity of care, economic barriers, geographic barriers, and sociocultural barriers, have a detrimental effect on the health and quality of life of individuals and are discussed in the following subsections.

Continuity of Care

Individuals who have a provider or facility where they receive routine care are more likely to receive preventive health care (AHRQ, 2010). These individuals usually have better health outcomes and experience reduced disparities. In 2008, the percentage of people with a specific source of ongoing care was significantly lower for poor people than for high-income people (77.5% compared with 92.1%). The AHRQ also notes that having a routine provider of care correlates with a greater trust in the provider and increased likelihood that the person coordinates care with the provider. In this regard, one role and responsibility of the nurse is to educate the community and patients on the importance of continuity of care with a routine healthcare provider and/or facility.

Economic Barriers

Undoubtedly, poverty poses the greatest risk to health status (Kavanagh, 2001). The United States has a long-standing reputation for providing the highest quality health care to persons in the highest socioeconomic strata. Likewise, the lowest quality health care is provided to those at the other end of the socioeconomic continuum (Jacob & Carnegie, 2002). As the largest segment of the healthcare industry, RNs can have a positive impact on the change required in this established system. Recognizing the stronghold that poverty currently has on the health care of citizens is a beginning to the much-needed work in the fight for equality.

Although stereotypes communicate to us that poverty is limited to certain groups, we understand that poverty affects people of all cultures and ethnicities. We must recognize the impact that poverty has on healthcare practices. If poverty were eradicated, there would be no homelessness, none who are uninsured, and no more choices between food and medicine. Until that time, nursing continues to face the challenge of meeting the needs of all people.

Geographic Barriers

Those living in rural areas have unique concerns regarding **access to care**. As many rural hospitals close due to a lack of financing, more communities find themselves struggling to find primary care providers who will work in those areas. State and national efforts attempt to provide more service to these areas, but the demand outweighs the supply.

Urban dwellers are not immune to geographic barriers. Large cities have economically depressed sections with fewer healthcare providers than the more affluent areas. Dependency on public transportation is another factor to be managed. Finally, most rural and many urban communities do not support a full range of healthcare services in one location. These variables affect patients' access to care and their continuation in prescribed treatment plans. It is imperative for the nurse to collaborate with other members of the healthcare team to become aware of various services available to enhance the health and quality of life of patients.

Sociocultural Barriers

The need for cultural and ethnic diversity in the nursing workforce has been discussed. Moreover, healthcare settings are challenged to provide an environment where people of various sociocultural backgrounds are respected. For example, having translators on site or within easy contact is critical for ensuring safe care to non-English-speaking clients. Written materials should also be provided in appropriate languages and at an appropriate reading level. It is not feasible or cost effective to provide educational materials and products to patients who will not use them because they are in a foreign language or too advanced. Specifically, consent forms for surgery and other procedures must be available in the client's language. To ignore the need for language-appropriate literature leads to patient harm, as well as disrespect for the uniqueness of others.

One subculture that has garnered much attention in recent years is the military patient population. The Department of Defense operates and finances health care through TRICARE, a comprehensive healthcare coverage program for members of the uniformed services, their families, and survivors. With national resources decreasing and demands for health care of our military population on the rise, nurses play a pivotal role in influencing the direction of care for this special group.

In an effort to address the needs of the military population and their families specifically, First Lady Michelle Obama led the "Joining Forces" national initiative to mobilize all sectors of the community to give service members, veterans, and their families the support they deserve, especially in regard to employment, education, and wellness. According to Joining Forces (White House, 2012), military service members, veterans, and their families have made significant contributions to the nation's safety and security. This contribution comes at great cost to each veteran and family. The profession of nursing has a long and established history of meeting and supporting the physical and mental health needs of our nation's military service members, veterans, and their families. The profession of nursing has pledged to inspire and prepare each nurse to recognize the unique health and wellness concerns of the population. One hundred fifty nursing organizations and 500 nursing schools pledged their support to help educate nurses on post-traumatic stress disorder (PTSD) and traumatic brain injury (TBI) in the coming years. Although each organization and nursing school has its unique mission and vision, various strategies to be employed include (1) increasing nurse awareness of PTSD and TBI,

(2) recognizing the signs and symptoms in patients, and (3) integrating PTSD and TBI content in nursing school curricula, to name a few. The ANA, American Academy of Nurse Practitioners, AACN, and National League for Nursing took the lead in seeking nationwide support from nursing organizations and schools of nursing.

CRITICAL THINKING QUESTIONS *

What barriers to health care do you see in your community? How are the underprivileged served in our current healthcare system? *

Societal Trends

At any time in history, societal trends affect the nursing profession. Major current movements include incivility, violence in the workplace, global aging, consumerism, complementary and alternative care, and disaster preparedness. Discussion of these issues allows us to see more clearly the social landscape and some of the challenges we face as a profession.

Incivility

Incivility, or "bullying," has been exposed in the media to a great extent in the past few years. This heightened attention is partly the result of media coverage of suicide attempts and homicides that were instigated by harassment at the physical, verbal, and electronic levels. Incivility is seen in every area of society, including high school, college, and even on the job. Nursing is not immune to this behavior. Greater light has been shed on the incidence and prevalence of bullying in nurse-to-nurse, faculty-to-student, and even student-to-faculty interactions. Rocker (2008) reports that some of the behaviors include criticism, humiliation in front of others, undervaluing of effort, and teasing. It is also reported that bullying contributes to burnout, school dropout, isolation, and even attempted suicides. Bullying is costly to organizations because it contributes to increased leave, nurse attrition, and decreased nurse productivity, satisfaction, and morale.

In light of this, it is vital that the nursing profession take an active step in preventing incivility not only in our communities, but also in nursing programs and places of employment. The ANA (2012) has taken such action by developing a booklet, *Bullying in the Workplace: Reversing a Culture*, to help nurses recognize, understand, and deal with bullying in the work environment. The ANA supports zero-tolerance policies related to workplace bullying. In addition, in its professional performance standards, the ANA (2015) indicates that nurses are required to take a leadership role in the practice setting and within the profession. Two of the competencies listed that demonstrate the expected performance related to this standard include communicating in a way that manages conflict and contributing to environments that support and maintain respect, trust, and dignity (p. 75).

Violence in the Workplace

The **violence** in our society is evident and appears to be increasing in frequency and severity. What is more alarming is our desensitization to the constant exposure by Internet, radio, and television. As nurses, we can easily put a face on violence. We see the man in the emergency department with a gunshot wound to the chest. Only 30 minutes before, he was leaving work for a weekend with family when someone decided that they needed his car more than this man needed his life. We see violence at the women's shelter when we rotate through that clinical site in community health nursing. We also see troubled individuals who take out their frustration on colleagues and supervisors by going on a shooting rampage, leaving a path of death and destruction. All of these examples affect nurses because we are caring for the ones who are injured and also providing care to the injurer. Nurses are required to be knowledgeable of how to act and provide competent care when violent incidents occur.

RNs can assume additional roles when addressing violence. The role of the nurse is not limited to providing care in the hospital or emergency department. To work aggressively to address violence, nurses can function in the role of a sexual assault nurse examiner (SANE) or forensic nurse (Littel, 2001). Forensic nurses are trained to recognize and collect evidence related to criminal acts of trauma or death (Santiago, 2012). The SANE RN must have advanced education and preparation in forensic examination of sexual assault victims. One result of the SANE programs is that victims of sexual assault consistently receive attention and compassion without delay (Littel, 2001).

Nurses must become socially aware and politically involved in preventing violence. We have to support legislation that proactively addresses violence and lobby for funding that provides nursing research into violence prevention and treatment. In every potential case, nurses have to use keen assessment skills to identify people at risk and to promote reporting, treatment, and rehabilitation.

Global Aging

In 2010, adults 62 years of age or older comprised 16.2% of the U.S. population (49.9 million) compared to 14.7% (41.2 million) in the year 2000. By 2030, it is estimated that the population of older adults will rise to 71 million (Howden & Meyer, 2011). By 2050 it is estimated that one in five Americans will be 65 years or older, with the greatest increases being in the group over 85 years (USDHHS, 2014).

However, this is not a trend unique to the United States. The Year of the Older Person—this is what the United Nations called the year 1999 to recognize and reaffirm **global aging**, the fact that our global population is aging at an unprecedented rate (U.S. Census Bureau, 2001). After World War II, fertility increased and death rates of all ages decreased. Not only are people in developed countries living longer and healthier, but so are those in the developing world. In the 1990s, developed countries had equal numbers of young (people 15 years or younger) and old (people 55 years or older), with approximately 22% of the population in each category. On the other hand, 35% of the people in developing countries were children compared with 10% who were older. Still, absolute numbers of older persons are large and growing. In the year 2000, more than half of the world's older people (59%, or 249 million people) lived in developing nations.

In the United States, a decrease in fertility, an increase in urbanization, better education, and improved health care all contribute to this social phenomenon. In addition, the older baby boomers who have turned 65 years of age have started to affect health care significantly with increasing numbers receiving Medicare benefits. The impact this will have on our healthcare system is daunting. According to the USDHHS (2014), more than 60% of older adults manage more than one chronic medical condition, such as diabetes, arthritis, heart failure, and dementia. Currently 46% of critical care patients and 60% of medical-surgical patients in U.S. hospitals are older adults. These acute care patients are challenging for nurses and resource intensive to the healthcare system because these vulnerable patients generally have multiple chronic conditions to treat simultaneously (Ellison & Farrar, 2015).

There is a need for clear health policy at a national level if we are to be prepared to care for the increasing number of aging citizens. Preventive health services for older adults are delineated as provisions made in the Affordable Care Act of 2010. Healthy People 2020 included objectives specifically for older adults that should be used by healthcare professionals, including nurses, to promote healthy outcomes, including improved health, function, and quality of life for this population. Issues that emerge as nurses promote these outcomes may include coordination of care and helping older adults manage their own care (USDHHS, 2014).

In response to the global aging phenomenon and the specialized set of skills required to care for older adults, most schools of nursing have either incorporated gerontology courses or increased the geriatric content throughout the curriculum. Geriatric Nurse Practitioner programs have grown in number, and some schools offer dual-track Adult/Geriatric Nurse Practitioner and Geriatric Psychiatric Mental Health Nurse Practitioner programs in graduate programs. Clinical experiences in nursing programs include many experiences with older persons. Still, as a nation, we lack an organized plan to make certain that healthcare needs will be met—not just for the aging, but also for those who come after them.

Consumerism

Since the American Hospital Association's development of A Patient's Bill of Rights in 1973, consumers have assumed more control of their healthcare experiences; this shift is called **consumerism**. The 1992 version of the document was replaced by the brochure *The Patient Care Partnership: Understanding Expectations, Rights, and Responsibilities* (American Hospital Association, 2003b). This brochure is available in several languages and can be accessed in its entirety via the American Hospital Association website at www.aha.org/advocacy-issues/communicatingpts/index.shtml. A summary of the original document is presented in **Box 5-1**. Gone are the days when patients blindly followed the instructions of their physicians. This is cause for celebration in the nursing arena because nursing has long sought to empower patients to take responsibility for their own health. Although pockets of medical paternalism may continue to exist, a shift has occurred and consumers of health care now hold healthcare providers to a higher standard than ever before.

In addition to *The Patient Care Partnership*, the American Hospital Association also developed a resource toolkit entitled *Strategies for Leadership: Improving Communications with Patients and Families: A Blueprint for Action* (2003a). The resource includes checklists to help hospitals assess their strengths and weaknesses related to communications with patients and families. The resource also includes case studies that illustrate initiatives that other hospitals have implemented to foster improved communication.

Information technology has given patients an enormous resource for gaining knowledge about diseases, medications, and treatment options, as well as support groups and other self-help resources. In today's environment, consumers of healthcare search for answers to their healthcare questions and compare provider and healthcare system outcomes online. Based on the information available, they are able to make informed choices related to health care.

KEY COMPETENCY 5-3

Examples of Applicable *Nurse of the Future: Nursing Core Competencies*

Patient-Centered Care:

Attitudes/Behaviors (A2b) Respects and encourages the patient's input relative to decisions about health care and services

Source: Massachusetts Department of Higher Education. (2010). *Nurse of the future: Nursing core competencies* (p. 9). Retrieved from http://www.mass.edu/currentinit /documents/NursingCoreCompetencies.pdf

---

BOX 5-1 THE PATIENT CARE PARTNERSHIP

What to expect during your hospital stay:

1. High-quality patient care
2. A clean and safe environment
3. Involvement in your care
   a. Discussing your medical condition and information about medically appropriate treatment choices
   b. Discussing your treatment plan
   c. Getting information from you
   d. Understanding your healthcare goals and values
   e. Understanding who should make decisions when you cannot
4. Protection of your privacy
5. Preparing you and your family for when you leave the hospital
6. Help with your bill and filing insurance claims

Complementary and Alternative Approaches

As the consumer's perspective grows in influence, and individuals take on greater responsibility in their healthcare decisions, they explore approaches to health care that can actually contrast with Western traditions. Different terminology has been used synonymously to define this growing field, such as *complementary care practices* and *alternative medicine*. According to the National Center for Complementary and Alternative Medicine (2012), "Complementary and alternative medicine is a group of diverse medical and healthcare systems, practices, and products that are not presently considered to be part of conventional medicine." Complementary medicine refers to an approach that combines conventional medicine with less conventional options, whereas alternative medicine is an approach used instead of conventional medicine. Major types of **complementary and alternative medicine** include the following:

- Alternative medical systems (built on complete systems of practice such as homeopathic medicine or naturopathic medicine)
- Mind–body interventions (techniques designed to enhance the mind's capacity to affect bodily function such as meditation, prayer, music, and support groups)
- Biologically based therapies (use of substances found in nature such as herbs, foods, and vitamins)
- Manipulative and body-based methods (based on manipulation or movement of one or more parts of the body such as chiropractic manipulation or massage)
- Energy therapies (involves the use of energy fields through either biofield therapies such as therapeutic touch, qi gong, or Reiki, or bioelectro-magnetic-based therapies such as magnetic therapy)

Alternative and complementary therapies affect the selection of traditional choices for treatment, and ignoring that they exist is not an option. People persist in the use of alternative and complementary therapies for obvious reasons: (1) the therapies have been found valuable, and (2) Western medicine has limited options. Many people are inclined not to divulge information about complementary therapy to their healthcare provider; however, some alternative therapies may interact with medications and may be contraindicated in certain circumstances, so it is imperative that healthcare providers seek out this information. Nurses should provide a safe, trusting atmosphere where patients feel free to discuss their healthcare routines and preferences.

Disaster Preparedness

Prior to the turn of this century, **disaster preparedness** was not a major topic of discussion in programs of nursing. Further, the key roles that professional nurses now play in preparing and responding to disasters were unexplored until recently. The World Trade Center attack in 2001 and the shock of Hurricane Katrina in 2005 opened the nation's eyes to our vulnerabilities and our strengths. As a result, disaster management has become common language in our schools, agencies, and communities.

Disaster management, plans designating responses during an emergency, are coordinated by local, state, and federal groups. Firefighters, police officers, and healthcare professionals are part of response teams. Disaster training is also available to other volunteers. We have learned that caring for large groups affected by disaster requires an organized, thoughtful, unbiased approach. Professional nurses carry the burden of being knowledgeable about potential disasters, educating the public about the risks, and responding when persons are affected.

Disaster resources are available from many organizations. The American Red Cross and the ANA make available policies, resources, and educational opportunities on disaster preparedness for nurses. In addition, the IOM (2009) provides guidance for entities establishing standards of care for disaster preparedness. The Centers for Disease Control and Prevention (CDC) Clinician Outreach and Communication Activity program formed in 2011 in response to the anthrax attacks in the United States. The mission of the outreach program is to help healthcare professionals provide optimal care by facilitating communication between clinicians and the CDC about emerging health threats, identifying clinical issues during emergencies to help inform outreach strategies, and disseminating evidence-based health information and public health emergency messages (CDC, 2012).

Trends in Nursing

The profession of nursing is currently facing some daunting challenges that include a projected nursing shortage, workplace issues, the education–practice gap, unclear practice roles, and changes in population demographics. Although it is true that each of these issues is not a new challenge to nursing practice, it is critical to now acknowledge the collective impact of all of these together in the contemplation of future directions in professional nursing practice.

Nursing is rich in history, resilient in its journey to develop as a profession and a discipline, and adaptive in its practice to meet the healthcare needs of the patient. Throughout the history of nursing, there are identifiable periods of time in which the practice and education of nurses responded to the evolving changes in health care and in society. Today, nursing is again at the crossroads of a major transition in its education and practice. An awareness of the merging of these issues creates urgency when contemplating the role, practice, and education of nurses.

Nurse Shortage

The shortage of nurses is not a new issue; the predicted **nursing shortage** has been prominent in the media for most of nursing's history and more recently in the past several years. The U.S. Bureau of Labor Statistics estimated that more than 1 million new and replacement nurses would be needed by 2016 (Dohm & Shniper, 2007). Buerhaus, Auerbach, and Staiger (2009) project the shortage of nurses in the United States could be as high as 500,000 in 2025. These projections are based on the following trends: an increase in population, a larger proportion of elderly persons, increases in technology, and advances in medical science (HRSA, 2002). Other issues affecting the projected supply of nurses include declines in the number of nursing school graduates, aging of the RN workforce, declines in relative earning, and emergence of alternative job opportunities, especially for women, who are the prominent gender in nursing.

History documents a cyclic pattern of nursing shortages, making it difficult to comprehend the seriousness of this shortage, especially viewed through the lens of history. The economic slowdown; the decreased vacancies in healthcare agencies, especially hospitals; and the uncertainty of the consequences of healthcare reform given the Affordable Care Act (2010) further complicate predictions related to the future nursing workforce. In the 2013–2014 academic year, schools of nursing documented that a significant number of qualified nursing school applicants (57,944) were denied admission to undergraduate nursing programs (AACN, 2014) due to lack of faculty and resource constraints that prohibit further increases in student enrollments. In recent years, employers in various parts of the United States have reported a decrease in the demand for RNs, and nursing students report that it is more challenging after graduation to find employment, sometimes taking 6 months to a year.

These findings have led many people to question whether the nursing shortage still exists. Experts claim that the recession might have given some hospitals a temporary reprieve from chronic shortages, but it is not curing the longer-term problem and might be making it worse (Robert Wood Johnson Foundation, 2009). The Tri-Council for Nursing (2010) released a joint statement cautioning stakeholders about declaring an end to the nursing shortage. The statement says, "The downturn in the economy has led to an easing of the shortage in many parts of the country, a recent development most analysts believe to be temporary." The council raises serious concerns about slowing the production of RNs given the projected demand for nursing services, particularly in light of healthcare reform. It further states that diminishing the pipeline of future nurses can put the health of many Americans at risk, particularly those from rural and underserved communities, and leave our healthcare delivery system unprepared to meet the demand for essential nursing services.

Where do we stand today? A report from the Bureau of Labor Statistics on employment projections identifies the registered nursing workforce as the top occupation in terms of job growth through 2020 (Bureau of Labor Statistics, 2012). The number of employed nurses is expected to grow from 2.74 million in 2010 to 3.45 million in 2020, and a need for 495,500 replacements in the nursing workforce is projected for 2020.

Data collected in the 2008 National Sample Survey of Registered Nurses (HRSA, 2010) document that the average age of the RN population is 46.8 years. It is significant to note that the average age of the RN population did not increase from the 2004 survey. The plateau in the average age reflects an increase in employed RNs younger than 30 years of age. Between 1988 and 2004, the percentage of employed nurses younger than 30 years fell from 18.3% to 9.1%. The trend of increasing enrollments in schools of nursing, especially baccalaureate programs, is credited for the increased employment of younger nurses (HRSA, 2010).

A recent report from the AACN shows an increase in the enrollment of generic baccalaureate students by 3.1% in 2011–2012 and by 17% in the past 5 years (AACN, 2012). There was no increase in 2012–2013, but this was followed by an increased enrollment of baccalaureate students, more than doubling to 6.6% in 2013–2014 (AACN, 2015a). Yet, the following statement is included with the documentation of increased enrollment: "Although the dramatic rise in enrollments and the increase in graduations over the past five years are encouraging, many more baccalaureate-prepared nurses will be needed to meet the health care needs of the population" (AACN, 2012, p. 3).

A national nurse shortage still exists. Although nursing school enrollments and graduations are increasing, and the statistics on younger nurses in the workforce are encouraging, the following factors must be considered in addressing the future of professional nursing practice. Baccalaureate and graduate programs in nursing report that 75,587 qualified applicants were not admitted into nursing programs because of lack of clinical space and faculty shortage. There is a prediction that more than 32 million Americans will soon gain new access to healthcare services, and the aging population is increasing and will require management of their chronic illnesses (AACN, 2012). This leaves us with questions such as: Who will provide these healthcare services? Who will care for the old? As people age and experience health problems, their needs are often more complex and acute, thereby demanding an even more highly skilled nursing force.

Nurse Faculty Shortage

In previous cycles of nursing shortages, the primary solution was to increase the enrollment in nursing programs. However, ample evidence supports the conclusion that a national **nursing faculty shortage** also exists. In a 2013–2014 survey, the AACN reported that the professoriate continues to age, and an exodus from the ranks of faculty looms before us due to retirement. The mean age of doctoral faculty holding the rank of professor is 61.6 years, for faculty holding the rank of associate professor it is 57.6 years, and for assistant professors it is 51.4 years. The national faculty vacancy rate is 6.9%. Of the reported vacancies, 89.6% involve doctoral-prepared faculty. This shortage is limiting student capacity in nursing programs across the nation (AACN, 2015b).

The number of nurses employed in nursing education has changed little since 1980, with 31,065 nurses working as faculty. When the number of nurse educators is compared to the increase in the number of RNs, the result is actually a decline (2.4%) in the percentage of nurses working in education (HRSA, 2010). The statistics associated with nursing faculty are concerning, especially in consideration of the nursing shortage and healthcare projections of nurse demand in the future.

Nursing Practice and Workplace Environment

Given the anticipated nursing shortage and the increased demand for nurses, it is important to address the issues associated with the practice of nursing and the environment where nurses work. It is understandable how the shortage of nurses affects the practicing nurse, especially in staff and patient ratios and workload and the resulting influences on nurse turnover rate. However, other issues associated with the nurse practice setting result in problematic quality outcomes, such as nurse job dissatisfaction, unsafe patient care, unhealthy workplace environment, and unclear role expectations.

It is evident that health care and healthcare delivery have changed significantly in the past two decades. Most of these changes have been associated with response to the increasing cost of care, the decreasing reimbursement to healthcare providers, increased use of technology in practice, and the knowledge explosion concerning disease management. A full discussion of each of these issues is beyond the scope of this chapter; however, it is important to note that most of the changes result from a focus on reducing the cost of health care. Cost containment strategies aim to determine the setting of the delivery of care, the length of stay in the hospital, the cost reimbursed to providers of care, and the designation of the appropriate provider of care.

Hospitals remain the most common employment setting for RNs in the United States, with 62.2% of employed RNs reporting hospitals as their primary place of employment (HRSA, 2010). Contrary to earlier predictions, the percentage of nurses working in hospitals increased from 2004 to 2008 (HRSA, 2010); however, note that the percentage of nurses working in home health services has also increased. Data from the national survey of RNs reflect that the percentage of nurses working in hospitals decreases with the increasing age of nurses. Only 50% of RNs age 55 years or older work in hospital settings.

Nurses in hospitals provide care for patients who are sicker, older, and have more complex physical, psychosocial, and economic needs (Brown, 2004; Clark, 2004). The combination of older patients with higher acuity, sophisticated technology, and shorter hospital stays creates a chaotic environment and demands that nurses assume greater responsibility (Cram, 2011). This chaos increases not only the risk of errors in patient care, but also the risk of health concerns for the nurse, such as the threat of infection, needle sticks, ever-increasing sensitivity to latex, back injuries, and stress-related health problems. In addition to these health risks, nurses are susceptible to workplace violence (e.g., physical violence, horizontal violence) and sexual harassment (Longo & Sherman, 2006; Ray & Ream, 2007; Smith-Pittman & McKoy, 1999; Valente & Bullough, 2004).

The issues associated with the hospital work environment have been shown to dominate problems and outcomes associated with nursing practice. Because of this environment, the profession of nursing has been challenged to evaluate its practice and outcomes. In fact, a majority of nurses completing surveys stated they perceived that the unsafe working environment interfered with their ability to provide quality patient care (ANA, 2011; Pellico, Djukic, Kovner, & Brewer, 2009). Staff nurses strongly desire a practice setting in which they feel that they have the ability to provide quality patient care (Schmalenberg & Kramer, 2008) and a work environment that facilitates clinical decision making.

Confounding the issues of the workplace environment are the shortage of qualified non-nurse healthcare workers, the supervision of unlicensed personnel, the appropriate delegation of care, mandatory overtime, and staffing ratios. The debate over the use of unlicensed personnel and the use of other licensed personnel in providing patient care is well documented in the literature (ANA, 1992, 1997, 1999; Zimmerman, 2006). Research studies indicate that a decrease in RN staff increases patient care errors, infection rates, readmission, and morbidity (Aiken, Clarke, Sloane, Sochalski, & Silber, 2002; Needleman, Buerhaus, Mattke, Stewart, & Zelevinsky, 2002; Sofer, 2005; Stanton & Rutherford, 2004).

Given that research indicates that a decrease in RN staff or the use of unlicensed personnel and other licensed personnel influences patient quality outcomes, what is a rationale for this practice? One answer that is quickly provided is the increased costs of a higher RN–patient ratio. Nurses represent about 23% or more of the hospital workforce. The salary of a licensed RN is higher compared to other nonphysician healthcare providers. Thus, the basic assumption is that to employ more unlicensed personnel or other licensed personnel reduces the cost of care. This assumption is not necessarily true when costs other than salary, such as costs of hiring, benefits, training, staff turnover, and responsibilities that must be assumed by a licensed care provider, are considered. Aiken et al. (2002) find that nurses in hospitals with low nurse–patient ratios are more than twice as likely to experience job-related burnout and dissatisfaction with their jobs when compared to nurses in hospitals with the highest nurse–patient ratios. Cooper (2004) and Kalisch and Kyung (2011) note that lower nursing staff ratios also indicate higher costs in a plethora of areas that reflect the actual reality of nursing practice. McCue, Mark, and Harless (2003) find that a 1% increase in non-nurse personnel increases the operating costs by 0.18% and diminishes profits by 0.021%. These data are significant in the overall budget considering the rising costs of health care and current emphasis on the association of quality and safety indicators with reimbursement.

Nurse Retention

There is a connection among nurse satisfaction, work environment, and nurse retention. The strongest predictor of nurse job dissatisfaction and intent to leave a job is personal stress related to the practice environment. The various causes of job stress include patient acuity, work schedules, poor physician–nurse interactions, new technology, staff shortages, unpredictable workflow or workload, and the perception that the care provided is unsafe (Groff-Paris & Terhaar, 2010). Surveys of practicing nurses document that job dissatisfaction, patient safety concerns, decreases in quality care, inadequate staffing, patient care delays, and mandated overtime are issues that negatively affect nursing practice (Aiken et al., 2002; Cooper, 2004; Pellico et al., 2009). Nurses have also reported their concern about their own health and safety issues, with job stress the most frequent health problem reported.

Despite the effort to address the issues of the chaotic and potentially harmful work environment, strategies to address these issues have fallen short of the target, and the dissatisfaction of hospital nurses persists. In national studies, 41% of nurses currently working report being dissatisfied with their jobs, 43% score high in a range of burnout measures, and 22% are planning to leave their jobs in the next year. Of the latter group, 33% are younger than age 30 years (Beecroft, Dorey, & Wentin, 2008; Laschinger, Finegan, & Welk, 2009). These factors help to fuel the shortage of nurses.

In 2008, 29.3% of RNs reported that they were extremely satisfied with their principal nursing positions, 50.5% were moderately satisfied, and 11.1% were dissatisfied (HRSA, 2010). Nurses working in academic education, ambulatory care, and home health settings reported the highest rate of job satisfaction (86.6%, 85.5%, and 82.8%, respectively). Almost 12% of RNs employed in hospitals reported moderate or extreme dissatisfaction (HRSA, 2010).

The retention of competent professional nurses in jobs is a major problem of the U.S. healthcare industry, particularly in hospitals and long-term care facilities. An average yearly nurse turnover rate is reported as 5–21% (PricewaterhouseCooper's Health Research Institute, 2007). Other research has found that during the first year of professional practice, new RNs experience turnover rates around 35–61% (Almada, Carafoli, Flattery,

French, & McNamara, 2004). Kovner and colleagues (2007) found that 13% of newly licensed RNs had changed principal jobs after 1 year, and 37% reported that they felt ready to change jobs (Huntington et al., 2012; Pellico et al., 2009). In a comprehensive report initiated by the AHRQ, the authors found that the shortage of RNs, in combination with an increased workload, poses a potential threat to the quality of care. In addition, every 1% increase in nurse turnover costs a hospital about $300,000 a year.

Complexity of Nursing Work

The healthcare workplace has changed over the past 20 years in response to economic and service pressures. However, some of these reforms have had undesirable consequences for nurses' work in hospitals and the use of their time and skills. As the pace and complexity of hospital care increases, nursing work is expanding at both ends of the complexity continuum. Nurses often undertake tasks that less qualified staff could do, while at the other end of the spectrum they are unable to use their high-level skills and expertise. This inefficiency in the use of nursing time can also negatively affect patient outcomes. Nurses' work that does not directly contribute to patient care, engage higher-order cognitive skills, or provide opportunity for role expansion can decrease retention of well-qualified and highly skilled nurses in the health workforce (Duffield, Gardner, & Catling-Paull, 2008).

The major barrier to making progress in patient safety and quality is the failure to appreciate the complexity of the work in health care today. Current research focusing on work complexity and related issues enables an increased understanding of RN decision making (the invisible, cognitive work of nursing) in actual care situations and demonstrates how both the knowledge and competencies of RNs as well as the complex environments in which RNs provide care contribute to patient safety, quality of care, and healthy work environments or lack thereof (Ebright, 2010).

Krichbaum et al. (2007) identify a nurse care-delivery experience they term "complexity compression" and note this experience occurs when nurses are expected to assume, in a condensed time frame, additional, unplanned responsibilities while simultaneously conducting their other multiple responsibilities. Nurses report that personal, environmental, practice, administrative, system, and technology factors, as well as autonomy and control factors, all contribute to this experience. Associated with complexity compression is the phenomenon of stacking. Stacking is the invisible, decision-making work of RNs about the what, how, and when of delivering nursing care to an assigned group of patients (Ebright, Patterson, Chalko, & Render, 2003). This process results in decisions about what care is needed, what care is possible, and when and how to deliver this care.

A commitment to understanding and appreciating the complexity involved in RN work is needed to guide the more substantive and sustained improvements required to achieve safety and quality. Attention to and action based on an understanding of the complexity of RN work and the value of safe, quality care; desired patient outcomes; and nurse recruitment and retention have the potential to achieve the goals of healthy work environments. Using complexity science to understand the work of nursing is becoming increasingly accepted as a very fitting approach to explaining healthcare organizational dynamics and the work of nursing (Lindberg & Lindberg, 2008).

Nursing Education

The healthcare system of the 21st century is complex, technologically rich, ethically challenging, and ever changing. The roles of all healthcare providers evolve continually, and boundaries of practice shift regularly. Knowledge explodes at unprecedented rates, and although the evidence base for practice grows stronger every day, healthcare providers must repeatedly make decisions and take action in situations that are characterized by ambiguity and uncertainty (Cowan & Moorhead, 2011).

Throughout the years, nursing education has made an effort to transition its curriculum and programs to accommodate the knowledge explosion and the advanced technology associated with health care. However, the transition within the programs of nursing has assumed a patchwork approach instead of significant reform. This is in part the result of the tradition associated with the history of nursing education, the inability to resolve the differences in prelicensure programs, and faculty propensity to be reluctant to "leave behind" what is no longer successful in a changing practice arena. In addition, nurse educators are caught in the "perfect storm" composed of a changing healthcare delivery system, changing practice models, nursing shortage, faculty shortage, changes in external standards of care and educational accreditation, university budget cuts, and changes in external funding that support new nursing programs.

In 2003, the IOM issued a report titled *Health Professions Education: A Bridge to Quality* (IOM, 2003a). This report, which focuses on knowledge that healthcare professionals need to provide quality care, states that students in the health professions are not prepared to address the shifts in the country's demographics nor are they educated to work in interdisciplinary teams. It further states that students were not able to access evidence for use in practice, determine the reasons for or prevent patient care errors, or access technology to acquire the latest information. Specifically, the report expresses concern with the adequacy of nursing education at all levels, yet focuses intensely on education at the prelicensure level. The report identifies five core competencies that all clinicians should possess: (1) provide patient-centered care, (2) work in interdisciplinary teams, (3) use evidence-based practice, (4) apply quality improvement and identify errors and hazards in care, and (5) utilize informatics (IOM, 2003a).

KEY COMPETENCY 5-4

Examples of Applicable *Nurse of the Future: Nursing Core Competencies*

Systems-Based Practice:

Knowledge (K2a) Understands the impact of macrosystem changes on planning, organizing, and delivering patient care at the work unit level

Attitudes/Behaviors (A2a) Appreciates the complexity of the work unit environment

Source: Massachusetts Department of Higher Education. (2010). *Nurse of the future: Nursing core competencies* (p. 19). Retrieved from http://www.mass.edu/currentInlt/documents/NursingCoreCompetencies.pdf

In 2005, the National Council of State Boards of Nursing (NCSBN) released five recommendations regarding prelicensure clinical instruction. These recommendations address the appropriate or desired setting of clinical experience, the scope of clinical experience, the qualifications of clinical faculty, the role of nursing faculty in clinical education, and the need for research. The NCSBN board has also done work associated with postgraduate nurse competence that includes clinical reasoning and judgment, patient care delivery and management skills, communication and interpersonal relationships, and recognizing limits and seeking help (Li, 2007).

Despite these changes, new standards of instruction, and new competencies for postgraduates, the educational preparation of nurses has remained virtually unchanged for more than 50 years. Nursing education remains content focused and teacher centered (Valiga & Champagne, 2011). Recently the results of two national studies reinforced the belief that nursing education must be reformed. The two reports, *Educating Nurses: A Call for Radical Transformation* (Benner, Sutphen, Leonard, & Day, 2010) and *The Future of Nursing: Leading Change, Advancing Health* (IOM, 2011), explore the issue of whether nurses are entering practice equipped with the knowledge and skills needed for today's practice and prepared to continue clinical learning for tomorrow's nursing, given the enormous changes in and complexity of current nursing practice and practice settings. In both reports the response is that nurses are not prepared for future healthcare change. Both reports challenge nursing education to make reforms in preparation of new graduates in terms of establishing new competencies and outcomes for graduates, new curriculum designs, new pedagogy, better evaluation models, and new models for clinical education, such as residency programs.

In response to the changes in healthcare delivery and the call for new roles in nursing, two new degrees have been introduced by the AACN since the turn of the century: the doctor of nursing practice and the clinical nurse leader (AACN, 2007). The **clinical nurse leader (CNL)** is an advanced generalist role prepared at the master's level of education. The CNL oversees the coordination of care for a group of patients, assesses cohort risk, provides direct patient care in complex situations, and functions as part of an interdisciplinary team (AACN, 2007). The lateral integration of care has been what is missing in the delivery of care to patients with complex needs. No single person oversees patient care laterally and over time and is able to intervene, facilitate, or coordinate care for the entire patient experience. The CNL will be instrumental in helping all disciplines see the interdependencies that exist between and among them (Begun, Hamilton, Tornabeni, & White, 2006).

The other new program within nursing is the **doctor of nursing practice (DNP)**. The need for this terminal practice degree is based on the series of reports from the IOM that address quality of health care, patient safety, and educational reform, as well as following the movement of other healthcare professions to the practice doctorate. After much national debate, it was determined that a practice doctorate was needed that encompasses any form of nursing intervention that influences healthcare outcomes for individual patients, management of care for individuals and populations, administration of nursing and health organization, and the development and implementation of health policy (AACN, 2004). It is clearly stated that this practice degree is not the same as the research doctoral degree and that graduates would be prepared to blend clinical, economic, organizational, and leadership skills and to use science in improving the direct care of patients, care of patient populations, and practice that supports patient care (Champagne, 2006).

The development of the DNP and the CNL programs of study represents a bold effort by the profession of nursing to address new roles of nursing and educational reform needed to prepare graduates to meet the healthcare needs of the future. Although questions and concerns related to the implementation of these new programs still exist, the evaluation of the implementation of these programs is mostly positive. One must applaud the spirit of evidence-based educational innovation.

Closing the Education and Practice Gap

The gap between education and practice looms larger as the healthcare setting continuously changes. In general, curriculums in nursing programs have not evolved to keep pace with changes in the practice setting; however, the current emphasis on integrating clinical simulation, the dedicated education unit, and nurse residency programs are steps in the right direction.

Evidence supports that a better-educated nurse is needed in practice. The initial educational preparation for the largest proportion of RNs is the associate degree. During the last national nurse survey in 2008, the initial educational level of RNs indicated that 20.4% were diploma, 45.4% were associate degree, and 34.2% were baccalaureate (HRSA, 2010). Leaders in nursing education must identify a way to move younger students to the desired graduate level of education more expediently.

Where do we go from here? The IOM report *The Future of Nursing: Leading Change, Advancing Health* provides us with a blueprint (IOM, 2011). The IOM and Robert Wood Johnson Foundation partnered to assess and respond to the need to transform nursing to ensure that the nursing workforce has the capacity, in terms of numbers, skills, and competence, to meet the present and future healthcare needs of the public. This transformation would enable nurses to be partners and leaders in advancing health for the future. The key messages of the study include: (1) nurses should practice to the full extent of their education and training, (2) nurses should achieve higher levels of education and training through an improved education system that promotes seamless academic

KEY COMPETENCY 5-6

Examples of Applicable *Nurse of the Future: Nursing Core Competencies*

Leadership:

Knowledge (K5) Explains the importance, necessity, and process of change

Skills (S5b) Anticipates consequences, plans ahead, and changes approaches to get best results

Attitudes/Behaviors (A5b) Values new ideas and interventions to improve patient care

Source: Massachusetts Department of Higher Education. (2010). *Nurse of the future: Nursing core competencies* (p. 18). Retrieved from http://www.mass.edu/currentinit/documents/NursingCoreCompetencies.pdf

CRITICAL THINKING QUESTIONS *

Based on the trends and recommendations presented in this chapter, what do you think nursing education will look like in 2025? What do you think the profession of nursing will look like in the year 2025? *

progression, (3) nurses should be full partners, with physicians and other health professionals, in redesigning health care in the United States, and (4) effective workforce planning and policy making require better data collection and an improved information infrastructure (IOM, 2011, p. 4). Recommendations include to: (1) remove scope-of-practice barriers, (2) expand opportunities for nurses to lead and diffuse collaborative improvement efforts, (3) implement nurse residency programs, (4) increase the proportion of nurses with a baccalaureate degree to 80% by 2020, (5) double the number of nurses with a doctorate by 2020, (6) ensure that nurses engage in lifelong learning, (7) prepare and enable nurses to lead change to advance health, and (8) build an infrastructure for the collection and analysis of interprofessional healthcare workforce data. It is imperative that professional nurses control their future and redefine their roles in practice; the recommendations and the strategies identified in this report provide the way.

Conclusion

Now, when you hear the word *nursing*, what image comes to mind? If the picture is blurry or confused by the expanding social context presented in this chapter—good! The cloudiness indicates that the tradition continues to be questioned. We have looked at some of the social phenomena and trends that help define nursing. Because those experiences change constantly, what we envision now will also be transformed. Are you ready to be a part of transforming professional nursing practice as we transition our profession into a future that continues to meet the needs of society?

References

Affordable Care Act. (2010). Read the law. Retrieved from http://www.healthcare.gov/law/full/

Agency for Healthcare Research and Quality. (2007). *Research news*. Washington, DC: Author.

Agency for Healthcare Research and Quality. (2010). 2010 national healthcare quality and disparities reports. Retrieved from http://www.ahrq.gov/qual/qrdr10.htm

Aiken, L., Clarke, S., Sloane, D., Sochalski, J., & Silber, J. (2002). Hospital nurse staffing and patient mortality, nurse burnout, and job dissatisfaction. *Journal of the American Medical Association*, 288(16), 1987–1993.

Almada, P., Carafoli, K., Flattery, J., French, D., & McNamara, M. (2004). Improving the retention rate of newly graduated nurses. *Journal for Nurses in Staff Development*, 20(6), 268–273.

American Association of Colleges of Nursing. (2004). AACN position statement on the practice doctorate in nursing. Retrieved from http://www.aacn.nche.edu/publications/position/DNPpositionstatement.pdf

American Association of Colleges of Nursing. (2007, February). *White paper on the education and role of the clinical nurse leader*. Washington, DC: Author.

American Association of Colleges of Nursing. (2008). Cultural competency in baccalaureate nursing education. Retrieved from http://www.aacn.nche.edu/leading-initiatives/education-resources/competency.pdf

American Association of Colleges of Nursing. (2012). *Enrollment and graduations in baccalaureate and graduate programs in nursing*. Washington, DC: Author.

American Association of Colleges of Nursing. (2014). Annual report 2014: Building a framework for the future. Retrieved from http://www.aacn.nche.edu/aacn-publications/annual-reports/AnnualReport14.pdf

American Association of Colleges of Nursing. (2015a). New AACN data confirm enrollment surge in schools of nursing. Retrieved from http://www.aacn.nche.edu/news/articles/2015/enrollment

American Association of Colleges of Nursing. (2015b). Nursing faculty shortage fact sheet. Retrieved from http://www.aacn.nche.edu/media-relations/FacultyShortageFS.pdf

American Hospital Association. (2003a). Strategies for leadership: Improving communications with patients and families. A blueprint for action. Retrieved from http://www.aha.org/advocacy-issues/communicatingpts/

American Hospital Association. (2003b). The patient care partnership: Understanding expectations, rights, and responsibilities. Retrieved from http://www.aha.org/aha/issues/Communicating-With-Patients/pt-care-partnership.html

American Nurses Association. (1992). *Position statement on registered nurse utilization of unlicensed assistive personnel*. Washington, DC: Author.

American Nurses Association. (1997). *Implementing nursing's report card: Study of RN staffing, length of stay, and patient outcomes*. Washington, DC: Author.

American Nurses Association. (1999). *Principles for nurse staffing*. Washington, DC: Author.

American Nurses Association. (2007). American Nurses Association recognizes the contributions of men in nursing with the (ANA) Luther Christman Award. *Wyoming Nurse, 20*(2), 13.

American Nurses Association. (2010). *Nursing's social policy statement: The essence of the profession*. Silver Spring, MD: Author.

American Nurses Association. (2011). NursingWorld.org health and safety survey. Retrieved from http://www.nursingworld.org/MainMenuCategories/WorkplaceSafety/Healthy-Work-Environment/Work-Environment/2011-HealthSafetySurvey.html

American Nurses Association. (2012). *Bullying in the workplace: Reversing a culture*. Silver Spring, MD: Author.

American Nurses Association. (2015). *Nursing: Scope and standards of practice* (3rd ed.). Silver Spring, MD: Author.

American Society of Registered Nurses. (2008). Men in nursing. Retrieved from http://www.asrn.org/journal-nursing/374-men-in-nursing.html

Armstrong, F. (2002). Not just women's business: Men in nursing. *Australian Nursing Journal, 9*(11), 24–26.

Beecroft, P., Dorey, F., & Wentin, M. (2008). Turnover intention in new graduate nurses: A multivariate analysis. *Journal of Advanced Nursing, 62*(11), 41–52.

Begun, J., Hamilton, J., Tornabeni, J., & White, K. (2006). Opportunities for improving patient care through lateral integration: The clinical nurse leader. *Journal of Healthcare Management, 51*(1), 19–25.

Benner, P., Sutphen, M., Leonard, V., & Day, L. (2010). *Educating nurses: A call for radical transformation.* San Francisco, CA: Jossey-Bass.

Berlin, L. E., Stennett, J., & Bednash, G. D. (2004). *2003–2004 enrollment and graduations in baccalaureate and graduate programs in nursing.* Washington, DC: American Association of Colleges of Nursing.

Betancourt, J. R., Green, A. R., Carrillo, J. E., & Ananeh-Firempong, O. (2003). Defining cultural competence: A practical framework for addressing racial/ethnic disparities in health and health care. *Public Health Report, 118*(4), 293–302.

Blais, K., Hayes, J. S., Kozier, B., & Erb, G. (2001). *Professional nursing practice: Concepts and perspectives* (4th ed.). Upper Saddle River, NJ: Pearson.

Brady, M. S., & Sherrod, D. R. (2003). Retaining men in nursing programs designed for women [Electronic version]. *Journal of Nursing Education, 42,* 159–163.

Brown, B. (2004). From the editor: Restoring caring back into nursing. *Nursing Administration Quarterly, 28,* 237–238.

Buerhaus, P., Auerbach, D., & Staiger, D. (2009, June 12). The recent surge in nurse employment: Causes and implications. *Health Affairs,* 657–668.

Bureau of Labor Statistics. (2012, January). Employment outlook, 2010–2020. Retrieved from http://www.bls.gov/opub/mlr/2012/01/mlr201201.pdf

Buresh, B., & Gordon, S. (2000). *From silence to voice: What nurses know and must communicate to the public.* New York, NY: Cornell University Press.

Buresh, B., & Gordon, S. (2006). *From silence to voice: What nurses know and must communicate to the public* (2nd ed.). New York, NY: Cornell University Press.

Cardillo, D. W. (2001). *Your first year as a nurse: Making the transition from total novice to successful professional.* Roseville, CA: Prima.

Centers for Disease Control and Prevention. (2012). Clinical outreach and communication activity (COCA). Retrieved from http://www.bt.cdc.gov/coca

Champagne, M. (2006). The future of nursing education: Educational models for future care. In P. Cowen & S. Moorhead (Eds.), *Current issues in nursing* (7th ed.). St. Louis, MO: Mosby Elsevier.

Chitty, K., & Campbell, C. (2001). The social context of nursing. In K. K. Chitty (Ed.), *Professional nursing: Concepts and challenges* (pp. 64–100). Philadelphia, PA: Saunders.

Chung, V. (2000). Men in nursing: Representing less than 1% of all working R.N.s, minority men are shattering stereotypes and making their mark on the nursing profession. *Minority Nurse,* Summer, 38–42.

Clark, J. (2004). An aging population with chronic disease compels new delivery systems focused on new structures and practice. *Nursing Administration Quarterly, 28,* 105–115.

Cooper, P. (2004). Nurse–patient ratios revisited [Editorial]. *Nursing Forum, 39*(2), 3–4.

Cowan, P., & Moorhead, S. (2011). Nursing education in transition. In P. S. Cowen & S. Moorhead (Eds.), *Current issues in nursing* (8th ed., pp. 72–74). St. Louis, MO: Mosby Elsevier.

Cram, E. (2011). Staff nurses working in hospitals: Who they are, what they do, and what are their challenges? In P. Cowen and S. Moorhead (Eds.), *Current issues in nursing* (8th ed., pp. 13–22). St. Louis, MO: Mosby Elsevier.

Dean, P. (2005). Transforming ethnocentricity in nursing: A culturally relevant experience of reciprocal visits between Malta and the Midwest. *Journal of Continuing Education in Nursing, 36*(4), 163, 167.

DeSantis, L., & Lipson, J. (2007). Brief history of inclusion of content on culture in nursing education. *Journal of Transcultural Nursing, 18*(7), 7s–9s.

Dohm, A., & Shniper, L. (2007, November). Occupational employment projections to 2016: Employment outlook: 2006-16. *Monthly Labor Review,* 86–125.

Duffield, C., Gardner, G., & Catling-Paull, C. (2008). Nursing work and the use of time. *Journal of Clinical Nursing, 17,* 3269–3274.

Ebright, P. (2010). The complex work of RNs: Implications for healthy work environments. *OJIN: The Online Journal of Issues in Nursing, 15*(1). doi:10.3912/OJIN.Vol15No01Man04

Ebright, P., Patterson, E., Chalko, B., & Render, M. (2003). Understanding the complexity of registered nurse work in acute care settings. *Journal of Nursing Administration, 33*(12), 630–638.

Ellison, D, & Farrar, F. C. (2015). Aging population. *Nursing Clinics of North America, 50*(1), 185–213.

Gibbs, D. M., & Waugaman, W. R. (2004). Diversity behind the mask: Ethnicity, gender, and past career experience in a nurse anesthesiology program [Electronic version]. *Journal of Multicultural Nursing and Health, 10,* 77–82.

Gordon, S. (2005). *Nursing against the odds: How health care cost cutting, media stereotypes, and medical hubris undermine nurses and patient care.* Ithaca, NY: Cornell University Press.

Gordon, S. (2010). *When chicken soup isn't enough: Stories of nurses standing up for themselves, their patients, and their profession.* Ithaca, NY: Cornell University Press.

Gordon, S., Buchanan, J., & Bretherton, T. (2008). *Safety in numbers: Nurse-to-patient ratios and the future of health care.* Ithaca, NY: Cornell University Press.

Grant, L. F., & Letzring, T. D. (2003). Status of cultural competence in nursing education: A literature review [Electronic version]. *Journal of Multicultural Nursing and Health, 9*(2), 6–13.

Groff-Paris, L., & Terhaar, M. (2010). Using Maslow's pyramid and the National Database of Nursing Quality Indicators to attain a healthier work environment. *OJIN: The Online Journal of Issues in Nursing, 16*(1), 1–8.

Health Careers Center. (2012). 2005 Mississippi men in nursing calendar. Retrieved from http://www.mshealthcareers.com/calendar/

Health Resources and Services Administration. (2002). *Projected supply, demand, and shortages of registered nurses: 2000–2020.* Washington, DC: Health Resources and Services Administration, Bureau of Health Professions, National Center for Health Workforce Analysis.

Health Resources and Services Administration. (2010, September). *The registered nurse population: Findings from the 2008 National Sample Survey of Registered Nurses.* Washington, DC: Health Resources and Services Administration, Bureau of Health Professions.

Howden, L. M., & Meyer, J. A. (2011). *Age and sex composition: 2010*. Washington, DC: U.S. Census Bureau. Retrieved from http://www.census.gov/prod/cen2010 /briefs/c2010br-03.pdf

Huntington, A., Gilmour, J., Tuckett, A., Neville, S., Wilson, D., & Turner, D. (2012). Is anybody listening? A qualitative study of nurses' reflections on practice. *Journal of Clinical Nursing, 20,* 1413–1422.

Institute of Medicine. (2003a). *Health professions education: A bridge to quality.* Washington, DC: National Academy Press.

Institute of Medicine. (2003b). *Unequal treatment: Confronting racial and ethnic disparities in health care.* Washington, DC: National Academy Press.

Institute of Medicine. (2009). Guidance for establishing standards of care for use in disaster situations. Retrieved from http://iom.nationalacademies.org/Reports/2009 /DisasterCareStandards.aspx

Institute of Medicine. (2011). *The future of nursing: Leading change, advancing health.* Washington, DC: National Academies Press.

Jacob, S. R., & Carnegie, M. E. (2002). Cultural competency and social issues in nursing and health care. In B. Cherry (Ed.), *Contemporary nursing: Issues, trends, and management* (pp. 239–262). St. Louis, MO: Mosby.

Kalisch, B., & Kyung, H. (2011). Nurse staffing levels and teamwork: A cross-sectional study of patient care units in acute care hospitals. *Journal of Nursing Scholarship, 43*(1), 82–88.

Kavanagh, K. H. (2001). Social and cultural dimensions of health and health care. In J. L. Creasia & B. Parker (Eds.), *Conceptual foundations: The bridge to professional nursing practice* (pp. 294–314). St. Louis, MO: Mosby.

Keogh, B., & O'Lynn, C. (2007). Male nurses' experiences of gender barriers: Irish and American perspectives. *Nurse Educator, 32*(6), 256–259.

Kovner, C., Brewer, C., Fairchild, S., Poornima, S., Hongsoo, K., & Djukic, M. (2007). Newly licensed RNs' characteristics, work attitudes, and intentions to work. *American Journal of Nursing, 107*(9), 58–70.

Krichbaum, K., Diemart, C., Jacox, L., Jones, A., Koenig, P., Mueller, C., & Disch, J. (2007). Complexity compression: Nurses under fire. *Nursing Forum, 42*(2), 86–95.

Laschinger, H., Finegan, J., & Welk, P. (2009). New graduate burnout: The impact of professional practice environment, workplace civility, and empowerment. *Nursing Economic$, 27*(6), 377–383.

Levine, K. (2012). When speaking the same language means speaking different languages. Retrieved from http://minoritynurse.com/when-speaking-the-same -language-means-speaking-different-languages/

Li, S. (2007). Assessing clinical competence and practice errors of newly licensed registered nurses. In P. Cowen & S. Moorhead (Eds.), *Current issues in nursing* (p. 93). St. Louis, MO: Mosby Elsevier.

Lindberg, C., & Lindberg, C. (2008). Nurses take note: A primer on complexity science. In C. Lindberg, S. Nash, & C. Lindberg (Eds.), *On the edge: Nursing in the age of complexity* (pp. 23–47). Bordentown, NJ: Plexus.

Littel, K. (2001). Sexual assault nurse examiner (SANE) programs: Improving the community response to sexual assault victims. Retrieved from http://www.vawnet .org/Assoc_Files_VAWnet/OVC_SANE0401-186366.pdf

Longo, J., & Sherman, R. (2006). Leveling horizontal violence. *Nursing Management, 38*(3), 34–37, 50–51.

Massachusetts Department of Higher Education. (2010). *Nurse of the future: Nursing core competencies*. Retrieved from http://www.mass.edu/currentinit/documents /NursingCoreCompetencies.pdf

McCue, M., Mark, B., & Harless, D. (2003). Nurse staffing, quality, and financial performance. *Journal of Healthcare Finance, 29*(4), 54–76.

Meyers, S. (2003). Real men choose nursing [Electronic version]. *Hospitals and Health Networks, 77*(6), 72–74.

National Advisory Council on Nurse Education and Practice. (2003). Third report to the Secretary of Health and Human Services and the Congress. Retrieved from http://www.hrsa.gov/advisorycommittees/bhpradvisory/nacnep/Reports /thirdreport.pdf

National Center for Complementary and Alternative Medicine. (2012). Complementary, alternative, or integrative health: What's in a name? Retrieved from http://nccam .nih.gov/health/whatiscam

National Council of State Boards of Nursing. (2005). Clinical instruction in prelicensure programs. Retrieved from https://www.ncsbn.org/3951.htm

Needleman, J., Buerhaus, P., Mattke, S., Stewart, M., & Zelevinsky, K. (2002). Nurse staffing levels and the quality of care in hospitals. *New England Journal of Medicine, 346*, 1715–1722.

Oregon Center for Nursing. (2002). Are you man enough ... to be a nurse? Retrieved from http://oregoncenterfornursing.org/resources/nursing-posters/

Pellico, L., Djukic, M., Kovner, C., & Brewer, C. (2009). Moving on, up, or out: Changing work needs of new RNs at different stages of their beginning nursing practice. *OJIN: The Online Journal of Issues in Nursing, 15*(1). doi:10.3912/OJIN. Vol15No01PPT02

PricewaterhouseCooper's Health Research Institute. (2007, July). What works: Healing the healthcare staffing shortage. Retrieved from http://www.pwc.com/extweb /pwcpublications.nsf/docid/674D1E79A678A0428525730D006B74A9

Purnell, L., & Paulanka, B. (2008). *Transcultural health care: A culturally competent approach* (3rd ed.). Philadelphia, PA: F. A. Davis.

Ray, M., & Ream, K. (2007). The dark side of the job: Violence in the emergency department. *Journal of Emergency Nursing, 33*(3), 257–261.

Riffkin, R. (2014). Americans rate nurses highest on honesty, ethical standards. Retrieved from http://www.gallup.com/poll/180260/americans-rate-nurses-highest -honesty-ethical-standards.aspx

Robert Wood Johnson Foundation. (2009, April 17). Has the recession solved the nursing shortage? Experts say no. Retrieved from http://www.rwjf.org/newsroom /product.jsp?id=41728

Rocker, C. F. (2008). Addressing nurse-to-nurse bullying to promote nurse retention. *The Online Journal of Issues in Nursing, 13*(3). doi:10.3912/OJIN.Vol13No03PPT05

Santiago, A. (2012). Forensic nursing careers. Retrieved from http://healthcareers .about.com/od/nursingcareers/a/ForensicNursing.htm

Schmalenberg, C., & Kramer, M. (2008). Essentials of a productive nurse work environment. *Nursing Research, 57*(1), 2–13.

Sigma Theta Tau International. (1998). *The Woodhull study on nursing and the media: Health care's invisible partner*. Indianapolis, IN: STTI Center Nursing Press.

Smith-Pittman, M., & McKoy, Y. (1999). Workplace violence in healthcare environments. *Nursing Forum, 34*(3), 5–13.

Sofer, D. (2005). You get what you pay for: News flash: Higher nurse–patient ratios still save lives. *American Journal of Nursing, 105*(11), 20.

Stanton, M., & Rutherford, M. (2004). How many nurses are enough? Hospital staff nursing and quality care research. *Accidents and Emergency Nursing, 15*(1), 1–2.

Sullivan Commission. (2004). Missing persons: Minorities in the health professions. A report of the Sullivan Commission on diversity in the health care workforce. Retrieved from http://health-equity.pitt.edu/40/

Tri-Council for Nursing. (2010). Joint statement from the Tri-Council for Nursing on recent registered nurse supply and demand projections. Retrieved from http://www.tricouncilfornursing.org/documents/JointStatementRecentRNSupplyDemand Projections.pdf

Trossman, S. (2003). Caring knows no gender: Break the stereotype and boost the number of men in nursing. *American Journal of Nursing, 103,* 65–68.

U.S. Census Bureau. (2001). *An aging world: 2001.* Retrieved from http://www.census.gov/prod/2001pubs/p95-01-1.pdf

U.S. Department of Health and Human Services. (2010). The registered nurse population: Initial findings from the 2008 National Sample Survey of Registered Nurses. Retrieved from http://bhpr.hrsa.gov/healthworkforce/rnsurveys/rnsurveyinitial2008.pdf

U.S. Department of Health and Human Services. (2014). Healthy people 2020: Older adults. Retrieved from https://www.healthypeople.gov/2020/topics-objectives/topic/older-adults

Valente, S., & Bullough, V. (2004). Sexual harassment of nurses in the workplace. *Journal of Nursing Care Quality, 19*(3), 234–241.

Valiga, T., & Champagne, M. (2011). Creating the future of nursing education: Challenges and opportunities. In P. Cowen & S. Moorhead (Eds.), *Current issues in nursing* (pp. 75–83). St. Louis, MO: Mosby Elsevier.

White House. (2012). *Joining forces.* Retrieved from http://www.whitehouse.gov/joiningforces

Zimmerman, P. (2006). Who should provide nursing care? In P. Cowen & S. Moorhead (Eds.), *Current issues in nursing* (7th ed., pp. 324–331). St. Louis, MO: Mosby Elsevier.

CHAPTER 6

Education and Socialization to the Professional Nursing Role

Kathleen Masters and Melanie Gilmore

Learning Objectives

After completing this chapter, the student should be able to:

1. Discuss the essentlal features of nursing.
2. Describe the stages of educational socialization.
3. Describe the process of socialization or formation in professional nursing.
4. Identify factors that facilitate professional role development.

Nursing continues to evolve into a profession with a distinct body of knowledge, specialized practice, and standards of practice. According to the American Nurses Association (ANA), "nursing is a learned profession built on a core body of knowledge that reflects its dual components of science and art" (2015b, p. 7), and as such is a scientific discipline as well as a profession. The science of nursing, based on the nursing process, is an analytical framework for critical thinking. Nursing practice also requires knowledge of the principles of biological, physical, behavioral, and social sciences. The art of nursing is based on respect for human dignity and caring, although it is important to note that a compassionate approach to care carries a mandate to provide competent care. The professional nurse is responsible for practice that incorporates this specialized body of knowledge and standards of practice with care that demonstrates respect and caring (ANA, 2015b).

Socialization to professional nursing is the process of acquiring the knowledge, skills, and sense of identity that are characteristic of the profession. It is a process by which a student internalizes the attitudes, beliefs, norms, values, and standards of the profession into his or her own behavior

Key Terms and Concepts

» Socialization
» Formation
» Professional values
» Novice
» Advanced beginner
» Competent
» Ethical comportment
» Proficient
» Salience
» Expert
» Role transition

pattern. Professional socialization has four goals: (1) to learn the technology of the profession—the facts, skills, and theory, (2) to learn to internalize the professional culture, (3) to find a personally and professionally acceptable version of the role, and (4) to integrate this professional role into all of the other life roles (Cohen, 1981).

Benner, Sutphen, Leonard, and Day (2010) make the case for using the term **formation** to describe this process that occurs over time because it better denotes "the development of perceptual abilities, the ability to draw on knowledge and skilled know-how, and a way of being and acting in practice and in the world" (p. 166). Whatever terminology is chosen, the process described in this chapter refers to the transformation of the layperson into a skilled nurse who is prepared to respond skillfully and respectfully to persons in need of nursing care, or, as described by Benner et al. (2010), "the lay student moves from *acting* like a nurse to *being* a nurse" (p. 177). This development of professional identity occurs initially through the formal educational process and culminates in the practice setting.

Professional Nursing Roles and Values

So, what is it that professional nurses do? The scope of nursing practice describes the "who," "what," where," "when," "why," and " how," of nursing practice (2015b, p. 2). The standards of professional nursing practice are authoritative statements that describe the duties that all registered nurses are expected to competently perform. The standards of professional nursing practice are composed of standards of practice and standards of professional performance. The standards of practice describe competent nursing care as demonstrated by use of the nursing process. The standards of professional performance describe a competent level of behavior in the professional nursing role (ANA, 2015, pp. 3–5). See Appendix A for list of the standards of professional nursing practice.

According to the ANA, there are seven essential features of nursing that include the provision of a caring relationship that facilitates health and healing, attention to the range of experiences and responses to health and illness within the physical and social environments, and integration of assessment data with knowledge gained from an appreciation of the patient or group. In addition, nursing includes the application of scientific knowledge to the processes of diagnosis and treatment through the use of judgment and critical thinking, advancement of professional nursing knowledge through scholarly inquiry, influence on social and public policy to promote social justice, and assurance of safe, quality, and evidence-based practice (2010, p. 9).

The American Association of Colleges of Nursing (2008, p. 7) lists the roles of the professional nurse as provider of care, designer/manager/coordinator of care, and member of a profession. As a provider of direct and indirect care, the nurse is a patient advocate and patient educator. In addition, the nurse provides care based on best, current evidence and from a holistic, patient-centered perspective. Professional nurses are members of the healthcare team delivering care in an increasingly complex healthcare environment. Nurses function autonomously and interdependently within the healthcare team to provide patient care and are accountable for the care provided and for the tasks delegated to others. The nurse as a professional implies the formation of a professional identity and accountability for the professional image portrayed. Nursing requires a broad knowledge base for practice as well as strong communication, critical reasoning, clinical judgment, and assessment skills. In addition, professional nursing requires the development of an appropriate value set and ethical framework for practice (2008, p. 9).

Professional values are beliefs or ideals that guide interactions with patients, colleagues, other professionals, and the public. Professional values are considered a component of excellence, and the existence of a code is considered a hallmark of professionalism. The development of professional values begins with professional education in nursing and continues along a continuum throughout the years of nursing practice. Professional values associated with nursing are outlined in the ANA's *Code of Ethics* (ANA, 2001, 2015a). The values of (1) commitment to public service, (2) autonomy, (3) commitment to lifelong learning and education, and (4) a belief in the dignity and worth of each person epitomize the caring, professional nurse.

Nursing is a helping profession directed toward health promotion and disease prevention for individuals, families, and communities. Caring is a concept central to the profession of nursing. Inherent in this value is a strong commitment to public service. The role of the nurse is focused on assessing and promoting the health and well-being of all humans. Registered nurses remain in nursing to promote, advocate, and strive to protect the health and safety of patients, families, and communities (ANA, 2015b).

Autonomy is the right to self-determination as a profession. The role of the professional nurse is to honor and assist individuals and families to make informed decisions about health care and provide information so that they can make informed choices. The professional nurse respects patients' rights to make decisions about their health care.

Commitment to lifelong learning and education is necessary in the dynamic healthcare arena that surrounds nursing practice in this century. Nurses need continuous education to maintain a safe level of practice and expand their level of competence as professionals. With new technologies and the rapid growth of medical and nursing knowledge, the nurse must actively and continuously seek to expand professional knowledge. Professional nursing

KEY COMPETENCY 6-1

Examples of Applicable *Nurse of the Future: Nursing Core Competencies*

Professionalism:

Knowledge (K4a) Describes factors essential to the promotion of professional development

Skills (S4a) Participates in life-long learning

Attitudes/Behaviors (A4a) Committed to life-long learning

Source: Massachusetts Department of Higher Education. (2010). *Nurse of the future: Nursing core competencies* (p. 13). Retrieved from http://www.mass.edu/currentinit/documents/NursingCoreCompetencies.pdf

CRITICAL THINKING QUESTIONS *

As a nursing student, do you share the values of commitment to public service, autonomy, commitment to lifelong learning and education, and the belief in the dignity and worth of each person? Do nurses with whom you have interacted demonstrate these values? *

involves a commitment to be resourceful, to respond to the dynamic challenges of delivering health care, to incorporate technology into their caring, and to remain visionaries as the future unfolds (ANA, 2010).

Human dignity is respect for the inherent worth and uniqueness of individuals and communities and is such a deeply held value in the profession of nursing that it is the topic of Provision 1 in the *Code of Ethics for Nurses* (ANA, 2015a). According to the International Council of Nurses' *Code of Ethics for Nurses* (2012), "inherent in nursing is respect for human rights, including cultural rights, the right to life and choice, to dignity and to be treated with respect. Nursing care is respectful of and unrestricted by considerations of age, color, creed, culture, disability or illness, gender, sexual orientation, nationality, politics, race or social status" (p. 1).

The Socialization (or Formation) Process

Socialization into a profession is a process of adapting to and becoming a part of the culture of the profession (Ousey, 2009). This process begins during the student's formal educational program and continues after graduation and licensure in the practice setting.

Socialization Through Education

Students new to the nursing profession begin to learn the role while still in the educational setting. Cohen (1981) used the theories of cognitive development to develop a model of professional nursing socialization through education. The model describes four stages students must experience as they begin to internalize the roles of a profession. In stage 1, Unilateral Dependence, the individual places complete reliance on external controls and searches for the one right answer (Cohen, 1981, p. 16). In essence, the student looks to the instructor for the right answers and is unlikely to question the authority. As the student gains foundational knowledge and skill, there begins the process of questioning the authority.

During stage 2, Negative/Independence, the student begins to pull away from external controls and is characterized by cognitive rebellion. The student begins to think critically and begins to question the instructor and relies more on his or her own judgments.

Stage 3, Dependence/Mutuality, marks the beginning of empathy and commitment to others (Cohen, 1981, p. 18). In this stage, the student begins to apply knowledge to practice and tests information and facts. "Students have a knowledge base upon which to anchor critical thought and can relate new material to their previous knowledge base" (Cohen, 1981, p. 18). In this stage, the student is actively engaged in the learning, thinking through problems. For this stage to emerge, the learning environment must support and value risk taking. The role of the teacher is that of coach, mentor, and senior learner. The mentor helps the student link theory to practice while in the clinical areas, thus helping the student to learn from experiences and to improve practices to support professional socialization.

Stage 4, Interdependence, occurs when neither mutuality nor autonomy is dominant. Learning from others and gaining the ability to solve problems independently are evident. This is the stage of the professional lifelong learner who demonstrates reflection in practice and is responsible for continued learning. Professional socialization toward the stage of interdependence requires a supportive educational climate that values autonomy, independent thinking, and authenticity. Students become professionals.

Professional Formation

Several models in the literature describe professional socialization. Regardless of the model embraced, socialization into the nursing profession or formation into a professional nurse must include new competencies for the 21st century. The Institute of Medicine (IOM, 2011) reported that nurses need requisite competencies including leadership, health policy, system improvement, research and evidence-based practice, and teamwork and collaboration to meet the needs of the current dynamic healthcare environment. Nursing educators must provide students with opportunities to develop the requisite skills that equip them for the profession as well as instill in them the desire to become lifelong learners because nurses currently need continuous education to maintain a safe level of practice and expand their level of competence as professionals.

Benner (1984) describes the development of the professional clinical practice of nurses. Benner's model identifies the stages of novice, advanced beginner, competent, proficient, and expert that are based on the nurse's experience in practice. With an understanding of this progression of knowledge and skills, educational programs have developed supportive curricula using a continuum of experiences to enhance skill and knowledge development. Healthcare environments have also incorporated this model to facilitate the nurse's professional practice by assessing the nurse's stage of development. This model is not limited to the student experience or to that of the new graduate nurse. Experienced nurses also benefit from experiences designed to move the nurse toward the stage of expert.

The first stage, **novice**, is characterized by a lack of knowledge and experience. In this stage, the facts, rules, and guidelines for practice are the focus. Rules for practice are context free, and the student task is to acquire

> **KEY COMPETENCY 6-2**
>
> Examples of Applicable *Nurse of the Future: Nursing Core Competencies*
>
> Professionalism:
>
> Knowledge (K4c) Understands the importance of reflection to advancing practice and improving outcomes of care
>
> Skills (S4b) Demonstrates ability for reflection in action, reflection for action, and reflection on action
>
> Attitudes/Behaviors (A4c) Values and is committed to being a reflective practitioner
>
> *Source:* Massachusetts Department of Higher Education. (2010). *Nurse of the future: Nursing core competencies* (p. 13). Retrieved from http://www.mass.edu/currentinit/documents/NursingCoreCompetencies.pdf

the knowledge and skills. The stage of novice is not related to the age of the student but rather to the knowledge and skill in the area of study. For example, learning how to give injections would be presented with the procedural guidelines, and the novice would then practice the skill. At this stage, much of the student's energy and attention are aimed at remembering the rules. Because the focus is on remembering rules, the student's practice is inflexible, the student is unable to use discretionary judgment, and the student is dependent on and has confidence in those with greater expertise rather than having confidence in his or her own judgment (Benner, 1984; Benner, Tanner, & Chelsea, 2009). This stage can be compared to an experience that most nursing students can relate to, the experience of learning to drive a car. Initially, the experience is characterized by halting progress as the student driver actively tries to gauge the pressure required on the gas pedal and the brake, remember how many feet before the corner to use the turn signal, and how many feet to keep between cars. Obviously, this analogy simplifies the stage of novice related to nurse formation, but most can remember the excitement and the frustrations of learning to drive a car, and also remember the transition when driving began to require less effort.

In the next stage, **advanced beginner**, the nurse can formulate principles that dictate action. For example, the advanced beginner grasps the rationale behind why different medications require different injection techniques. However, advanced beginners still lack the experience to know how to prioritize in more complex situations and might feel at a loss in terms of what they can safely leave out, making the patient care situation appear as a perplexing set of problems that they must figure out how to solve. The advanced beginner will still emphasize tasks that need to be accomplished as well as rules, but does not have the experience to adjust or adapt the rules to the situation. The nurse in the stage of advanced beginner still requires guidance. Given the complexity of nursing practice and the range of clinical experiences, new graduates can be described as advanced beginners (Benner, 1984; Benner et al., 2009).

Benner's stage 3, **competent**, is characterized by the ability to look at situations in terms of principles, analyze problems, and prioritize, and thus a nurse in this stage has the ability to plan as well as to alter plans as necessary. The nurse in this stage has improved time management and organizational skills as well as technical skills. The nurse in the competent stage will also demonstrate increased ability in diagnostic reasoning, which means he or she is able to make a clinical case for action to other members of the healthcare team. Movement from one stage to the next does not cross distinct boundaries, but the nurse at this stage has had experience in a variety of clinical situations and can draw on prior knowledge and experience; typically, the nurse will have 1–2 years of experience in a similar job situation. The competent stage of learning is important in the formation of the **ethical comportment** of the nurse. Ethical comportment refers to good conduct born out of an individualized relationship with the patient that involves engagement in a particular situation and entails a sense of membership in the relevant professional group. It is socially embedded, lived, and embodied in practices, ways of being, and responses to a clinical situation that promote the well-being of the patient (Day & Benner, 2002). Continued active learning and mentoring are important for movement to the proficient stage. Students who have the opportunity to have extended internships in a specialty area during their education can graduate entering this stage (Benner, 1984; Benner et al., 2009).

Stage 4, **proficient**, refers to the professional nurse who can grasp the situation contextually as a whole and whose performance is guided by maxims. This nurse has a solid grasp of the norms as well as solid experiences that shed light on the variations from the norm. Based on an intuitive grasp of the situation, the nurse recognizes the most salient aspects of the situation or the most salient recurring meaningful components of the situation. **Salience** is a perceptual stance or embodied knowledge whereby aspects of a situation stand out as more or less important (Benner, 1984); therefore, the nurse at this stage knows what can wait and what cannot. The nurse has moved into a place where he or she can engage in a clinical situation and connect with the patient and family in ways that are truly beneficial. Incorporated into practice is the ability to test knowledge against situations that might not fit and to solve problems with alternative approaches. In this stage, the professional tests the rules and theories and looks at cases that can lead to developing alternative rules and theories. One might say that this is the stage when the professional begins to "break the rules" because he or she sees that the rules do not always apply. Achieving this level of proficiency in nursing typically takes 3–5 years of practice with similar patient populations (Benner, 1984; Benner et al., 2009).

Benner's final stage, **expert**, means the nurse has moved beyond a fixed set of rules. The expert has an internalized understanding grounded in a wealth of experience as well as depth of knowledge. The expert nurse is able to skillfully manage multiple tasks simultaneously. The expert nurse has a grasp of the whole with an ability to move beyond the immediate clinical situation but remain attuned to the clinical situation at a level that allows a "mindful reading" of the patient responses even without conscious deliberation. The nurse may have difficulty explaining how he or she knows something because the recognition and assessment language are so linked with actions and outcomes that they are obvious to the expert nurse, although not obvious to others. The expert is always learning and always questioning using subjective and objective knowing. Benner (1984; Benner et al., 2009) proposes that not all nurses can obtain this stage; when it is obtained, it is only after extensive experience.

The typical career in nursing is not a linear process. There is considerable variation in progression of nurses related to degree attainment and career growth. In addition, with the focus of increasing the percentage of nurses with baccalaureate degrees and doctoral degrees in nursing (IOM, 2011), many nurses are returning to school for additional academic degrees in order to advance their careers. This often results in a change in the nurse's practice role. It can be stressful to transition from a role where the nurse is an expert to a new role where the nurse will not function at the same level of expertise. For example, when the expert pediatric nurse graduates from a pediatric nurse practitioner program, passes the certification exam, and begins to function in the advanced practice role, the nurse will not be an expert pediatric nurse practitioner. With experience in the new, advanced practice role, he or she will again transition through the stages of professional development. The same type of **role transition** occurs when the expert clinician changes practice roles to become a nurse educator or nurse researcher.

Facilitating the Transition to Professional Practice

Professional socialization requires that the student learn the technology of the profession, learn to internalize the professional culture, find a personally and professionally acceptable version of the role, and integrate this professional role into all of his or her other life roles (Cohen, 1981). Students are taught an ideal, theoretical, research-based practice that shelters them from the realities of the world where nursing practice consists of not only theory and research, but also human emotion and response, along with the policies and procedures of the particular working environment. This concept of idealism is important to the profession because it contributes to a high standard of professional practice. The perceived disconnect between education and practice is known as role discrepancy. Therefore, when students enter the practice environment, the culture of the classroom and the culture of clinical practice can seem worlds apart. *Reality shock* has been the traditional phrase to describe the transition from nursing student to registered nurse (Kramer, 1974).

Reality shock occurs when the perceived role (how an individual believes he or she should perform in a role) comes into conflict with the performed role (Catalano, 2009). Many new graduates experience this reality shock of knowing what to do and how to do it but encountering circumstances that prevent them from performing the role in that way. Role conflict exists when a nurse cannot integrate the ideal, the perceived, and the actual performed role into one professional role.

Role transition shock is the experience of moving from the known role of student to the role of practicing professional (Duchscher, 2009). For many nursing students, role conflict occurs when they transition from the role of student to that of registered nurse (Pellico, Brewer, & Kovner, 2009). The new graduate moves from a perceived role of what the professional nurse is and does to the actual performed role where his or her actions and beliefs might be challenged.

What do you think are the barriers to the process of professional socialization or formation? Do you think different environments might foster or hinder the process of professional socialization or formation? Do you think that personal characteristics of nurses might influence the process of professional socialization or formation? *

The reality shock or role transition shock that new graduates experience can be reduced to some extent. Many schools of nursing have implemented opportunities for externships or prolonged preceptor clinical experiences with a professional nurse before graduation. Research (Ruth-Sahd, Beck, & McCall, 2010) shows how participation in extern programs eases the gap between education and practice. One goal of this experience is to help the student assimilate the role of the professional nurse just before graduation. During this time, the student can experience a more realistic view of clinical practice in the real world environment. As one student commented, "All the lectures and assignments in nursing school cannot compare with the application of theory that this externship offered" (Ruth-Sahd et al., 2010, p. 83). Externships and preceptor clinical experiences can help nursing students begin the role transition from perceived role expectations to actual role expectations, thus easing the transition from student nurse to practicing professional.

In addition to programs before the graduation of the nurse, some hospitals are also offering nurse residency programs to facilitate the socialization into the profession. Hospitals offer formalized graduate nurse residency programs or internships that provide graduates with rotations through a number of clinical areas that include preceptor support. After the completion of such programs, new nurses gain a sense of belonging and the programs enhance socialization into the clinical workplace (McKenna & Newton, 2009). In addition to formal education, preceptors can assist students to develop skills of assertion, reflection, and critical thinking that are required to provide holistic, evidence-based care (Mooney, 2007).

Conclusion

The goal in the socialization of nurses today and for the future is to achieve caring with autonomy. The challenge for the profession is capitalizing on the strengths of everyone and finding a means of accommodating all individuals as a way of maintaining the viability of the profession (Leduc & Kotzer, 2009). Professional socialization of nurses in a profession that fully embraces caring for self and others reflects the internalization of what Roach (1991) refers to as "the five C's: compassion, competence, confidence, conscience, and commitment" (p. 132), representing a framework for human response from which professional caring is expressed.

Nursing education should be humanistic and caring, with caring experts as role models who contribute to the socialization of future generations of nurses and help them become caring experts in nursing practice. Through their research, Condon and Sharts-Hopko (2010) report that reflection can be an effective means of understanding human emotion and responses. One student stated, "I think the most important time is after the clinical training when I go home. I think about the information I get from the patient. What does it mean? What does it mean for the patient? I should connect to it" (Condon & Sharts-Hopko, 2010, p. 169). Regarding role development and socialization, it is important to remember that we learn what we live (Becker-Hentz, 2004).

Classroom Activity 1

Incorporate actual quotes from the nurses who were interviewed in Benner's book *From Novice to Expert* (1984) in class discussions to illustrate the differences among each of the stages: novice, advanced beginner, competent, proficient, and expert. This activity is simple but enlightening to students.

Classroom Activity 2

Read excerpts from the 2006 article *What Do Nurses Really Do?* by Suzanne Gordon (available at www.medscape.com/viewarticle/520714) in class to stimulate discussion, and ask the following questions:

- What do you think nurses actually do?
- What do you think about the current image of nurses?
- What do you think about the impact of the focus on caring over the knowledge of nurses?

Classroom Activity 3

As a follow-up to the previous activity, you may want to share a more recent Suzanne Gordon article, available at http://suzannecgordon.com/new-article-in-international-nursing-review/.

References

American Association of Colleges of Nursing. (2008). *The essentials of baccalaureate education for professional nursing practice*. Washington, DC: Author.

American Nurses Association. (2001). *Code of ethics for nurses with interpretive statements*. Washington, DC: Author.

American Nurses Association. (2010). *Nursing's social policy statement: The essence of the profession*. Silver Spring, MD: Author.

American Nurses Association. (2015a). *Code of ethics for nurses with interpretive statements*. Silver Spring, MD: Author.

American Nurses Association. (2015b). *Nursing: Scope and standards of practice* (3rd ed.). Silver Spring, MD: Author.

Becker-Hentz, P. (2004). *Understanding relationships: Learning what we live*. Unpublished manuscript.

Benner, P. (1984). *From novice to expert*. Menlo-Park, CA: Addison-Wesley.

Benner, P., Sutphen, M., Leonard, V., & Day, L. (2010). *Educating nurses: A call for radical transformation*. San Francisco, CA: Jossey-Bass.

Benner, P. E., Tanner, C. A., & Chelsea, C. A. (2009). *Expertise in nursing practice: Caring, clinical judgment, and ethics* (2nd ed.). New York, NY: Springer.

Catalano, J. (2009). *Nursing now!* (5th ed.). Philadelphia, PA: F. A. Davis.

Cohen, H. A. (1981). *The nurse's quest for a professional identity*. Menlo-Park, CA: Addison-Wesley.

Condon, E., & Sharts-Hopko, N. (2010). Socialization of Japanese nursing students. *Nursing Education Perspectives, 31*(3), 167–169.

Day, L., & Benner, P. (2002). Ethics, ethical comportment, and etiquette. *American Journal of Critical Care, 11*(1), 76–79.

Duchscher, J. E. B. (2009). Transition shock: The initial stage of role adaptation for newly graduated registered nurses. *Journal of Advanced Nursing, 65*(5), 1103–1113. doi:10.1111/j.1365-2648.2008.04898.x

Gordon, S. (2006). *What do nurses really do? Topics in advanced practice ejournal, 6*(1). Retrieved from http://www.medscape.com/viewarticle/520714

Institute of Medicine. (2011). *The future of nursing: Leading change, advancing health*. Washington. DC: National Academies Press.

International Council of Nurses. (2012). *The ICN code of ethics for nurses*. Geneva, Switzerland: Author. Retrieved from http://www.icn.ch/images/stories/documents/about/icncode_english.pdf

Kramer, M. (1974). *Reality shock, why nurses leave nursing*. St. Louis, MO: Mosby.

Leduc, K., & Kotzer, M. (2009). Bridging the gap: A comparison of the professional nursing values of students, new graduates and seasoned professionals. *Nursing Education Perspectives, 30*(5), 279–284.

Massachusetts Department of Higher Education. (2010). *Nurse of the future: Nursing core competencies*. Retrieved from http://www.mass.edu/currentinit/documents/NursingCoreCompetencies.pdf

McKenna, L., & Newton, J. M. (2009). After the graduate year: A phenomenological exploration of how new nurses develop their knowledge and skill over the first 18 months following graduation. *Contemporary Nurse: A Journal for the Australian Nursing Profession, 31*(2), 153–162.

Mooney, M. (2007). Professional socialization: The key to survival as a newly qualified nurse. *International Journal of Nursing Practice*, *30*, 75–80.

Ousey, K. (2009). Socialization of student nurses—the role of the mentor. *Learning in Health and Social Care*, *8*(3), 175–184.

Pellico, L. H., Brewer, C. S., & Kovner, C. T. (2009). What newly licensed registered nurses have to say about their first experiences. *Nursing Outlook*, *57*, 194–203.

Roach, M. S. (1991). Creating communities of caring. In National League for Nursing (Ed.), *Curriculum revolution: Community building and activism* (pp. 123–138). New York, NY: National League for Nursing Press.

Ruth-Sahd, L. A., Beck, J., & McCall, C. (2010). Transformative learning during a nursing externship program: The reflections of senior nursing students. *Nursing Education Perspectives*, *31*(2), 78–83.

CHAPTER 7

Advancing and Managing Your Professional Nursing Career

Mary Louise Coyne and Cynthia Chatham

Learning Objectives

After completing this chapter, the student should be able to:

1. Discuss the difference between a job and a career.
2. Articulate the importance of proactively managing his or her nursing career.
3. Discuss the benefits of a mentoring relationship.
4. Explore the impact of work-related stress.

Successful management of your professional nursing career does not occur by accident or default. Rather, it is a deliberate, purposeful, informed process requiring self-appraisal of your need for further professional growth and development, attentiveness to projected trends in healthcare delivery, dialogue with nurse colleagues who have demonstrated success in advancing their careers, exploration of nursing education programs that will support your career advancement, consideration of how to balance work and study demands and remain healthy, and investment of self to pursue these professional nursing career options. Be reflective and proactive in seizing opportunities to shape and refine your professional nursing career.

Key Terms and Concepts

» Career management
» Professional portfolio
» Mentoring
» Burnout
» Compassion fatigue

Nursing: A Job or a Career?

Your initial motivators for choosing to become a professional registered nurse (RN) may be far different from the reasons why you stay in professional nursing practice. Over time, nurses begin to appreciate that the practice of professional nursing as a career is a serious, sustained, and rewarding undertaking, dedicated to "the protection, promotion, and optimization of health and abilities, prevention of illness and injury, facilitation of healing, alleviation of suffering through the diagnosis and treatment of human response, and advocacy in the care of individuals, families, groups, communities, and populations" (American Nurses Association [ANA], 2015b, p. 1). Further, many seasoned nurses come to realize that a career in professional nursing requires academic preparation at the Bachelor of Science in Nursing (BSN) degree level or higher, engagement in lifelong learning to expand knowledge and clinical and management competencies, willingness to translate research evidence into practice on a continuous basis, and commitment to advance the health of patients and the profession of nursing.

Professional nursing is a career to be managed and not just a job where you "punch in and punch out." **Table 7-1** compares two views of nursing as a job and as a career. In advocating for **career management** in nursing, Daggett (2014) notes:

> A degree and a nursing license might be the ticket that gets you started on the journey, but without a destination, an itinerary, and a map, you will not travel very far. Like any important journey, a career requires research and planning; otherwise, you risk missing opportunities and critical milestones along the way. One should always assess the current location before planning future directions. Just as you track progress with a map while on a road trip, you should have a plan for managing your career, lest you find yourself wandering in the wilderness without making any true progress toward your career goals. (p. 168)

Purposefully manage your career—no one else can do this for you! Do not rely on healthcare employers to manage your career. Your best interests are yours and yours alone. Your career management and your short- and long-term goals are yours. For the career-oriented nurse, goals usually include: (1) pursuit of an academic program to obtain a BSN degree or graduate-level nursing education for advanced practice, administration, teaching, or research within a specified time frame, and/or (2) assuming a new position within a healthcare organization that has more responsibility and accountability in order to advance his or her nursing career.

Direction is needed to accomplish these goals. Without such a career map, nurses may wander aimlessly. Where am I going? How am I going? Part of career management is having the map to accomplish goals. Career mapping provides nurses with a clear direction including short-term stops to accomplish goals and a realistic time of arrival at the ultimate career destination. This may include position changes within an agency or a change in agencies. The map includes the skills obtained, the skills needed, and the resources needed to obtain skills (Hein, 2012). The pathway usually includes yearly goals as well as long-term goals. Without goals, nurses may leave the profession or risk beginning to view nursing as only a job that pays the bills.

CRITICAL THINKING QUESTIONS ✳

Do you view nursing as a career or a job? What are your professional goals related to nursing? ✳

TABLE 7-1	Do You View Nursing as a Job or a Professional Career?	
Factor	**View Nursing as a Job**	**View Nursing as a Career**
Academic preparation	Obtains the least amount needed for nursing licensure	Obtains a BSN and often pursues an advanced nursing degree: Master of Science in Nursing (MSN), Doctor of Nursing Practice (DNP), and/or Doctor of Philosophy (PhD)
Continuing education	Obtains the minimum continuing education (CE) units required for licensure and/or the job	Engages in formal and informal lifelong learning experiences across the nurse's professional career in order to: • Deepen and broaden knowledge and skill competencies • Improve the delivery of safe, cost-effective, quality-based patient care • Improve patient outcomes
Level of commitment	Continues with the job as long as it meets his or her personal needs; expects reasonable work for reasonable pay; responsibility ends with shift	Actively and joyfully engages in practicing the art and science of professional nursing as a member and, possibly, leader in professional nursing initiatives within the nurse's healthcare agency and in professional nursing organizations (local, regional, state, national, and/or international levels)

Trends That Impact Nursing Career Decisions

Healthcare agencies are constantly changing, with the goal of providing care to the community while containing costs. Although there is sufficient evidence demonstrating a professional nursing shortage in many areas across the United States, healthcare agencies are confronted with escalating costs, stringent cost containment initiatives, streamlined reimbursement systems, and a plethora of state and federal regulations that often constrain how well or poorly these agencies are able to deliver health care. In response to these budgetary constraints, many hospitals have responded by moving traditional inpatient care to outpatient settings, hiring fewer professional nurses, training more unlicensed assistive nursing personnel, cutting nursing salaries, hiring more RNs to part-time positions to avoid providing health and retirement benefits, and relying on fewer RNs to cover unfilled positions.

As you consider how to advance your nursing career, it is critical to examine projected trends in health care, particularly as they apply to (1) where health care is delivered, (2) the type of practitioners needed, and (3) the nursing educational preparation required to provide this care. The U.S. Department of Labor, Bureau of Labor Statistics (2015) reported that 90% of RNs worked in the following areas:

- 29.73% in general medical surgical hospitals
- 23.6% in specialty (except psychiatric and substance abuse) hospitals
- 15.43% in psychiatric and substance abuse hospitals
- 15.33% in outpatient care centers
- 13.46% in home healthcare services
- 8.99% in skilled nursing care facilities
- 7.47% in physicians' offices

In forecasting the future needs of the U.S. healthcare delivery system, the Institute of Medicine (IOM, 2010) projects that by 2020, the profession of nursing will need to double the number of nurses with a doctorate and increase the number of nurse practitioners in hospitals, home health, hospice, and nursing homes. In addition, the American Association of Colleges of Nursing (AACN, 2015b) reports that the nursing shortage may be easing in some parts of the country, but the demand for RNs prepared with baccalaureate, master's, and doctoral degrees continues to increase (p. 2).

Investigate where the shortages are in the location where you will be practicing, what types of practitioners are needed to meet these needs, and what type of advanced nursing education is required for these positions. Remember, you are in charge of making choices that best fit your short- and long-term career goals. You are your own best advocate in planning your nursing career!

Crafting the direction of your professional nursing career and executing the plan is transformational. The IOM (2011) report, *The Future of Nursing: Leading Change, Advancing Health*, provides a blueprint on how the entire profession must be transformed in order to advance the health of patients and simultaneously direct needed changes in the healthcare delivery system. In setting the agenda for nursing's future, the IOM Committee on Nursing identified four key messages and eight related recommendations that have potential for the greatest impact and for accomplishment within the next decade. The four key messages are:

- Nurses should practice to the full extent of their education and training.
- Nurses should achieve higher levels of education and training through an improved education system that promotes seamless academic progression.
- Nurses should be full partners, with physicians and other healthcare professionals, in redesigning health care in the United States.
- Effective workforce planning and policy making require better data collection and an improved information infrastructure (IOM, 2011, p. 4).

The eight recommendations are:

- Remove scope of practice barriers
- Expand opportunities for nurses to lead and diffuse collaborative improvement efforts
- Implement nurse residency programs
- Increase the proportion of nurses with a baccalaureate degree to 80% by 2020
- Double the number of nurses with a doctorate by 2020
- Ensure that nurses engage in lifelong learning
- Prepare and enable nurses to lead change to advance health
- Build an infrastructure for the collection and analysis of interprofessional healthcare workforce data (IOM, 2011, pp. 9–14)

The IOM report on the future of nursing is a great starting point for setting your professional nursing career goals and planning your career trajectory. Careful deliberation on these initiatives and recommendations provides insight into the questions that you might ask in setting your own professional nursing career goals. See **Box 7-1** for a list of questions to ask yourself as you plan your career goals.

BOX 7-1 QUESTIONS TO ASK AS YOU PLAN YOUR CAREER GOALS

- What is the *future of nursing* for me?
- Am I currently practicing to the *fullest extent of my nursing education and training*? (IOM, 2011, Initiative 1)
- What *changes* need to occur in my current practice in order to actualize this personal vision of my career?
- What are the projected employment trends and opportunities for nursing in my area?
- Have I achieved the *highest level of education and training* (IOM, 2011, Initiative 2) to support my desired career goals?
- What career path am I best equipped for and motivated to pursue to *lead change and advance health*? Should I pursue a BSN, MSN, DNP, or PhD, and if so, what specialization should I consider: a nurse practitioner, a nurse educator, a nurse anesthetist, a nurse–midwife, a nurse researcher, and/or a nurse executive?
- Have I sought out and had a dialogue with seasoned colleagues who have demonstrated success in advancing their nursing careers and elicited their input on trends in nursing practice and nursing education options?
- Have I explored nursing education program options at accredited academic institutions that will support my career advancement interests?
- Have I pursued ways to pay for advancing my nursing education through reimbursement at work, state and federal scholarships and traineeships, and/or public and private foundations?
- How will I balance work/family/study demands and remain physically, psychologically, and financially healthy?
- Lastly and perhaps most importantly, am I ready to take action in advancing my professional nursing career?

Showcasing Your Professional Self

Showcasing your nursing story is an important aspect of career management and includes how you present yourself in your **professional portfolio** and in the interview process. A résumé and cover letter will assist in getting an interview, but a complete professional portfolio may be what secures you the new position. A portfolio provides several advantages, including self-enlightenment, career enhancement, a record of growth and development, a record of performance over time, and a tool for planning, and it can act as a resource for others looking to create one (Masor, 2013, p. 41).

A professional portfolio, whether a print or electronic version, contains a cover letter; a résumé; examples of accomplishments cited but not elaborated upon in your résumé; selections of quality projects, papers, presentations, teaching tools/programs, patient or nursing care forms, policies, or procedures that you may have developed or co-developed across your career; and copies of licensure, certifications, awards, and professional organizational membership cards. In today's culture, being bilingual can be a definite advantage. Each language and dialect, if appropriate, should be included in your portfolio including competencies in reading, understanding, speaking, and writing. Awards received can be a testament to your diligence in a position and willingness to go beyond the job requirements. Being an officer in an organization shows leadership abilities (Schmidt, n.d.).

The portfolio will look different depending on the position you are seeking and the competencies you wish to showcase. Examples of some differences in the portfolio based on experience and desired position are below.

- If you are applying for a first-time position as a new RN, the portfolio can be used to showcase your competencies, intellectual skills, and teamwork while a student. New graduates, in particular, have to showcase themselves to stand apart from other applicants (Health eCareers Network, 2012).
- If you are applying for an advanced practice position, the IOM (2011) recommends that the portfolio be used as a means to document competencies and experience with patient populations.
- If you are applying for a staff position, you may consider providing a short case study describing the types of patients you have cared for and the specific skills and competencies you demonstrated in caring for this patient population.
- If you are applying for a management position, you may consider providing examples of leadership/management situations you have been engaged in, such as decision-making situations, schedules completed, and quality improvement initiatives.

Your cover letter should be directed to the human resources director, one page in length, word-processed, and printed on white stock paper with black ink, and should clearly identify the correct title of the position you are seeking, the length of time you have been an RN, a request for an interview, and your contact information.

Your résumé provides a brief overview of your professional career. Most résumés contain the following sections: identification, education, licensure and certifications, professional nursing employment history, professional committee engagement, and professional nursing organizations. Most résumés are one page in length and order entries from most recent to distant. See **Figure 7-1** for an example résumé.

First impressions made during the interview are also important. Arriving early and dressing professionally are a good beginning. Being prepared with answers for potential questions will only enhance the impression you make. Information concerning the job requirements, including duties, patient census and type, salary, and benefits, should be provided by the interviewer. Your follow-up questions assist you in understanding the expectations of the position. In "What Every Nursing Student Should Know When Seeking Employment: An Interview Tip Sheet for Baccalaureate and Higher Degree Prepared Nurses," the AACN (n.d.c) discusses characteristics of the organization that the applicant should assess. These eight hallmarks or characteristics are in the following list. Prior to your interview, refer to the brochure, which is available on the AACN website, for specific questions under each of the categories. The brochure is available at www.aacn.nche.edu/students/career-resource-center.

- Manifest a philosophy of clinical care emphasizing quality, safety, interdisciplinary collaboration, continuity of care, and professional accountability.
- Recognize the value of nurses' expertise on clinical care quality and patient outcomes.
- Promote executive-level nursing leadership.
- Empower nurses' participation in clinical decision making and organization of clinical care systems.
- Demonstrate professional development support for nurses.
- Maintain clinical advancement programs based on education, certification, and advanced preparation.
- Create collaborative relationships among members of the healthcare team.
- Utilize technological advances in clinical care and information systems.

It is illegal for employers to ask certain questions. Knowing those questions and, more importantly, knowing the questions that are allowed are key in preparation for the interview. HR World (2015) is a helpful website that can be used in preparing for your interview. Many interviewers use silence as a tool to evaluate the candidate. Use the silence to gather your thoughts and let the interviewer break the silence. At the conclusion of the interview, thank the interviewer for his or her time and ask about the timeline in filling the position. Send a follow-up note thanking the person for the interview and state that you are looking forward to a response.

CRITICAL THINKING QUESTION ✳

What kind of first impression do you make when searching for a new position? ✳

Figure 7-1   Example résumé

NAME

123 Street Name

City, State, Zip Code

(area code) phone number

email address

EDUCATION

2013   ***Bachelor of Science in Nursing*** (BSN), College of Nursing, Name of University, City, State.

LICENSURE AND CERTIFICATIONS

2013–2015   ***Registered Nurse.*** Multi-State License, Mississippi Board of Nursing.

2013–2015   ***Advanced Cardiac Life Support Provider*** (ACLS). American Heart Association.

2010–2015   ***Basic Life Support Provider*** (BLS). American Heart Association.

PROFESSIONAL NURSING EMPLOYMENT HISTORY

2013–2015   ***Primary Care Nurse,*** Adult Medical Intensive Care Unit, Memorial Hospital at

Gulfport, Gulfport, Mississippi. Responsible for providing comprehensive and

rapid assessments and management of critically ill adult patients requiring

intravenous and central lines, ventilator, tracheostomy and wound care;

member of Rapid Response Team.

PROFESSIONAL COMMITTEE ENGAGEMENT

2014–2015   ***Member.*** Electronic Health Record—Nursing Implementation Committee,

Memorial Hospital at Gulfport, Gulfport, Mississippi.

2013–2015   ***Member.*** Infection Control Committee, Memorial Hospital at Gulfport,

Gulfport, Mississippi.

PROFESSIONAL MEMBERSHIP

2013–2015   American Nurses Association

2012–2015   Gamma Lambda Chapter, Sigma Theta Tau International Honor Society

of Nursing

Mentoring

The IOM report on *The Future of Nursing* (2011) recommends **mentoring** to assist in increasing the readiness and retention of nurses to improve patient outcomes. Mentoring is a relationship between two nurses in which the more experienced nurse provides leadership and guidance to the nurse with less experience, often referred to as the "mentee" (Minority Nurse, 2013). Preceptors and mentors play different roles. A mentor provides counsel regarding career management, and the mentoring relationship may take place in the beginning of a nursing career, when changing positions, or when a nurse is furthering his or her education. The mentor–mentee relationship may be a long-term relationship. In contrast, a preceptor provides direct short-term coaching to a new graduate nurse, a newly hired nurse, or a nurse who transfers to another unit and orients the nurse to roles and responsibilities on the unit and within the organization. A mentor may also serve as a preceptor; however, a preceptor is not a mentor. It is not uncommon for mentees to become mentors guiding others in their pursuit of professional growth and development.

Being a mentor takes time and requires patience. The mentor must be reasonable, competent, committed to assisting the mentee in being successful in his or her career, adept at providing feedback, and open to sharing knowledge. Professional growth should be the outcome for both mentor and mentee. It is the responsibility of the person seeking career mentorship to find a mentor. The mentor may be a nursing faculty member, an experienced nurse within a healthcare organization or nursing school, or a nurse from a professional nursing organization. This relationship has benefits for both. The mentor receives confirmation from witnessing the career development and advancement of the mentee in professional nursing. The benefits of being mentored are many and include:

- Increased self-confidence
- Enhanced leadership skills
- Accelerated acclimation to the culture of the unit/facility
- Advancement opportunities
- Enhanced communication skills
- Reduced stress
- Improved networking ability
- Political savvy
- Legal and ethical insight

Problems with mentoring may occur with either person (Minority Nurse, 2015). The mentee may outgrow the mentor in knowledge and in the profession. The commitment in time and energy of the mentor may become overwhelming. The relationship may even become toxic if the mentor becomes inaccessible or harmful to the mentee and may even block the learning and progression of the mentee. If any of these become evident in the relationship, both must communicate and discuss the situation. They may agree to a separation or to repairing the relationship.

KEY COMPETENCY 7-1

Examples of Applicable *Nurse of the Future: Nursing Core Competencies*

Professionalism:

Attitudes/Behaviors (A4b) Values the mentoring relationship for professional development

Skills (S8g) Develops personal goals for professional development

Source: Massachusetts Department of Higher Education. (2010). *Nurse of the future: Nursing core competencies* (pp. 13, 15). Retrieved from http://www.mass.edu/currentinit/documents /NursingCoreCompetencies.pdf

Education and Lifelong Learning

The profession of nursing needs a more educated workforce for the sake of increasing healthcare quality and patient safety. The ANA standards of professional nursing practice, Standard 12, indicate that it is the responsibility of every nurse to seek "knowledge and competence that reflects current nursing practice and promotes futuristic thinking" (2015b, p. 76). The competencies associated with this standard reflect commitment to lifelong learning, the maintenance of a professional portfolio, and a commitment to mentoring. Every state board of nursing should require mandatory continuing education for all practicing RNs, but not all do. The call for a more educated professional nursing workforce to lead change and advance health has been mandated in the initiatives of the IOM (2011):

- "Increase the proportion of nurses with a baccalaureate degree to 80 percent by 2020." (Initiative 4)
- "Double the number of nurses with a doctorate by 2020." (Initiative 5)
- "Ensure that [all] nurses engage in lifelong learning." (Initiative 6)

In 2010, the U.S. Department of Health and Human Resources, Health Resources and Services Administration reported that the distribution of RNs by highest nursing or nursing-related educational preparation was as follows:

- 13.9% were diploma-prepared RNs.
- 36.1% of RNs had an associate degree in nursing (ADN).
- 36.8% had a BSN.
- 3.2% had a master's or doctoral degree.

In 2013, the ANA noted that of our 50 states, the District of Columbia, and 2 territories:

- 34% (18) had no mandatory continuing education (CE) requirement for RN licensure.
- 66% (35) had a mandatory CE requirement ranging from 14 to 30 CEs every 2 years or, in some cases, only if the RN was not engaged in practice during the previous renewal time.

The profession of nursing expects that nurses will practice the science of nursing with care. At the core of ADN and BSN academic programs are foundational science courses in biology, anatomy, physiology, microbiology, chemistry, pathophysiology, pharmacology, and statistics. These courses serve as the basis for translating research evidence into the science of nursing practice in courses such as adult health, pediatrics, obstetrics, psychiatric-mental health, and community health nursing. Although we readily acknowledge the essence of nursing as "caring for patients," we often do not embrace that nurses are also scientists committed to practicing the science of nursing with care and compassion toward patients. Caring is not enough. Science is not enough. Nursing is both an art and a science that is continuously evolving based on research findings, resulting in a deepening and broadening of the knowledge base fundamental to professional nursing practice. As nurses, we must be committed to and actively engaged in lifelong professional learning across our careers. Ongoing nursing education through CE programs, certification programs, and/or formal academic programs to pursue a BSN, an MSN, a DNP, and/or a PhD must be an expectation of professional nurses if we are to keep pace with the science of nursing, have credibility as a profession, and maintain our commitment to patients. It is only in this way that the profession of nursing will actualize the IOM mandates for leading change and advancing health.

Advancing your nursing career often means returning to school. In an unprecedented move advocating support for academic progression in nursing, the American Association of Community Colleges, the Association of Community College Trustees, the AACN, the National League for Nursing, and the National Organization for Associate Degree Nursing issued a powerful joint statement calling for nursing to work together in order to facilitate

> unity of nursing education programs and advance opportunities for academic progression, which may include seamless transition into associate, baccalaureate, master's, and doctoral programs. Collectively, we agree that every nursing student and nurse should have access to additional nursing education, and we stand ready to work together to ensure that nurses have the support needed to take the next step in their education. (AACN, 2015a, para. 3)

At the core of a seamless academic progression in nursing is respect for the academic integrity of educational programs provided by community colleges, colleges, and universities and efforts made to enable nursing students and nurses to readily progress from ADN to RN-BSN or RN-MSN to DNP or PhD programs. The AACN (n.d.a) website provides a user-friendly search engine called Nursing Program Search for academic programs in nursing at every level, such as RN-BSN, RN-MSN, LPN to BSN, entry-level BSN, accelerated BSN, BSN to DNP, BSN to PhD, entry-level MSN, MSN, CNL, MSN to DNP, DNP, and PhD programs.

If you are contemplating or have decided to return to school to pursue a BSN or an advanced graduate degree in nursing, be sure that you consider and investigate the following:

• Possess certainty about the specific courses that will successfully transfer and knowledge of the specific courses and their associated credit hours that need to be taken prior to admission.

- Prepare for and take any preliminary test required, such as the Graduate Record Examination, and know the expected scores for admission.
- Adhere to the application process, including admission dates.
- Be knowledgeable of the cost of the program in its entirety: tuition, books, and fees, such as online fees, clinical fees by course, and fees for validation credits of previously earned coursework that has been successfully completed. Some programs advertise that they give "life experience" credits. Be sure you receive in writing what these experiences are, whether you meet the criteria or if additional courses need to be taken or papers written describing these experiences, how many credit hours are awarded, and what the fees are for transferring these credits into your program of study.
- Be aware of tuition reimbursement options through work and the expected time commitment in return for tuition assistance.
- Be cognizant of and investigate opportunities and requirements for scholarships, loans, and/or traineeship programs awarded by the state government, the federal government, private foundations, and/or professional nursing organizations.

Information is power! In appraising your nursing career options, be informed about specialty areas available and of interest to you. The BSN degree is the sole academic portal of entry for graduate studies in nursing (MSN, DNP, and PhD) for such roles as nurse practitioner, nurse anesthetist, clinical nurse leader, nurse executive, nurse educator, and nurse researcher. There are several nursing career paths supported by graduate-level academic programs for you to consider:

- An *expert clinician* is an advanced practice registered nurse prepared at the graduate level, such as an adult, family, geriatric, or psychiatric-mental health nurse practitioner, nurse anesthetist, or nurse–midwife who provides safe, evidence-based, cost-effective care to a specific patient population (academic level: MSN, DNP).
- A *clinical nurse leader (CNL)* guides nurse colleagues and interdisciplinary teams in direct patient care situations to implement clinical practice guidelines and enable these patient populations to achieve positive outcomes (academic level: MSN, DNP).
- A *nurse executive* directs the infrastructure of the practice of nursing within an organization on clinical and fiscal levels and represents and advocates for nursing within the context of the business of health care (academic level: MSN, DNP, PhD).
- A *nurse educator* works in academic settings, guiding students to deepen and broaden their knowledge and practice of safe, quality-based professional nursing practice (academic level: MSN, DNP, PhD).
- A *nurse researcher* is dedicated to executing and translating evidence-based research into practice and expanding the body of knowledge fundamental to the art and science of nursing (academic level: MSN, DNP, PhD).

The Graduate Nursing Student Academy, established by the AACN (n.d.b), has established a series of webinars to inform you of areas of specialization and graduate degrees that may be of interest to you as you plan your career.

Professional Engagement

Professional engagement is a characteristic that discriminates between a person employed in a job and one pursuing a career. A professional nurse who is managing and advancing his or her career will actively engage in professional nursing initiatives within the nurse's healthcare agency and in professional nursing organizations.

Engagement in Your Healthcare Organization

As you are planning your nursing career path, seize opportunities now to actively engage in quality improvement activities that are currently underway within your healthcare organization. Examples of quality initiatives include, but are not limited to, committees within your agency that address nursing policy and procedures, quality improvement, core measures, clinical practice guidelines, safety, the Hospital Consumer Assessment of Healthcare Providers and Systems Hospital Survey of Customer Satisfaction, and the Medicare and Medicaid Survey Process for Nursing Homes or Home Health Agencies.

Engagement in programs to improve quality for patients, staff, and your organization will help you gain experience in clinical problem resolution, aid you in translating clinical practice guidelines and research evidence into practice, assist you with co-contributing to the creation of a milieu of safety and quality, and connect you in a collegial manner with the quality champions in your organization. If you are not sure how to get connected with these committees, start by meeting with your nurse manager and/or chief nursing officer and express your interest in serving on one or more of these committees. You will learn from your participation on these committees and you will maximize your visibility as an engaged, motivated employee.

Engagement in Professional Nursing Organizations

Engaging in professional nursing organizations connects students and RNs with membership and leadership opportunities. Some of the benefits of participating in these organizations include ongoing growth and development pertinent for your career and areas of specialization, receiving mentorship and guidance from seasoned members, obtaining reduced membership rates for students, and accessing scholarship and grant opportunities for members to supplement tuition in academic programs.

You may join many professional nursing organizations as a student or as an RN. These organizations include, but are not limited to, the ANA and its affiliate state nurses associations; Sigma Theta Tau International Honor Society of Nursing; American Organization of Nurse Executives; American Association of Nurse Practitioners; American Association of Nurse Anesthetists; American Association of Critical-Care Nurses; Association of Women's Health, Obstetric and Neonatal Nurses; and American College of Nurse-Midwives. A more thorough list of professional nursing organizations at national, state, and international levels is provided by the ANA (n.d.).

Expectations for Your Performance

Assessment of your performance as an RN is conducted on several levels, such as self-appraisal, work performance evaluations conducted by nurse managers on behalf of healthcare organizations, and collegial evaluations. Many performance appraisals for nurses and nursing students have their roots in professional documents such as *Nursing: Scope and Standards of Practice* (ANA, 2015b), *Nurse of the Future: Nursing Core Competencies* (Massachusetts Department of Higher Education, 2010), *The Essentials of Baccalaureate Education for Professional Nursing Practice* (AACN, 2008), and *The Essentials of Master's Education in Nursing* (AACN, 2011), as well as criteria established by specialty-based professional nursing organizations.

The core questions in most of these assessments are: "Am I currently practicing competently?" and "Am I currently practicing to the *fullest extent of my nursing education and training* in my current position?" (IOM, 2011, Initiative 1). It is important to know proactively the expectations of professional nurse competency in your specific setting so that you can meet and exceed them and continuously use them as indicators for identifying your strengths and areas that need further professional growth and development. Assessment of your performance as an RN is your own personal quality improvement program and is essential for professional growth and development. This should not be just an annual event, but an ongoing process of improving one's practice. Here are some suggestions for the evaluation of your performance as an RN:

- Conduct your own self-appraisal first in order to have a more informed dialogue with your nurse manager.
- Identify your areas of strength and areas in need of growth.

- Pursue continuing education to both enhance your strengths and narrow your limitations.
- Accept constructive feedback with respect, gratitude, and civility.
- If feedback does not make sense to you, ask the person to clarify what he or she said.
- Develop an ongoing plan of quality improvement for yourself.

CRITICAL THINKING QUESTIONS∗

Do you have the courage to ask for honest feedback? Do you have the courage to give honest feedback to a friend or colleague? How do you respond to negative feedback? ∗

Taking Care of Self

A nurse is a person who is present at birth, at death, and during the entire life span. A nurse makes life and death decisions. A nurse interacts with everyone in the healthcare community. A nurse interacts with people from every walk of life. A nurse must multitask during every shift. A nurse works every shift, weekends, and holidays. A nurse experiences stress unknown to most other professions. To prevent overwhelming stress, a nurse must take care of him- or herself by:

- Eating a balanced diet
- Getting enough sleep
- Avoiding addictive substances
- Exercising on a regular basis
- Paying attention to mental and spiritual health
- Being vigilant in coping with stress triggers at work and at home

Seig (2015) notes that "more than 40 percent of hospital nurses today suffer from the physical, emotional, or mental exhaustion characteristic of burnout. The result of unmanaged stress, burnout accounts for what is often a negative perception among nurses of their work and workplaces" (para. 1). Managing time is essential to preventing **burnout** and **compassion fatigue**. Francisco and Abarra (n.d.) present the following 12 tips for time management. Nurses can use these tips at work and during off time.

- Be organized.
- Make a list of the tasks you will need to do and post it in a place that you can easily see.
- Before making your rounds, make a checklist of the things you need to do for each patient.
- When doing rounds, always see your most critical patient first.
- Don't do other tasks when giving medications.
- Pay attention to time.
- Learn how to write quickly.
- Always bring easy-to-eat snacks.

KEY COMPETENCY 7-3

Examples of Applicable *Nurse of the Future: Nursing Core Competencies*

Professionalism:

Knowledge (K8b) Recognizes the relationship between personal health, self-renewal and the ability to deliver sustained quality care

Source: Massachusetts Department of Higher Education. (2010). *Nurse of the future: Nursing core competencies* (p. 15). Retrieved from http://www.mass.edu/currentinit/documents /NursingCoreCompetencies.pdf

- Be keen on details.
- Learn how to communicate.
- Learn to multitask.
- Be realistic.

Burnout and compassion fatigue may be the end result of stress not being managed. Burnout is progressive and involves disengagement and withdrawal. Compassion fatigue is acute and may present itself as over-involvement in patient care (Lombardo & Eyre, 2011). The two concepts may occur simultaneously. In caring for patients, the nurse may be depleted physically, emotionally, and spiritually. These indicators involve compassion fatigue. Burnout causes physical symptoms that lead to feelings of being constantly tired. Some observed signs are avoiding certain patients; not feeling compassion for your patients and their families; experiencing headaches, digestive problems, fatigue, mood swings, anxiety, and/or poor concentration; and/or feeling underappreciated and overworked. In response, nurses may not want to go to work and/or just go through the motions when at work.

The healthcare workplace is demanding, requiring many caregiving responsibilities from various members of the interdisciplinary team that must be accomplished and communicated within an abbreviated time. Sustained workplace stress can dramatically influence how we interact with colleagues, how professionally satisfied we are with current career choices, and employee retention rates.

Stress at work can be managed in a civil environment. Civility builds community and allows for efficient functioning units. Civility is defined as respect for others (Clark, 2010). A code of conduct establishes ways of behaving for interacting with people. The ANA (2015a) developed a *Code of Ethics for Nurses with Interpretive Statements* that requires nurses to communicate with respect when interacting with colleagues, patients, and students. Civil behavior is not always easy to accomplish; it requires courage and genuine concern for others. We have the choice to be colleagues who habitually respect and assist one another and who are instrumental in creating a milieu of civility and safety or to be colleagues who are engaged either overtly or subtly in lateral and vertical workplace violence exhibited by bullying, harassing, speaking ill of one another, demeaning one another, and excluding colleagues.

The first step toward managing stress and creating a civil milieu is to assess your work environment. Some of the characteristics of healthy collegial relationships include being a reliable and respectful colleague who works his or her scheduled days, arrives on time, shares equally in patient care and management responsibilities, provides care in a timely manner, and actively volunteers to help a colleague who needs assistance.

KEY COMPETENCY 7-4

Examples of Applicable *Nurse of the Future: Nursing Core Competencies*

Teamwork and Collaboration:

Knowledge (K7b) Identifies lateral violence as a barrier to teamwork and unit functioning

Attitudes/Behaviors (A7b) Recognizes behaviors that contribute to lateral violence

Skills (S7b) Practices strategies to minimize lateral violence

Source: Massachusetts Department of Higher Education. (2010). *Nurse of the future: Nursing core competencies* (p. 32). Retrieved from http://www.mass.edu/currentinit/documents/NursingCoreCompetencies.pdf

Self-care strategies that promote resilient nurses may include:

- Saying no to additional shifts and reducing overtime in order to conserve energy
- Taking a day off in order to renew energy
- Changing shift or unit in order to gain a new outlook on being a nurse

Consulting a social worker, a chaplain, your preceptor, and/or your mentor can provide you with resources for caring for self, managing burnout and compassion fatigue, and sustaining a resilient self.

Conclusion

You are responsible for actively managing and advancing your nursing career across your entire life span as a professional nurse. This means that you will need to make purposeful and strategic choices about your professional practice, academic preparation, and continuing education. Mentors, preceptors, and engagement in your healthcare organization and professional nursing organization serve as guides for advancing your professional path. Creating a healthy lifestyle and reducing the risk of burnout and compassion fatigue are essential for sustaining your personal and professional life.

Classroom Activity 1

Have students begin creating a career map that includes short-term and long-term goals and strategies to achieve those goals. The Nursing License Map (available at http://nursinglicensemap.com) may be useful in this activity if students want to compare educational requirements and salaries as they consider career goals.

Classroom Activity 2

Have students begin working on a professional portfolio that contains a cover letter and résumé, along with examples of accomplishments and selections of quality projects, papers, and presentations.

Classroom Activity 3

Have students register online for access to the ANA's New Graduate Profession Kit and then explore various parts of the toolbox that include taking care of your career, taking care of yourself, taking care of your profession, and taking care of your patients. The resources in this kit are available at: www.nursingworld.org/Content/New-Graduate/default.aspx

References

American Association of Colleges of Nursing. (2008, October 20). The essentials of baccalaureate education for professional nursing practice. Retrieved from http://www.aacn.nche.edu/education-resources/BaccEssentials08.pdf

American Association of Colleges of Nursing. (2011, March 21). The essentials of master's education in nursing. Retrieved from http://www.aacn.nche.edu/education-resources/MastersEssentials11.pdf

American Association of Colleges of Nursing. (2015a). Joint statement on academic progression for nursing students and graduates. Retrieved from http://www.aacn.nche.edu/aacn-publications/position/joint-statement-academic-progression

American Association of Colleges of Nursing. (2015b). Talking points: HRSA report on nursing workforce projections through 2025. Retrieved from http://www.aacn.nche.edu/media-relations/HRSA-Nursing-Workforce-Projections.pdf

American Association of Colleges of Nursing. (n.d.a). Students: Member program directory. Retrieved from https://www.aacn.nche.edu/students/nursing-program-search

American Association of Colleges of Nursing. (n.d.b). Students: Webinars. Retrieved from http://www.aacn.nche.edu/students/gnsa/webinars

American Association of Colleges of Nursing. (n.d.c). What every nursing student should know when seeking employment: An interview tip sheet for baccalaureate and higher degree prepared nurses. Retrieved from http://www.aacn.nche.edu/publications/hallmarks.pdf

American Nurses Association. (2013). States which require continuing education for RN licensure: 2013. Retrieved from http://www.nursingworld.org/MainMenuCategories/Policy-Advocacy/State/Legislative-Agenda-Reports/NursingEducation/CE-Licensure-Chart.pdf

American Nurses Association. (2015a). *Code of ethics for nurses with interpretive statements*. Retrieved from http://nursingworld.org/MainMenuCategories/EthicsStandards/CodeofEthicsforNurses/Code-of-Ethics-For-Nurses.html

American Nurses Association. (2015b). *Nursing: Scope and standards of practice* (3rd ed.). Silver Spring, MD: Author.

American Nurses Association. (n.d.). Nursing organizations. Retrieved from http://www.nurse.org/orgs.shtml

Clark, C. (2010). Why civility matters. Retrieved from http://www .reflectionsonnursingleadership.com/pages/vol36_1_clark2_civility.aspx

Daggett, L. M. (2014). Career management and care of the professional self. In K. Masters (Ed.), *Role development in professional nursing practice* (3rd ed., pp. 167–193). Burlington, MA: Jones & Bartlett Learning.

Francisco, M. E. V., & Abarra, J. (n.d.). 12 time management tips every nurse should know. Retrieved from http://www.nursebuff.com/2014/05/time-management -tips-for-nurses/

Health eCareers Network. (2012, December 11). 5 common career myths for nurses. Retrieved from http://www.healthecareers.com/article/5-common-career-myths -for-nurses/171657

Hein, R. (2012, December 5). Career mapping offers a clear path for both employees and employers. Retrieved from http://www.cio.com/article/2448964/careers-staffing /career-mapping-offers-a-clear-path-for-both-employees-and-employers.html

HR World. (2015). 30 interview questions you can't ask and 30 sneaky, legal alternatives to get the same info. Retrieved from http://www.hrworld.com/features/30-interview -questions-111507/

Institute of Medicine. (2010). Report brief: The future of nursing: Focus on education. Retrieved from http://www.iom.edu/~/media/Files/Report%20Files/2010/The -Future-of-Nursing/Nursing%20Education%202010%20Brief.pdf

Institute of Medicine. (2011). *The future of nursing*: *Leading change, advancing health*. Washington, DC: National Academy Press. Retrieved from http://www.nap.edu/ read/12956/chapter/1

Lombardo, B., & Eyre, C. (2011). Compassion fatigue: A nurse's primer. *Online Journal of Issues in Nursing, 16*. Retrieved from http://www.nursingworld.org /MainMenuCategories/ANAMarketplace/ANAPeriodicals/OJIN/TableofContents /Vol-16-2011/No1-Jan-2011/Compassion-Fatigue-A-Nurses-Primer.html

Masor, M. B. (2013). Let your light shine: Portfolio principles. In J. Phillips & J. M. Brown (Eds.), *Accelerate your career in nursing: A guide to professional advancement and recognition* (pp. 29–44). Indianapolis, IN: Sigma Theta Tau International Honor Society of Nursing.

Massachusetts Department of Higher Education. (2010). *Nurse of the future: Nursing core competencies*. Retrieved from http://www.mass.edu/currentinit/documents /NursingCoreCompetencies.pdf

Minority Nurse. (2013). Mentoring nurses toward success. Retrieved from http://minoritynurse.com/mentoring-nurses-toward-success/

Schmidt, K. (n.d.). Top 10 details to include on a nursing resume [Web log]. Retrieved from http://blog.bluepipes.com/top-10-details-to-include-on-a-nurse-resume/

Seig, D. (2015). 7 habits of highly resilient nurses. Retrieved from http://www .reflectionsonnursingleadership.org/Pages/Vol41_1_Sieg_7%20Habits.aspx

U.S. Department of Health and Human Services, Health Resources and Services Administration. (2010, March). The registered nurse population: Initial findings from the 2008 national sample survey of registered nurses. Retrieved from http://bhpr.hrsa.gov/healthworkforce/rnsurveys/rnsurveyinitial2008.pdf

U.S. Department of Labor, Bureau of Labor Statistics. (2015). Occupational employment and wages, May 2014, 29-1141 registered nurses. Retrieved from http://www.bls.gov/oes/current/oes291141.htm

Professional Nursing Practice and the Management of Patient Care

CHAPTER 8

Patient Safety and Professional Nursing Practice

Jill Rushing and Kathleen Masters

Learning Objectives

After completing this chapter, the student should be able to:

1. Explore various definitions of safety.
2. Describe the system approach to patient care safety.
3. Describe organizational culture in relationship to patient safety.
4. Describe the role of nurses in delivering safe health care.
5. Describe the relationships among critical thinking, clinical judgment, clinical reasoning, decision making, and mindfulness.
6. Explore the characteristics of critical thinking and the critical thinker.
7. Explore the process involved in critical thinking.
8. Explore strategies to develop critical thinking skills.

Although the concepts of quality and safety are intricately intertwined, this chapter will specifically focus on aspects of patient safety. The beginning of this chapter will review definitions of safety, the journey to decrease errors in health care, and approaches to improve safety. The latter portion of this chapter will explore safety from the perspective of the nurse's ability to critically think and make sound clinical decisions.

Patient Safety

Patient safety is paramount to nurses. Inherent in the standards of practice are nursing's goals of quality care and patient safety. The American Nurses Association (ANA, 2015b, p. 79) specifically addresses the requirements for nurses' responsibilities in relation to patient safety in professional nursing practice Standard 14, stating that the nurse "ensures that nursing practice is safe, effective, efficient, equitable, timely, and patient-centered."

Key Terms and Concepts

» Safety
» Error
» Culture of safety
» Just culture
» Patient handoff
» Never events
» Sentinel events
» Clinical judgment
» Clinical reasoning
» Mindfulness
» Critical thinking
» Reflective thinking
» Nursing process
» Concept mapping
» Journaling

The definition of **safety** provided by the Quality and Safety Education for Nurses (QSEN) (Cronenwett et al., 2007; QSEN, 2007) project refers to the minimization of risk of harm to patients and providers through both system effectiveness and individual performance. The Massachusetts Department of Higher Education (2010) uses the QSEN definition in the development of its safety competencies for the "nurse of the future."

In its landmark report, *To Err Is Human: Building a Safer Health System*, the Institute of Medicine (IOM, 2000) defined patient safety as freedom from accidental injury. In the same report, it estimated that at least 44,000 and possibly up to 98,000 people died each year as the result of preventable harm while receiving health care that was supposed to help them. Subsequent to this report, the IOM produced nine more reports regarding patient quality and safety. Why? Because the original report brought attention to the problems related to patient safety that permeate the healthcare system.

Culture of Safety

The IOM report (2000), while identifying alarming problems related to safety, was clear that the cause of the errors was defective system processes that either led people to make mistakes or failed to stop them from making a mistake, not the recklessness of individual providers. The report included recommendations such as the development of safer systems that would make it more difficult for humans to make mistakes.

The IOM report (2000) defined **error** as the failure of a planned action to be completed as intended or the use of a wrong plan to achieve an aim with the goal of preventing, recognizing, and mitigating harm. Adverse drug events and improper transfusions, surgical injuries and wrong site surgeries, suicides, restraint-related injuries or death, falls, burns, pressure ulcers, and mistaken patient identities were among the commonly occurring errors.

When errors occur, it is possible to analyze the event in two ways, a person approach or a system approach. Historically, in healthcare organizations errors were viewed from the person approach to safety or finding out who is at fault. This approach results in making the person who committed the error the target of blame, and creates an environment where providers fear admitting to mistakes and thus hide mistakes. This approach is counter to creating a **culture of safety** and transparency because it frequently results in disciplinary action. A safety culture, or culture of safety, is one that promotes trust and empowers staff to report risks, near misses, and errors (Hershey, 2015). Three key attributes in a culture of safety are trust of peers and management, reporting unsafe conditions, and improvement. Trust and reporting are increased when staff can observe improvements being made to correct unsafe conditions (Chassin & Loeb, 2013). Trust is lacking in many healthcare organizations, with many staff believing that error reporting will be held against them (Agency for Healthcare Research and Quality [AHRQ], 2014).

KEY COMPETENCY 8-1

Examples of Applicable *Nurse of the Future: Nursing Core Competencies*

Safety:

Knowledge (K5) Describes how patients, families, individual clinicians, health care teams, and systems can contribute to promoting safety and reducing errors

Skills (S5) Participates in analyzing errors and designing systems improvements

Attitudes/Behaviors (A5) Recognizes the value of analyzing systems and individual accountability when errors or near misses occur

Source: Massachusetts Department of Higher Education. (2010). *Nurse of the future: Nursing core competencies* (p. 34). Retrieved from http://www.mass.edu/currentinit /documents/NursingCoreCompetencies.pdf

This lack of trust leads to underreporting of errors and the potential for more errors (Hershey, 2015). In a culture of safety, the focus is on what went wrong, rather than who made the error. Patient safety initiatives can succeed when embedded in an organizational culture of safety (Rovinski-Wagner & Mills, 2014).

A system approach to safety includes viewing the error in the context of prevention of future errors by looking at all of the factors related to the incident. Nurses working in an organization with a system approach to safety are more likely to admit to errors or near misses because the identification of system issues will lead to patient safety. The system approach does not negate the accountability of the nurse for his or her actions, but allows for analysis of the error in a way that explores system problems to prevent future errors. This balance between not blaming individuals for errors and not tolerating careless or egregious behaviors is known as a **just culture** (Mitchell, 2008).

Measures of safety culture indicate that three areas of health care are in greatest need of improvement: a nonpunitive response to error, handoffs and transitions, and safe staffing (Hershey, 2015). If the healthcare system does include disciplinary action for error, then the basis of the punishment should be the type of behavior rather than the outcome of the error. The types of behavior that may result in error are human behavior, negligence, intentional rule violations, and reckless conduct. Human error does not change due to disciplinary action. There are arguments for and against punishment for negligence. Much can be learned to create safer systems to prevent future errors that result from human error and negligence. In the case of intentional rule violations, it is important to look at the latent issues creating a situation in which staff are violating rules intended to promote patient safety, rather than revert to discipline. However, in the case of reckless behavior, punishment is warranted (Marx, 2001).

A root cause analysis is one method to review error that has already occurred, and along with actions to eliminate risks, it is required by the Joint Commission for all sentinel events. A common approach to root cause analysis is a cause and effect diagram or fishbone diagram. During this process, the problem is clarified by completing an event flow diagram. Next, a list of causes is developed for each branch of the diagram. The diagram is completed as relationships among causal chains are identified and causal statements are developed. This process requires asking why the event happened in order to identify the underlying source of the error (Barnsteiner, 2012). This method considers elements of the total system rather than just the behavior of an individual involved in an error and can be used to review data over time to identify the system variables that contributed to errors during the identified period (Rovinski-Wagner & Mills, 2014).

An example of the use of an ongoing root cause analysis to increase patient safety is the Taxonomy of Error, Root Cause Analysis, and Practice-Responsibility (TERCAP) initiative by the National Council of State Boards

KEY COMPETENCY 8-2

Examples of Applicable *Nurse of the Future: Nursing Core Competencies*

Safety:

Knowledge (K3) Discusses effective strategies to enhance memory and recall and minimize interruptions

Skills (S3) Uses appropriate strategies to reduce reliance on memory and interruptions

Attitudes/Behaviors (A3) Recognizes that both individuals and systems are accountable for a safety culture

Source: Massachusetts Department of Higher Education. (2010). Nurse of the future: Nursing core competencies (p. 34). Retrieved from http://www.mass.edu/currentinit/documents/NursingCoreCompetencies.pdf

of Nursing (2013). The goal of the TERCAP initiative is to develop a data set to distinguish human and system errors from negligence or misconduct, while identifying the areas of nursing practice breakdown in relation to standards of nursing practice (Malloch, Benner, Sheets, Kenward, & Farrell, 2010). Practice breakdown categories include safe medication administration, documentation, attentiveness/surveillance, clinical reasoning, prevention, intervention, interpretation of authorized providers' orders, and professional responsibility/patient advocacy. System factors include communication, leadership/management, backup and support, environment, other health team members, staffing issues, and the healthcare team. Twenty-six state boards of nursing participate in TERCAP.

Another framework that is used to identify events or characteristics of a system that may allow potential errors is known as Reason's Adverse Event Trajectory or the Swiss Cheese Model (Reason, 2000). This model explains how faults in different layers of the system can lead to error through triggers that can set up a sequence of events. Multiple defenses that have been set in place to prevent errors may at times line up, allowing multiple triggers to align and, thus, allow an error to occur. The lining up of triggers has been illustrated as an arrow and the lining up of defenses the alignment of holes in Swiss cheese (thus, the name Swiss Cheese Model). When the defenses line up, the arrow or trigger goes through the defenses (holes) and an error may occur. When the defenses do not line up, then the trigger (arrow) is blocked and the error is averted.

Classification of Error

Errors may be classified by type. Types of errors include communication, patient management, and clinical performance before, during, or after interventions. Improper delegation is an example of a patient management error. The potential for communication error occurs during transitions in care and handoffs. Standardization in handoff processes with face-to-face communication is key to patient safety. Standardized change of shift checklists and SBAR (situation, background, assessment, recommendation) are two frequently used approaches to effective communication (Barnsteiner, 2012). A **patient handoff** is the transfer of responsibility for a patient from one clinician to another (Rovinski-Wagner & Mills, 2014, p. 118) and provides a frequent opportunity for error. Due to the vulnerability inherent in the patient handoff process, the Joint Commission has published expectations for handoffs in the National Patient Safety Goals. These expectations include an opportunity for questioning between the giver and receiver; provision of current information regarding patient care, treatment, services, conditions, and any changes; verification of information in the form of repeat-back or read-back; the recipient of information having the opportunity to review patient data; and limits on interruptions during handoffs to minimize opportunities for information transfer failures (Barnsteiner, 2012).

KEY COMPETENCY 8-3

Examples of Applicable *Nurse of the Future: Nursing Core Competencies*

Teamwork and Collaboration (Effect of Team on Safety and Quality):

Knowledge (K6a) Understands the impact of effective team functioning on safety and quality of care

Skills (S6a) Follows communication practices to minimize risks associated with transfers between providers during transitions in care delivery

Attitudes/Behaviors (A6) Recognizes the risks associated with transferring patient care responsibilities to another professional ("hand-off") during transitions in care

Source: Massachusetts Department of Higher Education. (2010). *Nurse of the future: Nursing core competencies* (p. 32). Retrieved from http://www.mass.edu/currentinit/documents/NursingCoreCompetencies.pdf

Errors may also be classified according to where the error occurs in the healthcare system. These errors include latent failure, arising from decisions affecting things such as organizational policies or allocation of resources, and active failure, referring to errors or harm at the "sharp" end or in direct contact with the patient. Organizational system failures are those errors related to management, organizational culture, and system process; technical failure refers to indirect failure of facilities or external resources. These terms also help identify the root cause of harm or error (Mitchell, 2008). An example of a potential error that results from management decisions is related to staffing levels on patient care units. There is a clear and documented relationship among insufficient staffing, excessive workloads, staff fatigue, and adverse events in health care, with nurses working shifts longer than 12.5 hours being three times more likely to make a patient care error (Joint Commission, 2011).

Errors that result from human factors can be classified as skill-based, rule-based, or knowledge-based error (Henriksen, Dayton, Keyes, Carayon, & Hughes, 2008). Skill-based errors occur when there is a deviation in the pattern of a routine activity; for example, a skill-based error could result if a nurse is interrupted during medication administration. Workarounds and shortcuts by the nurse are examples of rule-based and knowledge-based errors that occur due to mistakes in conscious thought. Workarounds occur when nurses create a quick way to solve a problem caused by some obstruction to providing care. Workarounds generally occur because nurses are busy or the process is time consuming or complicated. Workarounds may result in harm to patients when system defense mechanisms are bypassed. Strategies to eliminate workarounds include the addition of nurses in workflow planning as well as mechanisms within organizations for reporting and solving workflow issues in a timely manner (Barnsteiner, 2012).

Improving Patient Safety

Reports prepared by the IOM propelled the quality and safety movement in the healthcare system during the first decade of the 21st century. The ANA has contributed to patient safety through the development and dissemination of practice documents, such as *Nursing's Social Policy Statement* (2010b), the *Nursing: Scope and Standards of Practice* (2015b), and *Code of Ethics with Interpretive Statements* (2015a), as well as through credentialing and legislative efforts (Rowell, 2003). Other organizations such as the Joint Commission and the National Quality Forum (NQF) have also contributed to the effort to improve patient safety through the dissemination and development of standards and patient safety resources. In addition, the Centers for Medicare and Medicaid Services have linked quality indicators that relate to patient safety, such as pressure ulcer prevalence and hospital-acquired infections, with hospital payment, and some states have passed error-reporting laws. All of these efforts have begun to affect patient safety.

KEY COMPETENCY 8-4

Examples of Applicable *Nurse of the Future: Nursing Core Competencies*

Safety:

Knowledge (K1) Identifies human factors and basic safety design principles that affect safety

Skills (S1) Demonstrates effective use of technology and standardized practices that support safe practice

Attitudes/Behaviors (A1) Recognizes the cognitive and physical limitations of human performance

Source: Massachusetts Department of Higher Education. (2010). *Nurse of the future: Nursing core competencies* (p. 34). Retrieved from http://www.mass.edu/currentinit /documents/NursingCoreCompetencies.pdf

To Err Is Human: Building a Safer Health System

In addition to drawing attention to the problem of error in the healthcare system, *To Err Is Human: Building a Safer Health System* (IOM, 2000) also identified system approaches to the implementation of change in the recommendation section of the report. The nine recommendations were the development of user-centered designs, avoidance of reliance on memory, attending to work safety, avoidance of reliance on vigilance, training concepts for teams, involving patients in their care, anticipating the unexpected, designing for recovery, and improving access to accurate, timely information.

- The development of user-centered designs builds on human strengths and avoids human weaknesses. The first step is to make things visible to users so that users can determine what actions are possible during processes. A second step is to include affordances and natural mappings in relation to equipment and workspace, which includes clear communication of how the equipment is to be used, whether by design or through symbols indicating operations. Finally, user-centered design also includes what are known as constraints or forcing functions. Constraints make it hard to do the wrong thing. A forcing function makes it impossible to do the wrong thing; for example, using different tubing connections for intravenous lines and enteral lines makes it impossible to inadvertently switch the connections.

- Standardization reduces reliance on memory and allows even those unfamiliar with a device to use it safely. When devices or medications cannot be standardized, they should be clearly distinguishable. In addition, simplifying procedures minimizes the chance of error because less problem solving and fewer steps are required.

- Work conditions such as work hours, workloads, staffing ratios, and shift changes that affect the circadian rhythm of the nurse affect both patient safety and worker safety.

- People cannot remain vigilant for long periods, so the use of checklists and auditory and visual alarms can increase patient safety by avoiding reliance on vigilance. Avoiding long work shifts also helps decrease errors related to the limitations in vigilance of humans.

- Because healthcare professionals work in teams, the establishment of training programs for interprofessional teams is recommended. As team members, professionals must trust the judgment and expertise of colleagues.

- Patients and family members should be invited to be active partners in the care process. The healthcare team is able to provide better care when they are able to obtain accurate information from patients, and safety improves when patients and their caregivers know about their care.

- Whenever there are changes in an organization or technologies, healthcare professionals should anticipate the unexpected, which includes the possibility of an increase in error. Most organizations pilot new technologies prior to organization-wide implementation in order to test and modify as necessary to decrease the potential of unintended harm.

- Another recommendation includes the assumption that errors will occur and to design and plan for recovery from errors. An example of a strategy used to anticipate and plan for recovery from error is using simulation training to rehearse procedures for responding to adverse events.
- Finally, improving access to accurate, timely information such as the use of decision-making tools at the point of care will increase patient safety. Information coordinated across settings will also improve patient safety (Donaldson, 2008).

Crossing the Quality Chasm: A New Health System for the 21st Century

Building on the previous IOM report (2000), *Crossing the Quality Chasm: A New Health System for the 21st Century* (IOM, 2001) introduced performance expectations to create a system in which patients are assured care that is safe, timely, effective, efficient, equitable, and patient-centered. These expectations are known as the six aims for improving healthcare quality and are sometimes referred to in the literature as STEEEP.

In addition, the report outlined 10 rules for redesign to move the healthcare system toward the identified performance expectations. Most of the rules relate primarily to quality, but one of the rules is specific to safety. Rule number six states that safety is a system property. This means that patients should be safe from harm caused by the healthcare system and that reducing risk and ensuring safety require attention to system processes.

Keeping Patients Safe: Transforming the Work Environment of Nurses

Nurses are the healthcare professionals who spend the most time with patients and provide the majority of direct care to patients. The IOM (2004) report, *Keeping Patients Safe: Transforming the Work Environment of Nurses*, specifically addressed the link between the work environment of nurses and patient quality and safety. The report identified six major concerns related to direct care in nursing: monitoring patient status and surveillance, physiologic therapy, helping patients compensate for loss of function, emotional support, education for patients and families, and integration and coordination of care. Some of the key safety recommendations of this report included that the chief nursing executive should have a leadership role in the organization, the creation of satisfying work environments for nurses, evidence-based nurse staffing and scheduling to control fatigue, giving nurses a voice in patient care delivery, and designing work environments and cultures that promote patient safety.

Medication error is an area that affects nurses and is directly impacted by nurses because nurses are primarily responsible for medication administration in acute care settings. Medication errors make up the largest category of errors, with 3–4% of patients experiencing a serious error during hospitalization (IOM, 2006). Medication error accounts for over 7,000 deaths per year; on average, a patient in an inpatient setting will experience at least one medication error per day (Aspen, Walcott, Bootman, & Cronenwett, 2007). In response to these errors, the IOM (2006) made several recommendations to decrease medication error and increase patient safety. These recommendations included a paradigm shift in the patient–provider relationship in which the patient takes an active role in the health-care process and the provider does a better job of educating the patient about medications. Additional recommendations included using information technology to reduce medication errors, improving medication labeling and packaging, and policy changes to encourage the adoption of practices that will reduce medication errors.

Other Safety Initiatives

The goal of the NQF is to improve the quality of health care by setting national goals for performance improvement, endorsing national consensus standards for measuring and public reporting on performance, and promoting the attainment of national goals (2010, p. ii). The original set of the NQF–endorsed safe practices was released in 2003, and it was updated in 2006, 2009, and again in 2010 with the most current evidence. The endorsed safe practices "were defined to be universally applied in all clinical settings in order to reduce the risk of error and harm for patients" (2010, p. i). The NQF presents 34 practices that have been shown to decrease the occurrence of adverse health events. The practices are organized into seven categories for improving patient safety: creating and sustaining a culture of safety; informed consent, life-sustaining treatment, disclosure, and care of the caregiver; matching healthcare needs with service delivery capability; facilitating information transfer and clear communication; medication management; prevention of healthcare-associated infections; and condition and site-specific practices that include topics such as fall prevention, pressure ulcer prevention, and wrong site surgery (2010, p. v).

The NQF also endorses a list of 29 preventable, measurable, serious adverse events for public reporting. These events are known as **never events**. Never events are not expected, and Medicare has eliminated reimbursement for certain never events. Example never events include patient suicide, sexual assault on a patient, abduction of a patient, patient death associated with a fall, infant discharged to the wrong person, surgery performed on the wrong body part, and patient death or disability associated with the use of restraints or bedrails (Haviley, Anderson, & Currier, 2014, p. 15). These never events are organized into seven categories—six relating to provision of care (surgical or invasive procedure events, product or device events, patient protection events, care management events, environmental events, and radiologic events) and one category relating to four potential criminal events. The NQF acknowledges that a healthcare organization cannot eliminate all risk of adverse events; however, it can take measures to reduce risk (2010, p. 5).

The Joint Commission established the National Patient Safety Goals in order to promote improvements in patient safety. These goals are reviewed and updated annually and focus on system-wide solutions to problems identified in healthcare organizations (Barnsteiner, 2012). National Patient Safety Goals for 2015 include identifying patients correctly, using medications safely, improving staff communication, using alarms safely, preventing infection, identifying patient safety risks (suicide risk), and preventing mistakes in surgery (Joint Commission, 2014).

Never events are also **sentinel events**. A sentinel event is an unexpected occurrence involving death or serious physical or psychological injury or the risk thereof and is termed *sentinel* because the event signals the need for immediate investigation and response. Organizations are not required to report sentinel events to the Joint Commission, but those accredited by the Joint Commission are encouraged to do so. Examples of sentinel events include wrong patient, wrong site, wrong procedure, delay in treatment, operative or postoperative complication, retention of foreign body, suicide, medication error, perinatal death or injury, and criminal events. Between 2004 and 2011, nearly 5,000 sentinel events were reported to the Joint Commission (2012). State laws generally require the reporting of sentinel events.

With all of these reports and initiatives related to patient safety, have we made progress over the past decade? Progress toward IOM goals has been slow, but studies show that there has been some measurable progress in relation to patient safety. Healthcare organizations have responded to incentive programs, accreditation standards, and public opinion. Professional organizations have responded with revisions to professional standards that place more emphasis on healthcare quality and patient safety. Educators have responded by revising curricula to infuse quality and safety concepts into student didactic and clinical experiences guided by projects such as the QSEN initiative (QSEN, 2007) and *Nurse of the Future* (Massachusetts Department of Higher Education, 2010). Even with progress, the statistics are still staggering. According to Institute for Healthcare Improvement estimates, there are 40–50 incidents of patient harm per 100 hospital admissions (McCannon, Hackbarth, & Griffin, 2007).

When we talk about the reports and the data, we see the scope of the problem; however, when we see and hear patient stories, we understand the impact of healthcare error on patient lives. Numerous videos are available that relay the stories of patients who became victims of faulty systems and errors during their care. Some of the families of patient victims have used their devastating experience to try to improve the healthcare system and prevent other patients and families from suffering.

KEY COMPETENCY 8-5

Examples of Applicable *Nurse of the Future: Nursing Core Competencies*

Safety:

Knowledge (K4a) Delineates general categories of errors and hazards in care

(K4b) Describes factors that create a culture of safety

Skills (S4a) Participates in collecting and aggregating safety data

(S4b) Uses organizational error reporting system for "near miss" and error reporting

Attitudes/Behaviors (A4a) Recognizes the importance of transparency in communication with the patient, family, and health care team around safety and adverse events

(A4b) Recognizes the complexity and sensitivity of the clinical management of medical errors and adverse events

Source: Massachusetts Department of Higher Education. (2010). *Nurse of the future: Nursing core competencies* (p. 34). Retrieved from http://www.mass.edu/currentinit/documents/NursingCoreCompetencies.pdf

Critical Thinking, Clinical Judgment, and Clinical Reasoning in Nursing Practice

Nursing competence plays a large role in ensuring patient safety. In 2008, the Robert Wood Johnson Foundation and the IOM launched a 2-year initiative to respond to the need to assess and transform the nursing profession. The IOM report points out nurses are going to have a critical role in the future, especially in producing safe, quality care and coverage for all patients in our healthcare system (IOM, 2011). The AHRQ (2008) in collaboration with the Robert Wood Johnson Foundation developed a handbook for nurses on patient safety and quality. The handbook provides a wealth of information for nursing including background research and tools for improving the quality of care. In 2008, the American Association of Colleges of Nursing (AACN) revised *The Essentials of Baccalaureate Education for Professional Nursing Practice* based on early discussion of IOM reports and the necessity of building a safer healthcare system (AACN, 2008).

A majority of sentinel events occur in acute care settings, where new graduate nurses traditionally begin their professional nursing careers. The inability of a nurse to set priorities and work safely, effectively, and efficiently can delay patient treatment in a critical situation and result in serious life-threatening consequences. The ability of nurses to think critically and make sound clinical judgments is essential to providing safe, competent, and quality nursing care.

New realities of health care require nurses to master complex information, to coordinate a variety of care experiences, to use advanced technology for healthcare delivery and evaluation of patient outcomes, and to assist patients with managing and navigating an increasingly complex system of care. Some of the trends that have added to the complexities of the healthcare environment include increases in longevity, markedly shortened hospital stays (which are moving patients out of the hospital "quicker and sicker"), scientific advances and major advances in technology, increased diversity in the U.S. population, and an increased incidence of chronic diseases and infectious diseases (AACN, 2008).

The responsibilities of a professional registered nurse (RN) have increased significantly over the years. Nurses and nursing students must be able to function within the complicated environment of the healthcare system. The impact of advanced technology and the increased acuity level and complexity of patients, combined with the accountability and responsibility nurses have in the delivery of safe and effective care, make it essential, now more than ever, for nurses to possess the ability to think critically. In nursing, critical thinking is the ability to think in a systematic and logical manner, solve problems, make decisions, and establish priorities in the clinical setting. Critical thinking is the competent use of thinking skills and abilities to make sound clinical judgments and safe decisions.

Critical thinking in nursing is an essential component of professional accountability and quality nursing care. Concern for patient safety has grown as high rates of error and injury continue to be reported. To improve patient safety, nurses must be able to recognize changes in patient condition, perform independent nursing interventions, anticipate orders, and prioritize.

New nurses need to be prepared to practice safely, accurately, and compassionately, in varied settings, where knowledge and innovation increase at astonishing rates (Benner, Sutphen, Leonard, & Day, 2010). Nursing students must use a complex array of nursing skills and knowledge at the same time and practice thinking in changing situations, always for the good of the patient (Benner et al., 2010).

Recent studies indicate new nursing graduates have deficiencies in critical thinking ability including recognition of problems, reporting of essential clinical data, initiating independent nursing interventions, anticipating relevant medical orders, providing relevant rationale to support decisions, and differentiating urgency (Fero, Witsberger, Wesmiller, Zullo, & Hoffman, 2009). New graduate nurses practice at the novice or advanced beginner level (Benner, 1984). New graduate nurses are at the early stage of developing a skill set and applying critical thinking. For the novice, the beginning nursing student, the difficulty encountered in setting priorities is that all tasks, requests, and concerns seem to be of equal weight or importance and they must all be done (Benner et al., 2010). Determining which tasks are most important or urgent requires deliberate thought because the student has not yet learned to see the big picture or gained the skill to recognize quickly what is most urgent or most important in each clinical situation; this level of thinking is often difficult for the novice (Benner et al., 2010). For example, you are about to administer medications to a patient. What is the bigger picture? Why is the patient being given these medications? Alternatively, you have a patient who has just returned from surgery. What should be carried out in the first hours after surgery?

Thinking Like a Nurse

To prepare nursing students for the multifaceted role of professional nurse, the learning process involves components that will provide a solid foundation for developing clinical judgment and clinical reasoning skills. In other words, the student must learn to think like a nurse. What does it mean to think like a nurse? How does one begin to think like a nurse?

Clinical judgment is complex and includes critical thinking, problem solving, ethical reasoning, and decision making (ANA, 2010a, p. 78). According to Tanner (2006), clinical judgment is developed through reflection, thus enhancing critical thinking skills. What exactly is clinical judgment? According to Tanner, clinical judgment refers to "an interpretation or conclusion about a patient's needs, concerns, or health problems, and/or the decision to take action (or not), use or modify standard approaches, or improvise new ones as deemed appropriate by the patient's response" (2006, p. 204). How does that differ from clinical reasoning? Again according to Tanner, **clinical reasoning** refers to "the processes by which nurses and other clinicians make their judgments, and includes both the deliberative process of generating alternatives, weighing them against the evidence, and choosing the most appropriate, and those patterns that might be characterized as engaged, practical reasoning" including recognition of a pattern, an intuitive clinical grasp, or a response without evident forethought (2006, pp. 204–205).

Based on a review of nearly 200 studies, Tanner (2006, p. 204) proposed the following:

- Clinical judgments are more influenced by what nurses bring to the situation than by the objective data about the situation at hand.
- Sound clinical judgment rests to some degree on knowing the patient and his or her typical pattern of responses, as well as engagement with the patient and his or her concerns.
- Clinical judgments are influenced by the context in which the situation occurs and the culture of the nursing unit.
- Nurses use a variety of reasoning patterns alone or in combination.
- Reflection on practice is often triggered by a breakdown in clinical judgment and is critical for the development of clinical knowledge and improvement in clinical reasoning.

Tanner (2006, p. 209) concludes that thinking like a nurse is a form of engaged moral reasoning because nurses enter the care of the patient with a fundamental sense of what is good and right and a vision of what excellent care entails. Further, clinical reasoning should occur in relation to the particular patient and situation and be informed by the knowledge of the nurse and rational processes, but "never as a detached objective exercise, with the patient's concerns as a sidebar" (p. 210).

Another concept that is important to learning to "think like a nurse" is **mindfulness**. Weick and Sutcliffe (2007, p. 32) define mindfulness as "a rich awareness of discriminatory detail." In other words, when people act, they are aware of context, of ways in which details differ, and of deviations from their expectations. Mindfulness is similar to situation awareness but is different in the sense that mindfulness involves "the combination of ongoing scrutiny of existing expectations and continuous refinement and differentiation of expectations based on newer experiences" (p. 32). Mindfulness also involves a "willingness and capability to invent new expectations that make sense of unprecedented events, a more nuanced appreciation of context and ways to deal with it, and identification of new dimensions of context that improve foresight and current functioning" (p. 32).

Weick and Sutcliffe (2007) also note that certain conditions improve awareness. Awareness improves when attention is not distracted, when attention is focused on the present situation, when one is able to keep attention on the problem of interest, and when one is wary of fixing attention on preexisting categories. This pattern of awareness and attention is known as *mindfulness* and is used in many industries to facilitate quality and safety. In terms of nursing practice, mindfulness implies keeping attention focused in the present resulting in the ability to see salient aspects of the clinical situation and take decisive action to prevent harm.

What Is Critical Thinking?

Critical thinking is an integral part of nursing practice and promotes quality nursing care and positive patient outcomes. Although critical thinking is widely regarded as a component of clinical reasoning and decision making, it is difficult to define, and there is no single, simple definition that explains critical thinking. In nursing, critical thinking for clinical decision making is the ability to think in a systematic and logical manner, with openness to question and reflect on the reasoning process used to ensure safe nursing practice and quality care. It is providing effective care based on sound reasoning (Scriven & Paul, 2011). Critical thinking in nursing is an essential component of professional accountability and quality nursing care. Critical thinkers exhibit the following habits of mind: confidence, contextual perspective, creativity, flexibility, inquisitiveness, intellectual integrity, intuition, open-mindedness, perseverance, and reflection. In nursing, critical thinkers practice the cognitive skills of analyzing, applying standards, discriminating, information seeking, logical reasoning, predicting, and transforming knowledge (Scheffer & Rubenfeld, 2000).

There is a strong link between critical thinking and clinical judgment. The following definition offers a comprehensive description of elements incorporating critical thinking from a nursing prospective. Critical thinking and clinical judgment in nursing: (1) are purposeful, informed, outcome-focused thinking, (2) carefully identify key problems, issues, and risks, (3) are based on principles of nursing process, problem solving, and the scientific method, (4) apply logic, intuition, and creativity, (5) are driven by patient, family, and community needs, (6) call for strategies that make the most of human potential, and (7) require constant reevaluating (Alfaro-Lefevre, 2009). Thus, critical thinking, problem solving, and decision making are processes that are interrelated. Decision making and critical thinking need to occur concurrently to produce reasoning, clarification, and potential solutions.

CRITICAL THINKING QUESTION *

You are assigned to care for Ms. C., an 81-year-old patient who was admitted today with symptoms of increasing shortness of breath over the last week. She is currently receiving oxygen through a nasal cannula at 3 L/minute. You go into the room to assess her. You find that she is sitting up in bed at a 60-degree angle. She is restless and her respirations appear labored and rapid. Her skin is pale with circumoral cyanosis. You ask if she feels more short of breath. Because she is unable to catch her breath enough to speak, she nods her head "yes." Which action should you take first?

- Listen to her breath sounds.
- Ask when the shortness of breath started.
- Increase her oxygen flow rate to 6 L/min.
- Raise the head of the bed to 75 to 85 degrees

Based on knowledge you have learned, you realize the patient's symptoms indicate acute hypoxemia, so improving oxygen delivery is the priority. The other actions also are appropriate, but they are not as critical as the initial action. *

Competence in critical thinking is one of the expectations of nursing education. Critical thinkers are described as well informed, inquisitive, open minded, and orderly in complex matters. Critical thinking competence is an outcome for quality nursing care and for the development of clinical judgment. The ability to think critically is also described as reducing the research–practice gap and fostering evidence-based nursing (Wangensteen, Johansson, Bjorkstrom, & Nordstrom, 2010).

Learning to be a nurse requires more than memorizing facts. It requires that you learn to think like a nurse, to think through and reason at a greater depth, and to draw a more sophisticated or deeper understanding of what you are doing in clinical practice so that you provide safe, quality patient care. Nursing is not a careless, mindless activity. All acts in nursing are deeply significant and require the nurse's mind to be fully engaged. The following illustration shows nursing is both thinking and doing: The physician has ordered an intravenous (IV) line to be placed in a patient. How do you choose between a butterfly and an IV intracath? First, you have to consider why the line is being placed. You take into consideration whether it is a short-term, keep-open IV with limited medications; if so, then the butterfly IV is more comfortable and presents less of a threat of phlebitis. Doctors vary in their preferences as well, and this has to be considered. In addition, the condition of the patient and his or her veins makes a great deal of difference. For example, with older patients special skill is required. The veins look as though they are going to be easy to get because they look large, but they are very fragile. If you do not use a very slight tourniquet, the vein will pop open (Benner, 1984).

Characteristics of Critical Thinking

How do you know when critical thinking is taking place? Critical thinking has some of the following characteristics (Wilkinson, 2007):

- Critical thinking is rational and reasonable.
- Critical thinking involves conceptualization.
- Critical thinking requires reflection.
- Critical thinking involves cognitive (thinking) skills and attitudes (feelings).
- Critical thinking involves creative thinking.
- Critical thinking requires knowledge.

Critical thinking is rational and reasonable. It is based on reasons rather than preferences, prejudice, or self-interest. It uses facts and observations to draw conclusions. For example, suppose that during an election you decide to vote for the Democratic candidate because your family has always voted for Democrats. This decision is based on preference, prejudice, and, possibly, self-interest. By contrast, suppose you took time to reflect on what the candidates in the election said about the issues and based your choice on that. Even though you still might vote for the Democrat, you would be thinking rationally, using facts and observations to draw your conclusions (Wilkinson, 2007).

Critical thinking involves conceptualization. Conceptual thinking is the ability to understand a situation by identifying patterns or connections, focusing on key underlying issues, and integrating them into a conceptual framework. It involves using professional training and experience, creativity, and inductive reasoning that lead to solutions or alternatives that may not be easily identified. Conceptual thinking involves a willingness to explore and having an openness to a new way of seeing things or "looking outside of the box." Consider, for example, a case in which a patient with heart failure is coughing up yellow sputum. If the nurse suspects that the patient is short of breath from infection, he or she will evaluate other indicators of infection. The nurse will check the patient for an elevated temperature and will assess the last white blood cell count in the patient's chart to see if it is elevated. The nurse will also consider factors that may place the patient at risk for infection, such as immobility, poor nutrition, or immune suppression (Craven & Hirnle, 2007).

Critical thinking uses reflection. **Reflective thinking** is deliberate thinking and careful consideration. It is the process of analyzing, making judgments, and drawing conclusions. Reflective thinking involves creating an understanding through one's experiences and knowledge and exploring potential alternatives—assessing what you know, what you need to know, and how to bridge that gap. Processes of reflective thinking involve the following:

- Determine what information is needed (what you need to know) for understanding the issue.
- Examine what you have already experienced about an issue.
- Gather the available information.
- Synthesize the information and opinions.
- Consider the synthesis from different perspectives and frames of reference.
- Create some meaning from the relevant information and opinions.

CRITICAL THINKING QUESTION ✳

What do all of the following scenarios have in common?

- An elderly male becomes acutely confused and refuses to follow directions for his safety.
- A teen comes into an urgent care setting requesting information about sexually transmitted infections.
- A mother visits a school nurse and requests information about how the school handles sex education.
- A team leader needs to rearrange assignments when one team member goes home sick.
- Nursing staff in an intensive care unit need to develop an evacuation plan.

Answer: They all require critical thinking skills. ✳

CRITICAL THINKING QUESTION ✳

You will be taking care of a patient in a nursing home for the first time. Your assignment is to care for an older man who has heart disease. In addition, he has five other medical problems and takes 20 medications. While developing a plan of care for this patient, you can identify 8 to 10 nursing problems. You have no previous experience with nursing homes, and most of what you have heard and read about them is negative. Will you find yourself dreading the clinical day and expecting a negative experience before you even begin? ✳

Reflective thinking is important during complex problem-solving situations because it provides an opportunity to step back and think about how to actually solve problems and how problem-solving strategies are used for achieving set goals. Reflection allows students to observe and reflect, pulling together what they learn in the clinical and classroom settings in taking care of patients. Students can build and integrate knowledge and skills. Reflecting on a nursing experience or situation can assist nurses in critically reflecting on their practice. Choose a clinical situation and ask yourself some of the following questions:

- What was my role in this situation? Did I feel comfortable or uncomfortable? Why?
- What actions did I take? How did others and I respond? Was it appropriate?
- How could I have improved the situation for myself, the patient, and others involved? What can I change in the future?
- What have I learned through this situation?
- Did I expect anything different to happen? What and why?
- Has this situation changed my way of thinking in any way?
- What knowledge from theory and research can I apply in this situation?
- What broader issues, for example, ethical, social, or political, arise from this situation?

Through reflection, students manage to be more organized and effective because they have a better understanding of who the patient is and what his or her care needs are. Reflection on practice helps the student develop a self-improving practice (Benner et al., 2010).

Critical thinking involves cognitive (thinking) skills and attitudes (feelings). Critical thinking involves having thinking skills as well as the motivation to use them. It involves the willingness to utilize complex thought processes compared to easily understood ones. Critical thinkers do not oversimplify. Critical thinking is about being willing and able to think.

Critical thinking involves creative thinking. Creativity is part of the thinking process. When you brainstorm potential problem solutions or possible decisions, you are using creativity. Creative and critical thinkers combine ideas and information in ways that form new solutions or innovative ideas. A creative thinker is an open-minded thinker. Nurses can utilize creative thinking when encountering a patient situation in which traditional methods are not effective. For example, a pediatric nurse is caring for 9-year-old Pauline, who has ineffective respirations following abdominal surgery. The physician has ordered incentive spirometry breathing treatments, but Pauline is frightened by the equipment and she quickly tires during the treatments. The nurse offers Pauline a bottle of soap bubbles and a blowing wand. The nurse knows that the respiratory effort in blowing bubbles will promote alveolar expansion and suggests that Pauline blow bubbles between incentive spirometry treatments (Wilkinson, 2007).

Critical thinking requires knowledge. In most academic disciplines, the educational system uses an expert to deliver a body of knowledge to the unpracticed novice, who will later be expected to go out and apply the knowledge and rules learned in school to various work situations. In nursing, a specific educational knowledge base is required before applying that knowledge in patient care. It is important to know that the process is being applied correctly. In essence, to become a nurse you must learn the knowledge to think like a nurse. On the flip side of this, as the level of experience of the nurse increases, so will the scientific knowledge base that the nurse applies. For example, you are caring for a patient with heart failure. After obtaining the vital signs, what heart rate would prevent you from ambulating this patient? If you did not have knowledge regarding heart failure or did not know that the normal heart rate was 60–100 beats per minute, you could not make the good decision that ambulation should be postponed if the heart rate is above 100 beats per minute for this patient.

What Are the Characteristics of a Critical Thinker?

Nurses are required to think critically in all settings. Nurses' ability to think critically is one of their most important skills, and a commitment to think critically increases the nurse's ability to care for patients most effectively. A critical thinker has many characteristics, including the following:

- Critical thinkers are flexible—they can tolerate ambiguity and uncertainty.
- Critical thinkers base judgments on facts and reasoning, not personal feelings. They identify inherent biases and assumptions. Critical thinkers separate facts from opinions.
- Critical thinkers do not oversimplify.
- Critical thinkers examine available evidence before drawing conclusions.
- Critical thinkers think for themselves and do not simply go along with the crowd.
- Critical thinkers remain open to the need for adjustment and adaptation throughout the inquiry stages.
- Critical thinkers accept change.
- Critical thinkers empathize; they appreciate and try to understand others' thoughts, feelings, and behaviors.
- Critical thinkers welcome different views and value examining issues from every angle.
- Critical thinkers know that it is important to explore and understand positions with which they disagree.
- Critical thinkers discover and apply meaning to what they see, hear, and read.

KEY COMPETENCY 8-6

Examples of Applicable *Nurse of the Future: Nursing Core Competencies*

Leadership:

Knowledge (K2) Understands critical thinking and problem-solving processes

Skills (S2a) Uses systematic approaches in problem solving

Attitudes/Behaviors (A2) Values critical thinking processes in the management of client care situations

Source: Massachusetts Department of Higher Education. (2010). *Nurse of the future: Nursing core competencies* (p. 17). Retrieved from http://www.mass.edu/currentinit /documents/NursingCoreCompetencies.pdf

Approaches to Developing Critical Thinking Skills

As students develop in their nursing role, they learn and build critical thinking skills and apply them to real healthcare situations. Critical thinking requires conscious, deliberate effort. Critical thinking does not just come naturally; people tend to believe what is easy to believe or what those around them believe (Wilkinson, 2007). With effort and practice, everyone can achieve some level of critical thinking to become an effective problem solver and decision maker. As the elements of critical thought develop into a habit, nurses improve their ability to assess complex situations and engage in the practice of nursing. The objectives for critical thinking in nursing include the ability to ask pertinent questions, analyze multiple forms of evidence, and evaluate options before coming to a conclusion. Following are examples that can be used as approaches to developing critical thinking skills.

The Nursing Process

The ANA standards have set forth the framework necessary for critical thinking in the application of the nursing process. The **nursing process** is the tool by which all nurses can become equally proficient at critical thinking. The nursing process contains the following criteria: (1) assessment, (2) identifying the problem (nursing diagnosis), (3) planning, (4) implementation, and (5) evaluation. Through the application of each of these components, the nurse can become proficient at critical thinking. Nurses use critical thinking in each stage of the nursing process. This approach to critical thinking entails purposeful, informed, outcome-focused thinking, which requires identification of the nursing and healthcare needs of clients (Knapp, 2007).

The nursing process is a systematic, problem-solving approach to giving nursing care that allows the nurse to be accountable by using critical thinking before taking actions. Nurses provide effective care based on sound reasoning, which is the reasonable reflection on nursing problems before selecting one of a variety of solutions. This is accomplished by regularly employing the elements of critical thought, such as defining the problem, identifying the goal, and analyzing the evidence (Caputi, 2010).

Each of the following thinking skills is commonly used when a nurse gathers data (Caputi, 2010):

- Assessing systematically and comprehensively
- Checking accuracy and reliability
- Clustering related information
- Collaborating with coworkers
- Determining the importance of information
- Distinguishing relevant from irrelevant information
- Gathering complete and accurate data and then acting on those data
- Judging how much ambiguity is acceptable

KEY COMPETENCY 8-7

Examples of Applicable *Nurse of the Future: Nursing Core Competencies*

Professionalism:

Knowledge (K1b) Justifies clinical decisions

Skills (S1b) Exercises critical thinking within standards of practice

Attitudes/Behaviors (A1b) Shows commitment to provision of high quality, safe, and effective patient care

Source: Massachusetts Department of Higher Education. (2010). *Nurse of the future: Nursing core competencies* (p. 13). Retrieved from http://www.mass.edu/currentinit/documents/NursingCoreCompetencies.pdf

- Recognizing inconsistencies
- Using diagnostic reasoning

Each of the following thinking skills is commonly used when nurses provide care to patients (Caputi, 2010):

- Applying the nursing process to develop a treatment plan
- Communicating effectively
- Predicting and managing potential complications
- Resolving conflicts
- Resolving ethical dilemmas
- Setting priorities
- Teaching others

Assessment   The nursing assessment answers the questions of what is happening or what could happen. It involves systematically collecting, organizing, and analyzing information about the client. Once data or information has been collected and it is determined that the data are accurate and complete, the nurse performs data analysis or data interpretation. What are the client's actual and/or potential problems? A problem list is then developed based on the data, and the nurse prioritizes the client's problems. The nurse performs an ongoing assessment throughout the implementation of the nursing process.

Diagnosis   The nurse analyzes and derives meaning from the assessment information and selects a diagnosis. Diagnosis is the identification of a problem. It is a statement that describes a specific response to an actual or potential health problem. For example, a nursing diagnosis for a selected patient might be "decreased cardiac output related to inability of the heart to pump effectively, and occlusion and constriction of vessels impairing blood flow."

Planning   During planning, the nurse develops a plan to provide consistent, continuous care that meets the client's unique needs. Planning includes developing expected outcomes and working with the client to identify goals and to determine appropriate nursing actions and interventions that will reduce the identified problem. The nurse uses critical thinking to develop goals and nursing interventions for problems that require an individualized approach. Nurses use judgment to determine which interventions have a probability of achieving desired outcomes. To continue with the previous example, expected outcomes might include the following:

- Patient will be free of chest pain during my shift.
- Patient will maintain O_2 saturation of 90% during my shift.
- Vital signs will remain stable: T < 99.0°F, HR > 60 < 110 beats/min, R > 12 < 24 breaths/min, and SBP > 90 mm Hg while under my care.
- Patient will have no further weight gain and will have a decrease in edema during my shift.

KEY COMPETENCY 8-8

Examples of Applicable *Nurse of the Future: Nursing Core Competencies*

Patient-Centered Care:

Knowledge (K1) Identifies components of nursing process appropriate to individual, family, group, community, and population health care needs across the life span

Skills (S1a) Provides priority-based nursing care to individuals, families, and groups through independent and collaborative application of the nursing process

Attitudes/Behaviors (A1a) Values use of scientific inquiry, as demonstrated in the nursing process, as an essential tool for provision of nursing care

Source: Massachusetts Department of Higher Education. (2010). *Nurse of the future: Nursing core competencies* (p. 9). Retrieved from http://www.mass.edu/currentinit /documents/NursingCoreCompetencies.pdf

Implementation   Implementation is carrying out the plan of care and depends on the first three steps of the nursing process. These steps provide the basis for nursing actions performed during the implementation phase of the nursing process. The nurse carries out nursing interventions individualized to the patient, reassesses the client, and validates that the plan of care is accurate and successful. In this stage, to each patient care situation the nurse applies knowledge and principles from nursing and from related courses. The ability to apply, not just memorize, principles is a component of critical thinking (Wilkinson, 2007). For the patient with decreased cardiac output, the nurse could implement some of the following individualized interventions:

- Assess level of consciousness—confusion, anxiety.
- Provide reassurance to the patient.
- Monitor vital signs every 4 hours.
- Assess heart rate and rhythm; monitor telemetry or electrocardiography.
- Monitor for jugular vein distension.
- Monitor for chest pain.
- Monitor peripheral pulses; assess capillary refill.
- Auscultate lung sounds; monitor respiratory rate and rhythm; monitor oxygen saturation; assess for cough and sputum.
- Look at skin color and temperature.
- Monitor for fatigue and activity tolerance.
- Assess intake and output, daily weight, and edema in dependent areas.
- Assess abdomen for distension or bloating, ascites, and bowel function.
- Monitor lab and X-rays: complete blood count, prothrombin time/partial thromboplastin time, electrolytes, cardiac enzymes, arterial blood gases, and chest X-ray.
- Elevate head of bed to improve gas exchange.
- Administer oxygen as ordered to improve gas exchange.
- Administer morphine sulfate as prescribed to relieve chest pain, provide sedation and vasodilation, and monitor for respiratory depression and hypotension after administration.
- Administer diuretics as prescribed to reduce preload, enhance renal excretion of sodium and water, reduce circulating blood volume, and reduce pulmonary congestion; closely monitor potassium level, which might decrease as a result of diuretic therapy.
- Provide teaching: Identify precipitating risk factors of heart failure and prescribed medication regimen; notify physician if unable to take medications because of illness; avoid large amounts of caffeine; provide cardiac diet instruction; look for signs of exacerbation; monitor fluids; balance periods of activity and rest; avoid isometric activities that increase pressure in the heart.

Evaluation   During evaluation, the nurse compares the patient's current status to the patient goals. Were the goals achieved? The nurse analyzes outcomes to determine if the interventions worked, and if not, why? The information provided during evaluation can be used to begin another plan of care sufficient to meet patient needs. Continuing with the previous example, the evaluation might include the following:

- Patient denies chest pain on my shift. Patient rates pain 0 on pain scale.
- Patient's O_2 saturation dropped to 85% when oxygen at 3 L nasal cannula was removed. With oxygen on, patient's O_2 saturation remained at 92%.
- Vital signs were: T, 101.0°F; HR, 100–110 beats/min; R, 32 breaths/min and labored; BP, 90/50 mm Hg.
- Patient's weight was 241 pounds with 2+ edema in lower extremities.

Concept Mapping

Concept mapping is a visual representation of the relationships among concepts and ideas. The concepts are represented by boxes and linked with lines. In nursing, concept maps are used to organize and link information about a patient's health problems. This allows the nurse to see relationships among the patient's problems and helps plan interventions that can address more than one problem.

To begin a concept map, start in the center of the page with the main idea or central theme, and work outward in all directions, producing a growing organized structure composed of key words or pictures. Place words or pictures around the main idea to illustrate how they relate to each other and the central theme. Pictures, words, or a combination of both can be used to create a map.

Concept maps are useful for summarizing information, consolidating information from different sources, thinking through complex problems, and presenting information in a format that shows the overall structure of your subject. **Figure 8-1** illustrates mind mapping techniques used by students with a patient case.

Journaling

Keeping a journal of clinical experiences that were meaningful or troubling to you is a recommended way to help enhance and develop reasoning skills. Think about and record experiences that bother you, and consider what you could and would do differently in the future. This is a form of reflection and allows you to view your own thinking, reasoning, and actions. It helps create and clarify meaning and new understandings of a particular experience. When you encounter a similar situation, you should be able to recall what you did or

Figure 8-1   Mind mapping techniques

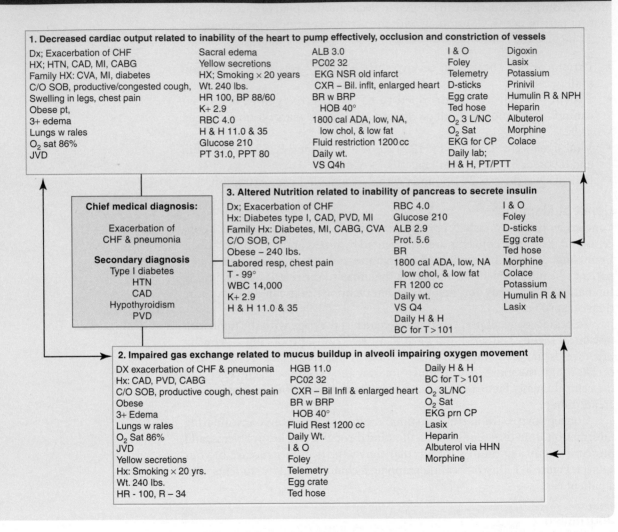

1. Decreased cardiac output related to inability of the heart to pump effectively, occlusion and constriction of vessels

Dx; Exacerbation of CHF	Sacral edema	ALB 3.0	I & O	Digoxin
HX; HTN, CAD, MI, CABG	Yellow secretions	PCO2 32	Foley	Lasix
Family HX: CVA, MI, diabetes	HX; Smoking × 20 years	EKG NSR old infarct	Telemetry	Potassium
C/O SOB, productive/congested cough,	Wt. 240 lbs.	CXR – Bil. inflt, enlarged heart	D-sticks	Prinivil
Swelling in legs, chest pain	HR 100, BP 88/60	BR w BRP	Egg crate	Humulin R & NPH
Obese pt,	K+ 2.9	HOB 40°	Ted hose	Heparin
3+ edema	RBC 4.0	1800 cal ADA, low, NA,	O₂ 3 L/NC	Albuterol
Lungs w rales	H & H 11.0 & 35	low chol, & low fat	O₂ Sat	Morphine
O₂ sat 86%	Glucose 210	Fluid restriction 1200 cc	EKG for CP	Colace
JVD	PT 31.0, PPT 80	Daily wt.	Daily lab;	
		VS Q4h	H & H, PT/PTT	

Chief medical diagnosis:

Exacerbation of
CHF & pneumonia

Secondary diagnosis
Type I diabetes
HTN
CAD
Hypothyroidism
PVD

3. Altered Nutrition related to inability of pancreas to secrete insulin

Dx; Exacerbation of CHF	RBC 4.0	I & O
Hx: Diabetes type I, CAD, PVD, MI	Glucose 210	Foley
Family Hx: Diabetes, MI, CABG, CVA	ALB 2.9	D-sticks
C/O SOB, CP	Prot. 5.6	Egg crate
Obese – 240 lbs.	BR	Ted hose
Labored resp, chest pain	1800 cal ADA, low, NA	Morphine
T - 99°	low chol, & low fat	Colace
WBC 14,000	FR 1200 cc	Potassium
K+ 2.9	Daily wt.	Humulin R & N
H & H 11.0 & 35	VS Q4	Lasix
	Daily H & H	
	BC for T > 101	

2. Impaired gas exchange related to mucus buildup in alveoli impairing oxygen movement

DX exacerbation of CHF & pneumonia	HGB 11.0	Daily H & H
Hx: CAD, PVD, CABG	PCO2 32	BC for T > 101
C/O SOB, productive cough, chest pain	CXR – Bil Infl & enlarged heart	O₂ 3L/NC
Obese	BR w BRP	O₂ Sat
3+ Edema	HOB 40°	EKG prn CP
Lungs w rales	Fluid Rest 1200 cc	Lasix
O₂ Sat 86%	Daily Wt.	Heparin
JVD	I & O	Albuterol via HHN
Yellow secretions	Foley	Morphine
Hx: Smoking × 20 yrs.	Telemetry	
Wt. 240 lbs.	Egg crate	
HR - 100, R – 34	Ted hose	

would do differently as well as the reasoning behind your actions (Raingruber & Haffer, 2001). Some suggestions you should try to address when **journaling** your nursing experience include the following:

- What happened? What are the facts?
- What was my role in the event?
- What feelings and senses surrounded the event?
- What did I do?
- How and what did I feel about what I did? Why?

- What was the setting?
- What were the important elements of the event?
- What preceded the event, and what followed it?
- What should I be aware of if the event recurs?

It is important that you write in your journal as soon as possible after an event to capture the essence of what happened in the clinical experience. The following is an example of a journal excerpt that illustrates reflection on events and the feelings elicited by those events over the course of many patient care encounters during the career of a nurse:

> I have learned, not so easily, that my job is not just about saving a life, trying to keep people well, or helping them get well when they are ill, but importantly, it also entails providing that same dedicated care to them as they take their last breaths in life. It is my job, my duty, and I have learned, my privilege. As I care for a dying patient, listening to the rise and fall of methodical machines imitating life, I hope I never am calloused to the point that I say, "I do this every day. It is just another patient." I want to appreciate that every individual's life has been remarkable in some way—which they are remarkable in some way. I want to make my patient's journey through this last chapter in their life a little easier, provide comfort, recognize their fears, hold their hand, and always realize this is not another patient, but a person.

Group Discussions and Reflection

Another way to enhance critical thinking skills is by using group discussions to explore alternatives and arrive at conclusions. Group discussions among nursing students and teachers can take place in the classroom or following clinical experiences. During discussions, students are encouraged to formulate alternatives to clinical or ethical decisions. Teacher and learner group discussions over clinical and ethical scenarios should encourage questions, analysis, and reflection. Group discussions can assist nursing students in connecting clinical events or decisions with information obtained in the classroom. This form of cooperative learning occurs when groups work together to maximize their own and each other's learning. For example, following a clinical experience, students and teacher use reflection and discussion on a certain clinical experience that a student encountered. Together they discuss different scenarios of "What if?," "What else?,"

CRITICAL THINKING QUESTIONS *

Think about a clinical experience that was troubling to you. Reflect on what bothered you about the experience. What could you have done differently? What were the reasons behind your actions? Try to create and clarify meaning or a new understanding of the particular situation. *

CRITICAL THINKING QUESTIONS *

Beginning nursing students often tend to focus primarily on their routines, such as to get their list of tasks done, such as assessments, ordered treatments, daily care, and charting. What if an unexpected situation occurred during the day? Do you think you would be able to reason, plan, and take appropriate action—think critically? *

KEY COMPETENCY 8-9

Examples of Applicable
*Nurse of the Future: Nursing
Core Competencies*

Professionalism:

Knowledge (K4c) Understands
the importance of reflection
to advancing practice and
improving outcomes of care

Skills (S4b) Demonstrates
ability for reflection in
actions, reflection for action,
and reflection on action

Attitudes/Behaviors (A4c)
Values and is committed
to being a reflective
practitioner

Source: Massachusetts Department of Higher
Education. (2010). *Nurse of the future:
Nursing core competencies* (p. 13). Retrieved
from http://www.mass.edu/currentinit
/documents/NursingCoreCompetencies.pdf

and "What then?" to encourage the formulation of alternatives or clinical decisions. Other examples of this process include the following:

- You are going into a patient's room—what are you going to do? When you go in there, what are you going to do? Walk yourself through it step by step.
- What are you going to do first? What should be done first? Which one takes importance and then where do you go from there?
- This is the patient, and this happens. What do you do next?
- These are your assessment findings. What else do you need to know?

You are working in an acute care clinical situation. After receiving report, you have started your morning routines. Everything is going as planned, and you are about to start preparing your medications. The wife of a patient reports that the oxygen is burning his nose and wants you to get an oxygen humidifier. All of a sudden, the daughter of another patient, Mr. Peary, rushes toward you and informs you that her father is spitting up blood. He looked fine when you observed him a few minutes ago. You walk rapidly toward the patient's room, thinking, "What am I going to do when I get there? I have to get the oxygen humidifier for room 202. His nose was burning, and his wife was waiting for me. What could be happening with Mr. Peary?"

You enter the room, and the first thing you think is: "He's lying flat," and you think to yourself, "I need to elevate his head. That is what I did on the respiratory unit where I recently worked." The daughter tells you that Mr. Peary coughed up some blood in the emesis basin. There is a small amount of bright red blood in it. You do not know what to do next. An RN stops by the room and tells you that the wife of the patient in room 202 is asking about the burning in her husband's nose again. Your mind does not seem to be able to think about anything. Do you feel scattered and things seem out of control at this point? Do you feel a little overwhelmed and cannot think what to do next? The RN says she will take over with Mr. Peary while you follow up with the patient in room 202. Later, you recall the situation and cannot believe you did not think to take Mr. Peary's blood pressure, count respirations, ask about pain, or listen to his lungs or anything else. All you did was just raise his head. You wonder why you missed so many things.

- What do you think was going on in the situation that influenced what was happening and caused you to lose your ability to think and plan what to do next?
- What would you do differently in this situation after having a chance to reflect on it? Prioritize the order in which you would have done things.
- If this had happened to you and no one helped you through it, what would you have done to mobilize yourself to think about what to do?

Conclusion

In nursing, critical thinking is the ability to think in a systematic and logical manner, solve problems, make decisions, and establish priorities in the clinical setting. Nurses need to develop critical thinking skills to make sound clinical judgments and to provide safe, competent patient care. Nursing requires constant decision making. What should I do first? What is the most important thing to do at this time? Prioritizing nursing actions involves recalling important nursing information as well as using complex problem-solving skills to make decisions in order to provide safe and effective patient care. Other tips for nurses at the bedside to improve safety include practicing mindfully, communicating clearly, reporting unsafe conditions and errors, responding to error justly, and recognizing personal limitations (Hershey, 2015, p. 149).

All of us want to believe that we will never be involved in an error that harms a patient. But as is evident, errors that result in patient harm do occur. This creates what has become known as the second victim, a term coined by Wu (2000) to describe the pain and suffering experienced after making a healthcare error. A nonjudgmental, supportive, and compassionate environment is recommended with the use of responses such as, "This must be difficult, are you okay?" or "Can we talk about it?" or "You are a good nurse working in a complex environment" (Hershey, 2015, p. 149). Creating a defensive environment does not allow the nurse at the sharp end of care to contribute to the safety process and therefore does nothing to increase patient safety. Thus, "responding to second victims with openness and compassion is not only the right thing to do, it is also the safe thing to do" (Hershey, 2015, p. 149).

CASE STUDY 8-1 ▪ JIM FULLER

Jim Fuller is a 40-year-old male patient. He is currently in the recovery room following an inguinal hernia repair under general anesthesia. His vital signs are: T, 99.0°F; BP, 120/80 mm Hg; HR, 80 beats/min; R, 18 breaths per minute.

Case Study Questions

1. Are Mr. Fuller's vital signs within normal limits? List normal adult ranges.

2. What factors might affect body temperature?

3. List sites where a nurse might take a patient's pulse. What sites are most commonly used?

4. What factors might influence respiratory rate?

Two hours postoperative, Mr. Fuller begins to complain of abdominal pain. Vital signs at this time are: T, 99.5°F; BP, 90/60 mm Hg; HR, 122 beats/min; R, 24 breaths/min.

Case Study Questions

1. What could Mr. Fuller's vital signs indicate?

2. What nursing interventions are indicated? What should the nurse assess in Mr. Fuller at this time?

3. What clinical signs associated with an elevated temperature might the nurse assess?

4. If Mr. Fuller's fever persists and increases, what might the nurse suspect is happening, and what might be done?

Classroom Activity 1

Critical thinking gives you the power to make sense of something by deliberately choosing how to respond to events that you encounter. You take in information, examine and ask questions about it, look at new perspectives, and identify a plan. You use problem-solving and decision-making strategies.

- Choose a decision that you need to make soon, and write it down.
- What goal or desired outcomes do you seek from this decision? Prioritize goals or desired outcomes, and write them down.
- Identify who and what will be affected by your decision, and indicate how your decision will affect them.
- Identify any available options you might have.
- Taking into account and evaluating your information, identify a plan or decide what you are going to do.
- After you have made your decision, evaluate the result.

Classroom Activity 2

You are receiving morning reports on the following patients from the night-shift nurse. After receiving the report, which patient would you choose to see first? As you make your decision, think about your thought processes and how you made your decision.

1. A woman who is scheduled to have a biopsy on a breast lump this morning, and who is scared and crying
2. An 85-year-old man who was admitted during the night because of increased confusion who remains disoriented this morning
3. A woman who had lung surgery the previous day, and who has two chest tubes in place with minimal drainage
4. A man who is scheduled to have a colon resection in 2 hours and is complaining of chills

Answer: You should have answered the client who is scheduled for surgery and is exhibiting symptoms of infection. This patient needs to be assessed immediately for infection, and the doctor notified. If an infection is present, the surgery needs to be postponed. The other patients are stable, and their needs do not have to be addressed immediately.

Classroom Activity 3

Numerous classroom and clinical activities related to safety are available on the QSEN website at http://qsen.org /teaching-strategies/strategy-search/. Choose activities from the website for students to complete that meet specific course objectives.

References

Agency for Healthcare Research and Quality. (2008). *Patient safety and quality: An evidence-based handbook for nurses* (Vols. 1–3). Rockville, MD: U.S. Department of Health and Human Services.

Agency for Healthcare Research and Quality. (2014). *2013 national healthcare quality report*. Rockville, MD: U.S. Department of Health and Human Services. Retrieved from http://www.ahrq.gov/research/findings/nhqrdr/

Alfaro-Lefevre, R. (2009). *Critical thinking and clinical judgment: A practical approach to outcome-focused thinking* (4th ed.). St. Louis, MO: Saunders Elsevier.

American Association of Colleges of Nursing. (2008). *The essentials of baccalaureate education for professional nursing practice*. Washington, DC: Author.

American Nurses Association. (2010a). *Nursing: Scope and standards of practice* (2nd ed.). Silver Spring, MD: Author.

American Nurses Association. (2010b). *Nursing's social policy statement: The essence of the profession*. Silver Spring, MD: Author.

American Nurses Association. (2015a). *Code of ethics with interpretive statements*. Silver Spring, MD: Author.

American Nurses Association. (2015b). *Nursing: Scope and standards of practice* (3rd ed.). Silver Spring, MD: Author.

Aspen, P., Walcott, J., Bootman, L., & Cronenwett, L. (2007). *Identifying and preventing medication errors*. Washington, DC: National Academies Press.

Barnsteiner, J. (2012). Safety. In G. Sherwood & J. Barnsteiner (Eds.), *Quality and safety in nursing: A competency approach to improving outcomes* (pp. 149–169). West Sussex, UK: Wiley.

Benner, P. (1984). *From novice to expert*. Menlo Park, CA: Addison-Wesley.

Benner, P. E., Sutphen, M., Leonard, V., & Day, L. (2010). *Educating nurses: A call for radical transformation*. San Francisco, CA: Jossey-Bass.

Caputi, L. (2010). Developing critical thinking in the nursing student. In L. Caputi (Ed.), *Teaching nursing: The art and science* (2nd ed., pp. 381–390). Glen Ellyn, IL: College of DuPage Press.

Chassin, M. R., & Loeb, J. M. (2013). High-reliability healthcare: Getting there from here. *Milbank Quarterly, 91*, 459–490.

Craven, R. F., & Hirnle, C. J. (2007). *Fundamentals of nursing: Human health and function* (5th ed.). Philadelphia, PA: Lippincott Williams & Wilkins.

Cronenwett, L., Sherwood, G., Barnsteiner, J., Disch, J., Johnson, J., Mitchell, P., … Warren, J. (2007). Quality and safety education for nurses. *Nursing Outlook, 55*(3), 122–131.

Donaldson, M. S. (2008). An overview of *To err is human*: Re-emphasizing the message of patient safety. In R. G. Hughes (Ed.), *Patient safety and quality: An evidence-based handbook for nurses* (Vol. 1, pp. 37–45). Publication No. 08-0043. Rockville, MD: Agency for Healthcare Research and Quality.

Fero, L., Witsberger, C., Wesmiller, S., Zullo, T., & Hoffman, L. (2009). Critical thinking ability of new graduate and experienced nurses. *Journal of Advanced Nursing, 65*(1), 139–148.

Haviley, C., Anderson, A. K., & Currier, A. (2014). Overview of patient safety and quality of care. In P. Kelly, B. A. Vottero, & C. A. Christie-McAuliffe (Eds.), *Introduction to quality and safety education for nurses* (pp. 1–37). New York, NY: Springer.

Henriksen, K., Dayton, E., Keyes, M. A., Carayon, P., & Hughes, R. (2008). Understanding adverse events: A human factors framework. In R. G. Hughes (Ed.), *Patient safety and quality: An evidence-based handbook for nurses* (Vol. 1, pp. 67–85). Publication No. 08-0043. Rockville, MD: Agency for Healthcare Research and Quality.

Hershey, K. (2015). Culture of safety. *Nursing Clinics of North America, 50,* 139–152.

Institute of Medicine. (2000). *To err is human: Building a safer health system.* Washington, DC: National Academies Press.

Institute of Medicine. (2001). *Crossing the quality chasm: A new health system for the 21st century.* Washington, DC: National Academies Press.

Institute of Medicine. (2004). *Keeping patients safe: Transforming the work environment of nurses.* Washington, DC: National Academies Press.

Institute of Medicine. (2006). *Preventing medication errors: Quality chasm series.* Washington, DC: National Academies Press.

Institute of Medicine. (2011). *The future of nursing: Leading change, advancing health.* Washington, DC: National Academies Press.

Joint Commission. (2011). Sentinel event alert issue 48: Health care worker fatigue and patient safety. Retrieved from http://www.jointcommission.org/sea_issue_48/

Joint Commission. (2012). Sentinel event: Patient safety systems chapter and the sentinel event policy. Retrieved from http://www.jointcommission.org/sentinel_event.aspx

Joint Commission. (2014). 2015 national patient safety goals. Retrieved from http://www.jointcommission.org/standards_information/npsgs.aspx

Knapp, R. (2007). Nursing education—the importance of critical thinking. Retrieved from http://www.articlecity.com/articles/education/article_1327.shtml

Malloch, K., Benner, P., Sheets, V., Kenward, K., & Farrell, M. (2010). Overview: NCSBN practice breakdown initiative. In P. E. Benner, K. Malloch, & V. Sheets (Eds.), *Nursing pathways for patient safety* (pp. 1–29). St. Louis, MO: Mosby.

Marx, D. (2001). *Patient safety and the "just culture": A primer for health care executives. Medical event reporting system-transfusion medicine.* New York, NY: Columbia University.

Massachusetts Department of Higher Education. (2010). *Nurse of the future: Nursing core competencies.* Retrieved from http://www.mass.edu/currentinit/documents /NursingCoreCompetencies.pdf

McCannon, C. J., Hackbarth, A. D., & Griffin, F. A. (2007). Miles to go: An introduction to the 5 million lives campaign. *Joint Commission Journal of Quality and Patient Safety, 33,* 477–484.

Mitchell, P. (2008). Defining patient safety and quality care. In R. G. Hughes (Ed.), *Patient safety and quality: An evidence-based handbook for nurses* (Vol. 1, pp. 1-6). Publication No. 08-0043. Rockville, MD: Agency for Healthcare Research and Quality.

National Council of State Boards of Nursing. (2013). Practice errors and risk factors (TERCAP). Retrieved from https://www.ncsbn.org/113.htm

National Quality Forum (NQF). (2010). *Safe practices for better healthcare 2010: A consensus report.* Washington, DC: Author.

Quality and Safety Education for Nurses. (2007). Competencies: Pre-licensure KSAS. Retrieved from http://qsen.org/competencies/pre-licensure-ksas/

Raingruber, B., & Haffer, A. (2001). *Using your head to land on your feet: A beginning nurse's guide to critical thinking*. Philadelphia, PA: F. A. Davis.

Reason, J. (2000). Human error: Models and management. *British Medical Journal*, *320*, 768–770.

Rovinski-Wagner, C., & Mills, P. D. (2014). Patient safety. In P. Kelly, B. A. Vottero, & C. A. Christie-McAuliffe (Eds.), *Introduction to quality and safety education for nurses* (pp. 95–130). New York, NY: Springer.

Rowell, P. (2003). The professional nursing association's role in patient safety. *Online Journal of Issues in Nursing*, *8*(3). Retrieved from http://www.nursingworld.org /MainMenuCategories/ANAMarketplace/ANAPeriodicals/OJIN/TableofContents /Volume82003/No3Sept2003/AssociationsRole.aspx

Scheffer, B. K., & Rubenfeld, M. G. (2000). A consensus statement on critical thinking in nursing. *Journal of Nursing Education*, *39*(8), 352–359.

Scriven, M., & Paul, R. (2011). *Defining critical thinking*. Retrieved from http://www .criticalthinking.org/pages/defining-critical-thinking/410

Tanner, C. A. (2006). Thinking like a nurse: A research based mode of clinical judgment in nursing. *Journal of Nursing Education*, *4*(6), 204–211.

Wangensteen, S., Johansson, I. S., Bjorkstrom, M. E., & Nordstrom, G. (2010). Critical thinking dispositions among newly graduated nurses. *Journal of Advanced Nursing*, *66*(10), 2170–2181.

Weick, K. E., & Sutcliffe, K. M. (2007). *Managing the unexpected: Resilient performance in an age of uncertainty* (2nd ed.). San Francisco, CA: Jossey-Bass.

Wilkinson, J. (2007). *Nursing process and critical thinking* (4th ed.). Upper Saddle River, NJ: Pearson.

Wu, A. (2000). Medical error: The second victim: The doctor who makes the mistake needs help too. *British Medical Journal*, *320*, 726–727.

CHAPTER 9

Quality Improvement and Professional Nursing Practice

Kathleen Masters

Learning Objectives

After completing this chapter, the student should be able to:

1. Explore the link between quality and safety.
2. Discuss the relationship of transparency and reporting to healthcare quality.
3. Describe nursing-sensitive measures.
4. Discuss the need for continuous quality improvement (CQI) in the provision of patient care.
5. Discuss the role of the nurse in quality improvement.

The overall quality of health care and patient safety is improving, particularly for hospital care and for measures that are being publicly reported by the Centers for Medicare and Medicaid Services (CMS). According to the Agency for Healthcare Research and Quality (AHRQ), hospital care was safer in 2013 than it was in 2010, with 17% less harm to patients and an estimated 1.3 million fewer hospital-acquired conditions and 50,000 fewer deaths. We have come a long way; however, quality is still far from optimal with millions of patients harmed by the care they receive and with only 70% of recommended care being delivered across a broad array of quality measures (AHRQ, 2015, pp. vi–vii).

Key Terms and Concepts

- » Quality
- » Quality improvement
- » Care bundle
- » Benchmarking
- » Healthcare transparency
- » Core measures
- » Accountability measures
- » Composite measures
- » Nursing-sensitive measures
- » Continuous quality improvement (CQI)

Healthcare Quality

Many reports such as the one just cited refer to quality and safety together. But what do we mean in health care when we speak about quality? According to the Institute of Medicine (IOM, 2001), **quality** is the degree to which health services for individuals and populations increase the likelihood of desired health outcomes and are consistent with current professional knowledge. Because professional knowledge is continually increasing, quality is a moving target; because quality is a moving target, there will always be room for quality improvement.

What is quality improvement? **Quality improvement** refers to the use of data to monitor the outcomes of care processes and uses improvement methods to design and test changes to continuously improve the quality and safety of healthcare systems (Cronenwett et al., 2007; Massachusetts Department of Higher Education, 2010, p. 36; Quality and Safety Education for Nurses [QSEN], 2007). Quality improvement focuses on systems, processes, satisfaction, and cost outcomes, usually within a specific organization. Quality improvement models assume that the process is continuous and that quality can always be improved, whereas quality assurance models seek to ensure that current quality exists (Owens & Koch, 2015).

Building on the previous IOM report, *To Err Is Human* (2000), *Crossing the Quality Chasm: A New Health System for the 21st Century* (IOM, 2001) introduced performance expectations to create a system where patients are assured care that is safe, timely, effective, efficient, equitable, and patient-centered. Safe care refers to avoiding harm to patients from care that is supposed to help them. Timely care includes reducing delays for those who receive care and for those who provide care. Effective care refers to the provision of services based on evidence to all who could benefit and refraining from providing services to those not likely to benefit. Efficient care refers to avoiding waste. Equitable refers to providing care that does not vary in quality based on characteristics such as ethnicity, gender, socioeconomic status, or geographic location. Patient-centered care refers to providing care that is responsive to patient preferences, needs, and values, and ensuring that patient values guide clinical decisions. These six aims are referred to as STEEEP.

In addition, the report outlined principles or rules for redesign to move the healthcare system toward the identified performance expectations. The 10 rules for redesign follow:

- Care is based on continuous healing relationships with patients receiving care whenever and wherever it is needed.
- Care can be customized according to the patient's needs and preferences even though the system is designed to meet the most common types of needs.
- The patient is the source of control, and as such should be given enough information and opportunity to exercise the degree of control the patient chooses regarding decisions that affect him or her.
- Knowledge is shared and information flows freely so that patients have access to their own medical information.
- Decision making is evidence based; that is, it is based on the best available scientific knowledge and should not vary illogically between clinicians or locations.

- Safety is a system property, and patients should be safe from harm caused by the healthcare system.
- Transparency is necessary where systems make information available to patients and families that enable them to make informed decisions when selecting a health plan, hospital, or clinic, or when choosing alternative treatments.
- Patient needs are anticipated rather than the system merely reacting to events.
- Waste of resources and patient time is continuously decreased.
- Cooperation among clinicians is a priority to ensure appropriate exchange of information and coordination of care (IOM, 2001).

This IOM report and the quality reports that followed set the quality standard for the healthcare system. Because patient safety and quality health care cannot be separated, the report addressed both. Recommendations in this report have impacted healthcare professional education, innovation in the realm of information technology for use in health care, accreditation, and regulation, as well as policies to align payment for healthcare services with outcomes and purchasing of health care with outcomes.

Another organization that has contributed to the quality movement is the Institute for Healthcare Improvement (IHI). In 2001, the IHI and the Voluntary Hospital Association collaborated to determine specifically how to achieve good outcomes with high levels of reliability in critical care units. The result of this collaborative initiative was the development of the concept of care bundles. A **care bundle** is defined by IHI as a small set of evidence-based interventions for a defined population of patients and care setting. Several bundles have been developed, but the original two bundles developed from the initiative were the IHI ventilator bundle and the IHI central line bundle. The use of bundles has significantly increased quality of care and improved patient outcomes (Owens & Koch, 2015, p. 35).

One of the best-known initiatives of the IHI was the 100,000 lives campaign when hospitals were challenged to extend or save 100,000 lives from January 2005 to June 2006 by deploying rapid response teams; delivering reliable, evidence-based care for acute myocardial infarction; preventing adverse drug events; preventing central line infections; preventing surgical site infections; and preventing ventilator-associated pneumonia. The goal of the next campaign was to prevent harm to 5 million lives from 2006 to 2008 by preventing pressure ulcers; reducing methicillin-resistant *Staphylococcus aureus*; preventing harm from high-alert medications; reducing surgical complications; delivering reliable, evidence-based care for congestive heart failure to reduce readmission; and getting boards of directors involved by defining and spreading new and leveraged processes for hospitals' boards of directors, so that they could become far more effective in accelerating the improvement of care (Berwick, 2014).

One of the most significant drivers of the quality movement in the healthcare system in the United States has been the implementation of pay for performance and more recently value-based purchasing. In a pay-for-performance approach, there is financial benefit for healthcare providers to report measures and give quality care. Value-based purchasing combines quality and payment but also includes strategies to direct purchasers to high-performing institutions and health plans. Examples of these approaches include hospitals not being paid for secondary diagnoses related to preventable adverse events, such as harm from fall, hospital-acquired infection, or wrong site surgery and the systems that make these types of data available to consumers (Johnson, 2012, p. 116).

Measurement of Quality

Quality improvement is data driven. One must have data to measure the effectiveness of care or the outcomes of care in order to know how good the care was that was provided to the patient. Another requirement for data to be useful is that language is consistent across institutions. For example, if one institution reports a fall only if the patient lands on the floor and another institution reports a fall based on the patient falling even though she is caught before landing on the floor, fall data will be measuring different phenomena in the two institutions (Johnson, 2012, p. 119). For data to be meaningful, the measures must be valid. For data to be comparable across multiple institutions, the data must reflect measures of the same phenomena. Data collected can then provide information related to how much care varies among nurses, units, and organizations as well as from the standard that is based on current professional knowledge.

Measures are the most useful when they can be compared with measures that are considered the standard or best practice measures, thus allowing institutions to compare outcomes. Commonly, benchmarks are national or state averages and may include highest and lowest score by category (Johnson, 2012, p. 122). **Benchmarking** may be defined as seeking out and implementing best practice or seeking to attain an attribute or achievement that serves as a standard for other institutions to emulate. Benchmarking may be either internal or external. Internal benchmarking may have the limitation of small numbers of units for comparison, whereas external benchmarking allows comparison with large numbers and top performers. Using benchmarking, data are compared to determine level of performance and use a systematic method to identify a problem, select best practices, determine how best practice fits the unit or organization, initiate a change process, and evaluate outcomes (Vottero, Block, & Bonaventura, 2012, p. 224).

Benchmarking begins with identification of the quality indicator that will be measured. Quality indicators are classified as structure, process, or

KEY COMPETENCY 9-1

Examples of Applicable *Nurse of the Future: Nursing Core Competencies*

Quality Improvement:

Knowledge (K1) Describes the nursing context for improving care

Skills (S1a) Actively seeks information about quality initiatives in their own care settings and organization

(S1b) Actively seeks information about quality improvement in the care setting from relevant institutional, regulatory and local/national sources

Attitudes/Behaviors (A1) Recognizes that quality improvement is an essential part of nursing

Source: Massachusetts Department of Higher Education. (2010). *Nurse of the future: Nursing core competencies* (p. 36). Retrieved from http://www.mass.edu/currentinit/documents/NursingCoreCompetencies.pdf

outcome indicators. Structure indicators reflect attributes of the care environment and may include things like staffing or availability of technology. Process indicators include the evidence-based interventions or actions that help achieve outcomes. Outcome indicators include the end results of care delivery such as hospital-acquired infection or pressure ulcer (Vottero et al., 2012, pp. 222–223).

Healthcare Quality Reporting

Healthcare transparency tends to improve care because the public availability of data allows patients to make informed choices about where they want to receive healthcare services. Healthcare transparency, as defined by the IOM (2001), is making information on the healthcare system's quality, efficiency, and consumer satisfaction with care, which includes safety data, available to the public so that patients and families can make informed decisions when choosing care and to influence the behavior of providers, payers, and others to achieve better outcomes. Numerous websites are available that allow consumers to access information related to provider and healthcare system safety and quality. Some of the best-known sites include:

- CMS: www.hospitalcompare.hhs.gov
- CMS Home Health Compare: www.medicare.gov/homehealthcompare/
- The Joint Commission Quality Check: www.qualitycheck.org/consumer /searchQCR.aspx
- The Leapfrog Group Hospital Safety: www.hospitalsafetyscore.org
- United Health Foundation: www.americashealthrankings.org
- IPRO: www.ipro.org/for-consumers
- IPRO Why Not the Best?: www.whynotthebest.org
- The Commonwealth Fund: www.commonwealthfund.org

In 1998, the Joint Commission launched the first national program for the measurement of hospital quality, initially only requiring the reporting of nonstandardized data on performance measures. In 2002, accredited hospitals were required to collect and report data for at least two of four core measure sets; these data were made publicly available by the Joint Commission in 2004 (Chassin, Loeb, Schmaltz, & Wachter, 2010).

From this beginning, we now have a healthcare quality landscape in which the National Quality Forum (NQF) has endorsed more than 600 quality measures and CMS has begun to financially penalize hospitals based on performance (Chassin et al., 2010). The Joint Commission has collaborated with CMS to align common measures to provide hospitals with some relief related to numerous data collection requirements. The system in place allows the same data sets to be used to satisfy multiple data requirements. For example, the Joint Commission and CMS common measures as well as Joint Commission–only measures are used in the CMS Quality Reporting Programs, and the

CMS Hospital Compare website reflects measures that CMS and the Joint Commission have in common (Joint Commission, 2014a).

In 2002, the Joint Commission introduced the **core measures** program. Core measures are standardized performance indicators. Because the indicators are standardized, they allow for comparison of the measures across healthcare organizations and over time (Haviley, Anderson, & Currier, 2014, p. 6). Measurement of performance indicator data reporting has been integrated into the accreditation process by the Joint Commission through what is known as the ORYX initiative. The initiative was one of the Joint Commission's first steps to focus the accreditation process on an ongoing picture of performance to facilitate focus on CQI related to patient care, treatment, and service issues versus looking at data only once every 3 years during the accreditation visit (Joint Commission, 2013). In 2002, the Joint Commission also introduced the first National Patient Safety Goals.

For several years hospitals were required to report on four mandatory measure sets: acute myocardial infarction, heart failure, pneumonia, and surgical care improvement. In 2012, the Joint Commission also reclassified process performance measures into accountability and nonaccountability measures. **Accountability measures** are evidence-based care processes closely linked to positive patient outcomes (Joint Commission, 2014a, p. 13). Accountability measures are quality indicators that must meet four criteria and that are designed to identify measures that produce the greatest positive impact on patient outcomes when hospitals demonstrate improvement. The four criteria used to determine if an indicator is an accountability measure are as follows:

- *Research:* Strong scientific evidence demonstrates that performing the evidence-based care process improves health outcomes.
- *Proximity:* Performing the care process is closely connected to the patient outcome.
- *Accuracy:* The measure accurately assesses whether the care process has actually been provided.
- *Adverse effects:* Implementing the measure has little or no chance of inducing unintended adverse consequences (Joint Commission, 2014b).

Measures that meet all four criteria can be used by organizations for purposes of accountability such as public reporting and accreditation. Those measures that are not designated as reportable accountability measures are still useful for quality improvement within individual healthcare organizations (Joint Commission, 2014a).

Composite measures combine the results of related measures into a single percentage rating calculated by adding up the number of times recommended evidence-based care was provided to patients and dividing this sum by the total number of opportunities to provide this care. Composite accountability measures are derived from 44 accountability measures within the 10 sets of measures. The current 10 sets of measures are heart attack care, heart failure care, pneumonia care, surgical care, children's asthma care, inpatient psychiatric services, venous thromboembolism care, stroke care, immunization, and perinatal care.

Beginning in 2015, hospitals now have greater flexibility in meeting the performance measure requirements. Data reporting requirements are intended to support healthcare organizations in their quality improvement efforts and are available to the public on the Joint Commission website at www.qualitycheck.org. The public availability of performance measure data permits comparisons of hospital performance at the state and national levels by consumers (Joint Commission, 2014c).

Measures of Nursing Care

Quality measurement can be viewed in terms of structure, process, and outcome. Structure refers to the context of healthcare delivery and includes things such as buildings, staffing, and equipment. Process refers to the delivery of care, which includes the interactions between providers and patients. Finally, outcomes refer to the effect of health care on the health status of patients and populations. Using this framework, appropriate structure is required to support processes that will lead to desired outcomes (Donabedian, 1966). It stands to reason, then, that if the outcome measured has not achieved the desired standard, some attention should be given to the structures and processes in place that impact the outcome in order to achieve the desired standard. This framework is proving successful for increasing the quality of care provided to patients. It is important to note, however, that although tremendous strides have been made, most of the measures captured in the standardized data sets described previously relate to outcomes of medical care processes rather than reflecting the impact of nursing care. The following sections describe some ongoing efforts to capture data that reflect the contribution of nursing to patient outcomes.

CAHPS Hospital Survey

The Hospital Consumer Assessment of Healthcare Providers and Systems (HCAHPS, pronounced "H-CAPS") survey, also known as the CAHPS Hospital Survey, is the only national survey that includes a measure of nursing quality. The survey asks a core set of questions with four of the questions relating specifically to nursing. The standardized questions allow for comparisons of patient care experiences. For example, one question asks the patient about how often they got help as soon as they wanted after pushing the call button. The following questions also are included in the category, *how often did nurses communicate well with patients?*

- How often did nurses treat you with courtesy and respect?
- How often did nurses listen carefully to you?
- How often did nurses explain things in a way you could understand? (U.S. Department of Health and Human Services, 2011).

These are simple questions, yet one can see that they relate to quality in terms of the timeliness of care and the provision of patient-centered care. Standardized questions allow for comparisons of patient care experiences across settings.

National Voluntary Consensus Standards for Nursing-Sensitive Care

Another effort to identify nursing-sensitive indicators to measure quality was born in 2003 when the Robert Wood Johnson Foundation (RWJF) funded eight research projects to examine and evaluate existing indicators of nursing performance. The projects found that data typically did not include the specific variables that quantify aspects of nurses' activities or contributions to quality of care. The studies also highlighted the need for "nursing-sensitive" measures. **Nursing-sensitive measures** were identified as patient-related processes or outcomes—or structural variables that serve as proxies to these processes and outcomes—that reflect the nurse-quality relationship (RWJF, 2011, p. 4).

RWJF turned to the NQF to endorse the compilation of nursing-sensitive measures through a consensus development process. In 2004, the NQF endorsed 15 voluntary consensus standards for nursing-sensitive care that could be used for performance measurement. These initial nursing-sensitive measures were referred to as the "NQF-15" and included measures in three domains: patient-centered measures, nursing-centered measures, and system-centered measures (NQF, 2004). The original list of measures included three measures related to smoking cessation that have since been retired from the list. The current list includes 12 endorsed measures:

- *Death among surgical inpatients with treatable serious complications ("failure to rescue"):* The percentage of major surgical inpatients who experience hospital-acquired complications and die
- *Pressure ulcer prevalence:* The percentage of inpatients who have a hospital-acquired pressure ulcer
- *Falls prevalence:* The number of inpatient falls per inpatient day
- *Falls with injury:* The number of inpatient falls with injury per inpatient day
- *Restraint prevalence:* The percentage of inpatients who have a vest or limb restraint
- *Urinary catheter–associated urinary tract infection for intensive care unit (ICU) patients:* The rate of urinary tract infections associated with use of urinary catheters for ICU patients
- *Central line catheter–associated bloodstream infection rate for ICU and high-risk nursery patients:* The rate of bloodstream infections associated with the use of central line catheters for ICU and high-risk nursery patients
- *Ventilator-associated pneumonia for ICU and high-risk nursery patients:* The rate of pneumonia associated with the use of ventilators for ICU and high-risk nursery patients

- *Skill mix:* The percentage of registered nurse, licensed vocational/practical nurse, unlicensed assistive personnel, and contracted nurse care hours to total nursing care hours
- *Nursing care hours per patient day:* The number of registered nurses per patient day and the number of nursing staff hours (registered nurse, licensed vocational/practical nurse, unlicensed assistive personnel) per patient day
- *Practice Environment Scale of the Nursing Work Index (composite plus five subscales):*
  - Nurse participation in hospital affairs
  - Nursing foundations for quality care
  - Nurse manager ability, leadership, and support of nurses
  - Staffing and resource adequacy
  - Collegiality of nurse–physician relations
- *Voluntary turnover of nursing staff:* The number of nurses who leave their jobs of their own volition during the month, by category (NQF, 2004, p. 14; RWJF, 2011, pp. 15–16)

The NQF report also identified a number of areas in which adequate measurements simply did not exist, and called for further research about such topics as the relationship between nursing variables such as staffing (turnover, experience, etc.) and patient outcomes, the contribution of nurses to pain management, and the relationship between patient outcomes and process measures for nursing-centered interventions, including measures that describe the distinctive contributions of nurses such as assessment, problem identification, prevention, and patient education. The original work was intended to be a starting point rather than an ending point in identification of nursing-sensitive measures. "The *2009 Implementation Guide for the National Quality Forum (NQF) Endorsed Nursing-Sensitive Care Performance Measures* provided detailed specifications for the 12 national voluntary consensus standards for nursing-sensitive care endorsed by the NQF" (Joint Commission, 2014d); however, the work to identify a comprehensive set of nursing-sensitive measures is far from complete. Once rigorous studies that demonstrate reliability and validity related to a nursing-sensitive measure have been completed, they can be submitted to the NQF for possible endorsement.

National Database of Nursing Quality Indicators (NDNQI)

In 1997, the American Nurses Association (ANA) also began identifying nursing-sensitive measures. These data are now part of a repository known as the National Database of Nursing Quality Indicators (NDNQI). Some of the measures included in the NDNQI are also NQF-approved measures, but other measures are not included in the NQF approved measures list. The NDNQI provides reporting on structure, process, and outcome on 19 nursing-sensitive indicators at the unit level. Because the data from the NDNQI are unit-level data, they can be compared to other units in the organization or to similar units in other geographical locations. Because the data are unit based, the data have been used to demonstrate linkages between unit staffing levels and patient outcomes to demonstrate the contributions of nursing to quality patient care. Measures include patient falls, nursing hours per patient day, staff mix, restraints, hospital-acquired pressure ulcers, nurse satisfaction, nurse education and certification, and pediatric pain assessment, among others (Montalvo, 2007). The NDNQI is currently owned and operated by Press Ganey, a healthcare improvement organization.

Quality Improvement Process and Tools

Continuous quality improvement (CQI) is defined as a structured organizational process that involves personnel in planning and implementing the continuous flow of improvements in the provision of quality health care that meets or exceeds expectations. There are two typical pathways in the quality improvement process. The first process occurs as data that are regularly collected are monitored. If the data indicate that a problem exists, then an analysis is done to identify possible causes and a process is initiated to pilot a change. The second pathway involves the identification of a problem outside of the routine data monitoring system (Johnson, 2012).

In addition to data, CQI generally have a common set of characteristics that include a link to key elements of the organization's strategic plan, a quality council composed of the organization's leadership, training programs for personnel, mechanisms for the selection of improvement opportunities, the formation of process improvement teams, staff support for process analysis and redesign, policies that motivate and support staff participation in process improvement, and the application of current and rigorous techniques of scientific method and statistical process control (Sollecito & Johnson, 2013, pp. 4–5). Collaboration and evidence-based practice are also key elements of successful quality improvement programs (Caramanica, Cousino, & Petersen, 2003).

There are several quality improvement tools that can assist in monitoring measures. Common tools include histograms, control charts, run charts, and scattergrams. These tools can assist in the identification of problems by visually showing the frequency of events and events outside of set parameters (Johnson, 2014, p. 124). Once problems are identified, the root cause analysis technique can be used to systematically identify the reason for the problem. A common approach to root cause analysis is to use a cause and effect diagram known as the Ishikawa or fishbone diagram, which assists in identifying problems such as system issues with multiple dimensions. The problem statement is the "head of the fish," and the related processes or categories that are potential causes of the problem are clarified by completing an event flow diagram that consists of the main bones of the fish. Next, subcategories of causation or contributing factors are developed that create each of the smaller bones or branches of the diagram.

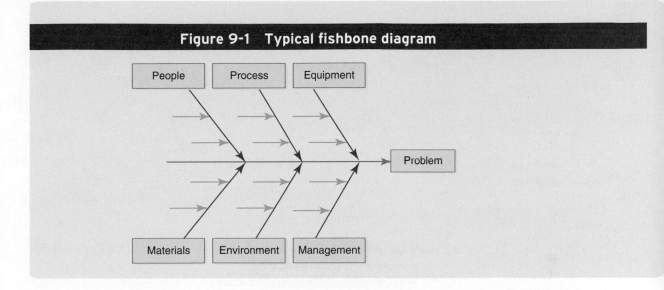

Figure 9-1 Typical fishbone diagram

The diagram is completed as relationships among causal chains are identified and causal statements are developed. This process requires asking why the event happened in order to identify the underlying source of the error (Barnsteiner, 2012). After all possible causes are identified, the team chooses the top two possible causes and then initiates a change process using one of several selected quality improvement methodologies. See **Figure 9-1** for a typical fishbone diagram.

Popularized by William Edwards Deming, the Deming cycle of Plan, Do, Check, Act or, as he later modified it, the Plan, Do, Study, Act (PDSA) process is the most commonly used quality improvement methodology in health care (see **Figure 9-2**). The basic premise of the PDSA is to encourage innovation by experimenting with a change, studying the results, and making refinements as necessary to achieve sustained desired outcomes (Strome, 2013, p. 63). The process includes questions and activities that guide each phase. Examples include:

- *Plan:* Begin with planning the changes to a process that are to be implemented and tested.
  - What is the objective?
  - What is the test of change?
- *Do:* Carry out the plan and make the desired changes to the process.
  - Conduct the test.
  - Document unexpected observations and problems.
- *Study:* Review the impact and outcomes of the implemented changes.
  - Analyze the data.
  - Were the outcomes as expected?
  - What was learned from the test?

Figure 9-2   Plan, Do, Study, Act (PDSA) cycle

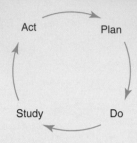

- *Act:* Determine if the changes can be implemented as is or if further cycles are necessary for refinement.
  - What modifications should be made?
  - What is the next test? (Johnson, 2012, p. 126; Strome, 2013, p. 64)

Six Sigma is another quality improvement methodology frequently used in health care. The goal of Six Sigma is to decrease the defects or errors from the current level within an organization. Six Sigma uses an approach that "emphasizes the use of information and statistical analysis to rigorously and routinely measure and improve an organization's performance, practices, and systems" (Strome, 2013, p. 71). Approaches to Six Sigma vary by organization, but initiatives generally have five elements in common. The common elements include intent, strategy, methodology, tools, and measurements. Six Sigma initiatives are undertaken with the intent of achieving significant improvement in a short time and can be applied at a corporate level or aimed strategically at an individual project. Several Six Sigma methodologies exist, but the most common one used in health care is what is known as DMAIC (Define, Measure, Analyze, Improve, Control). Tools involved in Six Sigma are numerous, but fall into three categories: requirements gathering, statistical analysis, and experimentation. Finally, the most common measurements used in Six Sigma include defects/errors per unit, defects per million opportunities, and Sigma level (Strome, 2013, p. 71).

The five phases of the Six Sigma methodology using the DMAIC, discussed in the following list, must always be followed in precisely the same order, but they provide a rigorous approach that is effective in identifying opportunities for improvement.

- *Define:* Clearly identify and state the problem that is the focus of the quality improvement initiative and outline the scope of the project. Determine the critical requirements and key benefits. Agree on the process to be improved and the plan to achieve the improvements.

- *Measure:* Review all available data, measure the extent of the quality problem, and obtain baseline performance information.
- *Analyze:* Use tools (such as a fishbone diagram) to study the root cause of the problem and develop potential solution alternatives.
- *Improve:* Develop alternative processes to help achieve the desired outcomes. Evaluate the alternatives based on each one's potential impact on the outcome, using statistical analysis to determine the highest likelihood of achieving the desired performance.
- *Control:* Sustain improvements through ongoing measurement and by conducting ongoing communication, reviews, and training (Strome, 2013, p. 72).

Another framework that is used to improve quality by identifying events or characteristics of a system that may allow potential errors to be averted is known as Reason's Adverse Event Trajectory or the Swiss Cheese Model (Reason, 2000). This model is used to prevent error by explaining how faults in different layers of the system can lead to error through triggers that can set up a sequence of events. Multiple defenses that have been set in place to prevent errors may at times line up, allowing multiple triggers to align and, thus, allow an error to occur. The lining up of triggers has been illustrated as an arrow and the lining up of defenses the alignment of holes in Swiss cheese (thus, the name Swiss Cheese Model). When the defenses line up, the arrow or trigger goes through the defenses (holes) and an error may occur. When the defenses do not line up, the trigger (arrow) is blocked and the error is averted.

Regardless of the methodology chosen for a quality improvement initiative, there are some general commonalities among processes. In all successful quality improvement initiatives, the problem must be defined, opportunities for improvement must be identified, and improvement activities executed. Outcomes must be evaluated, and finally, change must be sustained (Strome, 2013, p. 130).

KEY COMPETENCY 9-3

Examples of Applicable *Nurse of the Future: Nursing Core Competencies*

Quality Improvement:

Knowledge (K3) Explains the importance of variation and measurement in providing quality nursing care

Skills (S3) Participates in the use of quality improvement tools to assess performance and identify gaps between local and best practices

Attitudes/Behaviors (A3a) Appreciates how standardization supports quality patient care

(A3b) Recognizes how unwanted variation compromises care

Source: Massachusetts Department of Higher Education. (2010). *Nurse of the future: Nursing core competencies* (p. 36). Retrieved from http://www.mass.edu/currentinit/documents/NursingCoreCompetencies.pdf

---

The Role of the Nurse in Quality Improvement

As early as the 1860s, Florence Nightingale measured patient outcomes in relation to environmental conditions and proposed standardization in the presentation of hospital statistics (Kovner, Brewer, Yingrengreung, & Fairchild, 2010; Owens & Koch, 2015). Today, nurses continue to have a role in quality improvement.

The ANA standard of professional performance number 14 states that the registered nurse contributes to quality nursing practice with competencies that include the nurse's role in various quality improvement activities such as collecting data to monitor quality and collaboration with the interprofessional team to implement quality improvement plans and interventions (ANA, 2015, p. 79). Knowing that the registered nurse participates in quality improvement activities, the American Association of Colleges of Nursing (AACN, 2008) includes statements in *The Essentials of Baccalaureate Education for Professional Nursing Practice* related to the expectations of nurses graduating from programs of nursing in the realm of quality improvement. According to the AACN (2008), a graduate of a baccalaureate nursing program will "understand and use concepts, processes, and outcome measures...be able to assist or initiate basic quality and safety investigations; be able to assist in the development of quality improvement action plans; and assist in monitoring the results of these action plans..." (p. 13).

The role of the nurse in quality improvement builds on the ability of the nurse to collect and analyze patient data, something all nursing students learn early in their programs of study. The novice nurse and the expert nurse alike participate in quality improvement initiatives. The novice nurse will be involved in data collection and assisting with improvement interventions whereas the expert nurse may be leading the quality improvement initiative, but all nurses should be prepared for this nursing role.

The nurse's role in quality improvement is especially important in hospitals that promote a culture of patient safety. Registered nurses at the bedside use quality improvement techniques that were once employed only by quality assurance personnel. Nurses actively monitor outcomes of patient care processes utilizing spreadsheets, flow diagrams, computer programs, and control charts to record data and monitor data when analyzing a clinical problem or situation. Trended data collected by nurses are provided by the risk management department or performance improvement council and disseminated to the units.

In addition to the processes of data monitoring, analysis, and change that occur as a part of the routine quality improvement cycle, nurses are frequently involved in the identification of a problem outside of the routine data monitoring system. Nurses may initiate the process of quality improvement based on observations of clinical issues in daily practice. These observations may lead to the conduct of health record audits to compare care provided to standards or evidence-based clinical practice guidelines. The results of such a health record audit lead to the development of a quality improvement plan to align practice with current best practice. The recommendations may be based on a variety of guidelines depending on the setting and patient population. Examples of possible guidelines for use in the audit include IHI care bundles or Best Practice Guidelines from the Registered Nurses' Association of Ontario. Based on the results of the health record audit, the nurse will present the data visually (as a control chart or histogram, for example) and collaborate with appropriate stakeholders to develop the quality improvement plan. The resulting quality improvement implementation plan will need to include a specific plan for sustainability and evaluation to be successful. An example template for a health record audit matrix based on guideline recommendations is provided in **Table 9-1**. In the example template, an *x* indicates that the guideline recommendation was documented in the health record. A blank indicates that there was no documentation of the recommended activity. The matrix may alternatively be marked with Y and N

KEY COMPETENCY 9-4

Examples of Applicable *Nurse of the Future: Nursing Core Competencies*

Quality Improvement:

Knowledge (K2) Understands that nursing contributes to systems of care and processes that affect outcomes

Skills (S2) Participates in the use of quality improvement processes to make processes of care interdependent and explicit

Attitudes/Behaviors (A2) Recognizes that team relationships are important to quality improvement

Source: Massachusetts Department of Higher Education. (2010). *Nurse of the future: Nursing core competencies* (p. 36). Retrieved from http://www.mass.edu/currentinit/documents/NursingCoreCompetencies.pdf

TABLE 9-1 Example of Health Record Audit Matrix Template					
Diagnosis (Diagnosis flow sheet/tab)	Health Record #1	Health Record #2	Health Record #3	Health Record #4	Health Record #5
Recommendation 1.1	x	x		x	x
Recommendation 1.2	x	x	x		x
Recommendation 2.1		x	x		x
Recommendation 2.2	x	x	x	x	x

for yes and no because just as with a cause and effect diagram, there is no one correct way to create this document. The quality improvement tools should be developed in the format that best fosters data collection, analysis, and planning, evaluating, and sustaining quality outcomes.

Quality improvement is also tied into a nurse's performance evaluation. Individual nurse and team goals for quality and safety are important components of each staff member's annual review. As nursing leadership and staff foster a culture of safety and quality, they emphasize reporting near misses and unintended outcomes as a means to identify and fix weak links in processes of care (Caramanica et al., 2003). But nurses have identified challenges to their role in quality improvement processes, including adequacy of resources, engaging nurses from management to the bedside in the process, the increasing number of quality improvement activities, the administrative burden of quality improvement initiatives, and the lack of preparation of nurses in traditional nursing education programs for their role in quality improvement (Draper, Felland, Liebhaber, & Melichar, 2008). Thirty-nine percent of new graduates report that they are not prepared to adequately implement quality improvement initiatives or use quality improvement techniques, despite having the content in their prelicensure programs (Kovner et al., 2010).

Conclusion

Why is it important for nurses to be involved in quality improvement efforts? Nurses are at what is known as the sharp end of health care, meaning that nurses have significant, direct contact with patients at the bedside. Because of this closeness to clinical activity, nurses recognize the need for change, see the effects when the best care is not provided, and see the impact of changes. Thus, nurses are able to bring both clinical expertise and first-hand experience to discussions about quality improvement efforts within their organizations (Haviley et al., 2014, p. 22). More than ever before, quality improvement is considered a core responsibility of the professional nurse.

Classroom Activity 1

Provide students with a list of measures and have students search some of the websites listed under the Healthcare Transparency heading to find safety and quality information about your local hospitals. Discuss the results in the context of quality outcomes and consumer choice.

Classroom Activity 2

Provide students with case studies that describe nursing errors, such as the historical case studies in Emrich (2010). Have students work in groups to either identify the root cause of the error using a fishbone diagram and then engage in a PDSA process to plan a small-scale quality improvement initiative or identify how to prevent errors such as these using the Swiss cheese framework.

Classroom Activity 3

Provide small groups of students with chart audit results and appropriate clinical guidelines. The students should work together as a team to develop a quality improvement plan.

Classroom Activity 4

The IHI is a quality improvement organization that is dedicated to sharing information to improve healthcare safety. IHI Open School has free online courses and experiential learning opportunities available at www.ihi .org/education/ihiopenschool/Pages/default .aspx. Choose activities from the website for students to complete that meet specific course objectives.

> ## Classroom Activity 5
>
> Numerous classroom and clinical activities related to quality and quality improvement are available on the QSEN website at www.qsen.org/teaching-strategies /strategy-search/. Choose activities from the website for students to complete that meet specific course objectives.

References

Agency for Healthcare Research and Quality. (2015). *2014 national healthcare quality and disparities report.* AHRQ Publication No. 15-0007. Rockville, MD: Author.

American Association of Colleges of Nursing. (2008). *The essentials of baccalaureate education for professional nursing practice.* Washington, DC: Author.

American Nurses Association. (2015). *Nursing: Scope and standards of practice* (3rd ed.). Silver Spring, MD: Author.

Barnsteiner, J. (2012). Safety. In G. Sherwood & J. Barnsteiner (Eds.), *Quality and safety in nursing: A competency approach to improving outcomes* (pp. 149–169). West Sussex, UK: Wiley.

Berwick, D. M. (2014). *Promising care: How we can rescue health care by improving it.* San Francisco, CA: Jossey-Bass.

Caramanica, L., Cousino, J. A., & Petersen, S. (2003). Four elements of a successful quality program, alignment, collaboration, evidence-based practice, and excellence. *Nursing Administration Quarterly, 27*(4), 336–343.

Chassin, M. R., Loeb, J. M., Schmaltz, S. P., & Wachter, R. M. (2010). Accountability measures—Using measurement to promote quality improvement. *New England Journal of Medicine, 363,* 683–688. doi:10.1056/NEJMsb1002320

Cronenwett, L., Sherwood, G., Barnsteiner, J., Disch, J., Johnson, J., Mitchell, P., … Warren, J. (2007). Quality and safety education for nurses. *Nursing Outlook, 55*(3), 122–131.

Donabedian, A. (1966). Evaluating the quality of medical care. *Milbank Memorial Fund Quarterly, 44*(3 Supp), 166–206.

Draper, D. A., Felland, L. E., Liebhaber, A., & Melichar, L. (2008). *The role of nurses in hospital quality improvement* (Vol. 3). Washington, DC: Center for Studying Healthcare System Change.

Emrich, L. (2010). Practice breakdown: Medication administration. In P. E. Benner, K. Malloch, & V. Sheets (Eds.), *Nursing pathways for patient safety* (pp. 30–46). St. Louis, MO: Mosby.

Haviley, C., Anderson, A. K., & Currier, A. (2014). Overview of patient safety and quality of care. In P. Kelly, B. A. Vottero, & C. A. Christie-McAuliffe (Eds.), *Introduction to quality and safety education for nurses* (pp. 1–37). New York, NY: Springer.

Institute of Medicine. (2000). *To err is human: Building a safer health system*. Washington, DC: National Academies Press.

Institute of Medicine. (2001). *Crossing the quality chasm: A new health system for the 21st century*. Washington, DC: National Academies Press.

Johnson, J. (2012). Quality improvement. In G. Sherwood & J. Barnsteiner (Eds.), *Quality and safety in nursing: A competency approach to improving outcomes* (pp. 113–132). West Sussex, UK: Wiley.

Joint Commission. (2013). ORYX non-core measure information. Retrieved from http://www.jointcommission.org/oryx_non-core_measure_information/

Joint Commission. (2014a). America's hospitals: Improving quality and safety: Annual report 2014. Retrieved from http://www.jointcommission.org/accreditation/top _performers.aspx

Joint Commission. (2014b). Facts about accountability measures. Retrieved from http://www.jointcommission.org/accountability_measures.aspx

Joint Commission. (2014c). Facts about ORYX® for hospitals (national hospital quality measures). Retrieved from http://www.jointcommission.org/facts_about _oryx_for_hospitals/

Joint Commission. (2014d). National Quality Forum (NQF) endorsed nursing-sensitive care performance measures. Retrieved from http://www.jointcommission.org /national_quality_forum_nqf_endorsed_nursing-sensitive_care_performance _measures/

Kovner, C. T., Brewer, C. S., Yingrengreung, S., & Fairchild, S. (2010). New nurses' views of quality improvement education. *Joint Commission Journal of Quality and Patient Safety*, *36*(1), 29–35.

Massachusetts Department of Higher Education. (2010). *Nurse of the future: Nursing core competencies*. Retrieved from http://www.mass.edu/currentinit/documents /NursingCoreCompetencies.pdf

Montalvo, I. (2007). The national database of nursing quality indicators (NDNQI). *Online Journal of Issues in Nursing*, *12*(3). doi:10.3912/OJIN.Vol12No03Man02

National Quality Forum. (2004). *National voluntary consensus standards for nursing-sensitive care: An initial performance measure set*. Washington, DC: Author.

Owens, L. D., & Koch, R. W. (2015). Understanding quality patient care and the role of the practicing nurse. *Nursing Clinics of North America*, *50*, 33–43.

Quality and Safety Education for Nurses. (2007). Competencies: Prelicensure KSAS. Retrieved from http://qsen.org/competencies/pre-licensure-ksas/

Reason, J. (2000). Human error: Models and management. *British Medical Journal*, *320*, 768–770.

Robert Wood Johnson Foundation. (2011). Measuring the contributions of nurses to high-value health care: Special report. Retrieved from http://www.rwjf.org/content /dam/farm/reports/program_results_reports/2011/rwjf70343

Sollecito, W. A., & Johnson, J. K. (2013). *McLaughlin and Kaluzny's continuous quality improvement in health care* (4th ed.). Burlington, MA: Jones & Bartlett Learning.

Strome, T. L. (2013). *Healthcare analytics for quality and performance improvement*. Hoboken, NJ: Wiley.

U.S. Department of Health and Human Services. (2011). *National strategy for quality improvement in health care*. Washington, DC: Author.

Vottero, B. A., Block, M. E., & Bonaventura, L. (2012). Benchmarking quality performance. In P. Kelly, B. A. Vottero, & C. A. Christie-McAuliffe (Eds.), *Introduction to quality and safety education for nurses* (pp. 221–247). New York, NY: Springer.

CHAPTER 10

Evidence-Based Professional Nursing Practice

Kathleen Masters

Learning Objectives

After completing this chapter, the student should be able to:

1. Describe the importance of evidence-based nursing care.
2. Identify barriers to the implementation of evidence-based nursing practice.
3. Identify strategies for the implementation of evidence-based nursing practice.
4. Describe how and where to search for evidence.
5. Identify methods to evaluate the evidence.
6. Discuss approaches to integrating evidence into practice.
7. Identify models of evidence-based nursing practice.

Evidence-Based Practice: What Is It?

Evidence-based practice—it is more than a recent buzzword in nursing. Evidence-based practice is a mechanism that allows nurses to provide safe, high-quality patient care based on evidence grounded in research and professional expertise rather than tradition, myths, hunches, advice from peers, outdated textbooks, or even what the nurse learned in school 5, 10, or 15 years ago. Advances in information technology have facilitated the dissemination of research and other types of evidence, making them widely available. Only three decades ago nurses had to hand search indexes and hard copy journals to access research results, but nurses now have access to the most current evidence from professional journals and best practice guidelines available via the Internet.

Evidence-based practice provides a strategy to ensure that nursing care reflects the most up-to-date knowledge available. Nursing practice that is based on evidence is now the accepted standard for practice as well as one of

Key Terms and Concepts

» Evidence-based practice
» PICO(T)
» Clinical practice guidelines

the six core competencies for all registered nurses identified in the Quality and Safety Education for Nurses (QSEN) project (Cronenwett et al., 2007). Nurses are accountable for interventions they provide to patients. Evidence-based practice provides a systematic approach for decision making and provides a framework for the nurse to use to incorporate best nursing practices into the clinical care of patients (Pugh, 2012).

According to the American Association of Colleges of Nursing (AACN, 2008), professional nursing practice is grounded in the translation of current evidence into practice (p. 15). One of the skills expected of prelicensure graduates of nursing programs is the ability to base an individualized care plan on patient values, clinical expertise, and evidence (QSEN, 2015). In addition, Standard 13 of the standards of professional nursing practice indicates that the nurse will integrate evidence and research findings into practice (American Nurses Association [ANA], 2015, p. 77).

Most nurses want to provide care for their patients based on the most current evidence, but for many nurses, trying to integrate evidence-based practice into patient care in the clinical environment raises questions. The goal of this chapter is to answer those questions. So, to begin with, what exactly is evidence-based practice?

Evidence-based practice is a framework used by nurses and other healthcare professionals to deliver optimal health care through the integration of best current evidence, clinical expertise, and patient/family values (QSEN, 2015). Houser (2008, p. 14) describes this triad of evidence-based practice using the illustration of a three-legged stool. Just as each leg of the stool is necessary for the function of the stool, each of the three components—best current evidence, clinical expertise, and incorporation of patient/family values—are all necessary for the effective use of evidence-based practice.

Another question one might ask is, how is evidence-based practice relevant and applicable to nursing practice? Evidence-based practice is relevant to nursing practice because it does the following:

- Helps resolve problems in the clinical setting
- Results in effective patient care with better patient outcomes
- Contributes to the science of nursing through the introduction of innovation to practice
- Keeps practice current and relevant by helping nurses deliver care based on current best research
- Decreases variations in nursing care and increases confidence in decision making
- Supports Joint Commission readiness because policies and procedures are current and include the latest research
- Supports high-quality patient care and achievement of magnet status (Beyea & Slattery, 2006; Spector, 2007)

It takes approximately 17 years for clinical research to be integrated into patient care practices. Nurses and other healthcare providers can minimize the time from discovery to implementation through the process inherent in evidence-based practice that, in turn, will lead to improved patient outcomes. Because of the link between evidence-based practice and improved patient outcomes, the Institute of Medicine (IOM, 2008) has promoted the goal that by the year 2020, 90% of all health decisions will be based on evidence.

The evidence-based practice process enhances practice by encouraging reflection about what we know; it is applicable to virtually every area of nursing practice including patient assessment, diagnosis of patient problems, planning, patient care interventions, and evaluation of patient responses. In addition, evidence can be used as the foundation for policies and procedures and as the basis for patient care management tools such as care maps, pathways, and protocols (Houser, 2011, p. 9).

The seven steps involved in the evidence-based practice process address the question of how to begin.

- Cultivate a spirit of inquiry and culture of evidence-based practice among nurses and within the organization.
- Identify an issue and ask the question.
- Search for and collect the most relevant and best evidence to answer the clinical question.
- Critically appraise the evidence and synthesize the evidence.
- Integrate evidence with clinical expertise and patient preferences to make the best clinical decision.
- Evaluate the outcome of any evidence-based practice change.
- Disseminate the outcomes of the change (Melnyk & Fineout-Overholt, 2014).

> **KEY COMPETENCY 10-1**
>
> Examples of Applicable *Nurse of the Future: Nursing Core Competencies*
>
> Evidence-Based Practice:
>
> Knowledge (K2) Describes the concept of evidence-based practice (EBP), including the components of research evidence, clinical expertise, and patient/family values
>
> Skills (S2) Bases individualized care on best current evidence, patient values, and clinical expertise
>
> Attitudes/Behaviors (A2) Values the concept of EBP as integral to determining best clinical practice
>
> *Source:* Massachusetts Department of Higher Education. (2010). *Nurse of the future: Nursing core competencies* (p. 37). Retrieved from http://www.mass.edu/currentinit /documents/NursingCoreCompetencies.pdf

Barriers to Evidence-Based Practice

Because evidence-based practice is now the standard for professional nursing practice, one would think that practice based on evidence is commonplace; however, this is not the case. Practicing nurses cite many barriers to evidence-based practice. Common barriers to implementing evidence-based practice include the following:

- Lack of value for research in practice
- Difficulty in changing practice
- Lack of administrative support
- Lack of knowledgeable mentors
- Insufficient time
- Lack of education about the research process
- Lack of awareness about research or evidence-based practice

- Research reports and articles not readily available
- Difficulty accessing research reports and articles
- No time on the job to read research
- Complexity of research reports
- Lack of knowledge about evidence-based practice
- Lack of knowledge about the critique of articles
- Feeling overwhelmed by the process
- Lack of sense of control over practice
- Lack of confidence to implement change
- Lack of leadership, motivation, vision, strategy, or direction among managers (Beyea & Slattery, 2006; Revell, 2015; Spector, 2007)

Additional barriers to using evidence-based practice include the overwhelming information available in the research literature that is sometimes contradictory, as well as the perception that evidence-based practice is equivalent to "cookbook medicine." In addition, there may be a perceived lack of authority for clinicians to make changes in practice or peer pressure to maintain the status quo (Houser, 2011).

Promoting Evidence-Based Practice

Despite barriers, nurses are making a difference in patient outcomes through the use of evidence-based practice. Strategies that can be useful in the promotion of evidence in practice generally fall into two categories: strategies for individual nurses and organizational strategies.

Strategies for individual nurses include the following:

- Educate yourself about evidence-based practice through avenues such as online sites, original research articles, evidence reports, conferences, and participation in professional organizations that provide resources related to evidence-based practice (Revell, 2015).
- Conduct face-to-face or online journal clubs that can be used to educate yourself about the appraisal of evidence, share new research reports and guidelines with peers, and provide support to other nurses.
- Share your results through posters, newsletters, unit meetings, or a published article to support a culture of evidence-based nursing practice within the organization and the profession.
- Adopt a reflective and inquiring approach to practice by questioning the rationale for approaches to care that do not result in desired patient outcomes and continuously asking yourself and others within your organization questions such as, "What is the evidence for this intervention?" or "How do my patients respond to this intervention?" (Beyea & Slattery, 2006; QSEN, 2015).

CRITICAL THINKING QUESTIONS∗

How do I know what I know about nursing practice? Are my nursing decisions based on myths, traditions, experience, authority, trial and error, ritual, or scientific knowledge? ∗

Strategies for overcoming barriers and increasing adoption of evidence-based practice within an organization include:

- Specific identification of the facilitators and barriers to evidence-based practice. This will require administrative support by providing the time and the funds for necessary resources as well as enhancement of job descriptions to include criteria related to evidence-based practice.
- Education and training to improve knowledge and strengthen beliefs related to the benefits of evidence-based practice. This may require offering incentives such as a paid registration to a conference for the best clinical question in a unit-wide contest.
- Creation of an environment that encourages an inquisitive approach to patient care. Achievement of this environment may require the development of a center of evidence-based practice, access to electronic resources in the workplace, providing opportunities for nurses to collaborate with nurse researchers or faculty with nursing research expertise, and providing opportunities to disseminate the results of evidence-based practice projects (Houser, 2011, p. 12).

Whichever strategies are incorporated, it is important to note that multifaceted interventions are much more likely to be effective in facilitating evidence-based practice within an organization. It is also important to note that once evidence-based practice projects are complete, passive dissemination of results within an organization is ineffective in changing practice.

> ### CRITICAL THINKING QUESTIONS ✳
> How is new evidence disseminated to the bedside nurse in the organization in which you practice as a nursing student? How does the organization promote evidence-based practice? Do the nurses in the organization use current evidence in practice? ✳

Searching for Evidence

Competencies expected of the nurse include reading original research and evidence reports related to the practice area and the ability to locate relevant evidence reports and guidelines (QSEN, 2015). In order to find the evidence, the nurse must learn to ask clinical questions and search electronic indexes and other resources.

Asking the Question

Nurses must learn to ask questions in a format that facilitates searching for evidence. Developing a question that accurately reflects the practice to be evaluated, in a format that focuses the search for evidence, is a good place to begin (Tracy & Barnsteiner, 2014). It has been suggested that all nurses should learn how to use the PICO(T) format to ask clinical questions. **PICO(T)** is simply an acronym that assists in the formatting of clinical questions. Using this format helps the nurse to ask pertinent clinical questions, focus on asking the right questions, and choose relevant guidelines.

P = Patient, Population, or Problem
- How would I describe a group of patients similar to mine?
- What group do I want information on?

I = Intervention or Exposure or Topic of Interest
- Which main intervention am I considering?
- What event do I want to study the effect of?

C = Comparison or Alternate Intervention (if appropriate)
- What is the main alternative to compare with the intervention?
- Compared to what? Better or worse than no intervention at all, or than another intervention?

O = Outcome
- What can I hope to accomplish, measure, improve, or affect?
- What is the effect of the intervention? (Levin, 2006a)

Some researchers also add the element of time or time frame to the PICO question format and refer to the format as PICOT, although the time frame might not be applicable to all questions.

T = Time or Time Frame
- How much time is required to demonstrate an outcome?
- How long are participants observed?

After determining the patient, intervention, comparison, and outcome of interest, the nurse then combines these four elements into a single question in combinations such as the following examples:

- In (patient or population), what is the effect of (intervention or exposure) on (outcome) compared with (comparison)? (Levin, 2006b)
- For (patient or population), does the introduction of (intervention or exposure) reduce the risk of (outcome) compared with (comparison intervention)? (Levin, 2006b)

Electronic Resources

Because the PICO(T) question may have already been asked and answered by other nurses, beginning the search with sites that provide systematic reviews or guidelines is helpful (Tracy & Barnsteiner, 2014, p. 136). Electronic resources are available that can assist the nurse in uncovering the most current evidence for practice in the form of systematic reviews and guidelines. Some of the most commonly used include these:

- National Library of Medicine: www.nlm.nih.gov
- Cochrane Library: www.cochrane.org
- National Guideline Clearinghouse: www.guideline.gov

- Joanna Briggs Institute: www.joannabriggs.org
- Agency for Healthcare Research and Quality (AHRQ): www.effectivehealthcare .ahrq.gov
- Centre for Health Evidence: www.cche.net
- Registered Nurses' Association of Ontario: http://rnao.ca/bpg/guidelines
- McGill University Health Centre's Clinical and Research Resources: www .mcgill.ca/nursing/outreach/today/links/clinical

The Cochrane Library is a collection of databases that contain high-quality, independent evidence to inform healthcare decision making. Cochrane reviews represent the highest level of evidence on which to base clinical treatment decisions. In addition to the Cochrane systematic reviews, the Cochrane Library also offers other sources of information, including the Database of Abstracts of Reviews of Effects, Cochrane Controlled Trials Register, Cochrane Methodology Register, NHS Economic Evaluation Database, Health Technology Assessment Database, and Cochrane Database of Methodology Reviews.

Another site with high-quality evidence is the National Guideline Clearinghouse. As a part of the AHRQ, the National Guideline Clearinghouse includes structured summaries containing information about each guideline, including comparisons of guidelines covering similar topics that show areas of similarity and differences; full text or links to full text; ordering details for full guidelines; annotated bibliographies on guideline development, evaluation, implementation, and structure; weekly email updates; and guideline archives. Guidelines may be searched by topic or by organization.

The Registered Nurses' Association of Ontario provides high-quality best practice guidelines specifically focused on nursing care. Many of these guidelines are also available via the National Guideline Clearinghouse site. The guidelines are available online in full text and free of charge.

Electronic Indexes

Reviews may also be indexed, but if no reviews or guidelines are found relevant to your PICO(T) question, then individual articles must be searched (Tracy & Barnsteiner, 2014, p. 136). Electronic indexes provide options for narrowing or broadening a topic to identify relevant literature. Most electronic indexes provide citation information and will indicate if the selected articles are available locally in print form or if the items are available in an electronic format. Three of the most common electronic indexes used in health care are the Cumulative Index to Nursing and Allied Health Literature (CINAHL), available at www.cinahl.com; MEDLINE, available at www.nlm.nih.gov; and PubMed, a web-based format of MEDLINE available at www.pubmed.gov.

KEY COMPETENCY 10-2

Examples of Applicable
*Nurse of the Future: Nursing
Core Competencies*

Evidence-Based Practice:

Knowledge (K3) Describes
reliable sources for locating
evidence reports and clinical
practice guidelines

Skills (S3) Locates
evidence reports related to
clinical practice topics and
guidelines

Attitudes/Behaviors (A3)
Appreciates the importance
of accessing relevant clinical
evidence

Source: Massachusetts Department of Higher
Education. (2010). *Nurse of the future:
Nursing core competencies* (p. 37). Retrieved
from http://www.mass.edu/currentinit
/documents/NursingCoreCompetencies.pdf

Evaluating the Evidence

Regardless of the source, the nurse needs to evaluate the quality of the evidence. By evaluating the rigor of the evidence, we can have confidence that the evidence is accurate. This is important because it could contribute to a decline rather than an improvement in patient outcomes if we base changes to care on inaccurate research evidence (Sellers & McCrea, 2014). Begin by asking such questions as the following:

- What is the source of the information?
- When was it developed?
- How was it developed?
- Does it fit the current clinical environment?
- Does it fit the current situation?

Levels of Evidence

Best evidence for practice includes empirical evidence from randomized controlled trials, evidence from descriptive and qualitative research, and information from case reports, scientific principles, and expert opinion. When insufficient research is available, healthcare decision making is derived principally from nonresearch evidence sources such as expert opinion and scientific principles (Titler, 2008).

Several classification systems exist to evaluate the level or strength of the evidence. The AHRQ serves as the recognized authority regarding the assessment of clinical research in the United States. Standard levels of evidence include the classifications listed here (Melnyk & Fineout-Overholt, 2014):

1. Meta-analysis or systematic reviews of multiple well-designed controlled studies
2. Well-designed randomized controlled trials
3. Well-designed nonrandomized controlled trials (quasi-experimental)
4. Observational studies with controls (retrospective, interrupted time, case-control, cohort studies with controls)
5. Systematic review of descriptive and qualitative studies
6. Single descriptive or qualitative study
7. Opinions of authorities and/or reports of expert committees

Using this classification system, the strongest evidence comes from the first level, representing systematic reviews that integrate findings from multiple well-designed controlled studies. The weakest evidence is represented by the seventh level and is based on expert opinion (Polit & Beck, 2008).

In addition, grading the strength of a body of evidence should incorporate three domains: quality, quantity, and consistency. Quality has to do with the extent to which a study minimizes bias in the design, implementation, and analysis. Quantity refers to the number of studies that have evaluated the research question, as well as the sample size across the studies and the strength of the findings. The category of consistency refers to both the similarity and differences of study designs that investigate the same research question and report similar findings (AHRQ, 2002; LoBiondo-Wood & Haber, 2014).

Appraisal of Research

Prior to applying evidence in clinical practice, there must be an appraisal process. Key issues to address in an appraisal include the credibility of the study, including the researcher's credentials and experience; any evidence of bias due to a conflict of interest of the researcher or the journal; the statement of a blind peer review; and dates included in the journal to indicate the timeliness of publication. In addition, appraisals should include questions about the design of the study, sample size, sampling procedures, reliability and validity of instrumentation, and appropriate statistical analysis (DelMonte & Oman, 2011).

The Critical Appraisal Skills Programme (CASP, 2010) is a resource that provides checklists that help the user to interpret research evidence. The checklists are specific to various types of research including randomized controlled trials, systematic reviews, cohort studies, case-control studies, and qualitative studies. The checklists provide frameworks to determine the strength and reliability of research reports. CASP tools are available free of charge at www.casp-uk.net (Sellers & McCrea, 2014, p. 350).

Appraisal of Clinical Practice Guidelines

In addition to the appraisal of research, the nurse will need skill in the appraisal of guidelines to practice based on evidence. **Clinical practice guidelines** are developed to guide clinical practice and represent an effort to put a large body of evidence into a manageable form. Clinical practice guidelines are usually based on systematic reviews and give specific recommendations for clinicians. Guidelines usually attempt to address all the issues relevant to a clinical decision, including risks and benefits.

The IOM (2011), at the request of the U.S. Congress, developed a set of eight standards for the development of rigorous and trustworthy clinical practice guidelines. To evaluate the effects of the standards on clinical practice guideline development and healthcare quality and outcomes, the IOM has encouraged the AHRQ to pilot test the standards and assess their reliability and validity. The standards are:

- *Standard 1:* Establishing transparency related to funding and development processes.
- *Standard 2:* Management of conflict of interest.
- *Standard 3:* Guideline development group composition should be multi-disciplinary and balanced including a variety of experts and patient populations.

KEY COMPETENCY 10-3

Examples of Applicable *Nurse of the Future: Nursing Core Competencies*

Evidence-Based Practice:

Knowledge (K4) Differentiates clinical opinion from research and evidence summaries

Attitudes/Behaviors (A4) Appreciates that the strength and relevance of evidence should be determinants when choosing clinical interventions

Source: Massachusetts Department of Higher Education. (2010). *Nurse of the future: Nursing core competencies* (p. 37). Retrieved from http://www.mass.edu/currentinit/documents/NursingCoreCompetencies.pdf

- *Standard 4:* Use of systematic reviews that meet standards.
- *Standard 5:* Establishing evidence foundations for and rating strength of recommendations.
- *Standard 6:* Articulation of recommendations maintains a standardized form.
- *Standard 7:* External review by stakeholders.
- *Standard 8:* Updating should occur when new evidence suggests the need for modification of clinically important recommendations.

In addition to the relatively new IOM standards, there is an ongoing collaboration that has focused on improving the quality and effectiveness of clinical practice guidelines for over a decade. The group has established a framework for determining the quality of guidelines for diagnoses, health promotion, treatments, or clinical interventions. The instrument can be used with new, existing, or updated guidelines and is known as the Appraisal of Guidelines for Research and Evaluation (AGREE) instrument. The instrument, first published in 2003 by the AGREE Collaboration, has been revised and is now known as AGREE II (AGREE Next Steps Consortium, 2009). The AGREE II replaces the original instrument and is the preferred tool. The full version of the AGREE II instrument and training materials are available online at no cost at www.agreetrust.org. The AGREE instrument is composed of six categories comprising the 23 items listed here as well as 2 final items that require an overall judgment about the practice guideline:

- Scope and purpose
  - Overall objectives of the guideline are specifically described.
  - The health questions covered by the guideline are specifically described.
  - The population (patients, public, etc.) to whom the guideline is meant to apply is specifically described.
- Stakeholder involvement
  - Guideline development group includes individuals from all relevant professions.
  - The views and preferences of the target population (patients, public, etc.) have been sought.
  - Target users of the guideline are clearly defined.
- Rigor of development
  - Systematic methods were used to search for evidence.
  - The criteria for selecting the evidence are clearly described.
  - The strengths and limitations of the body of evidence are clearly described.
  - The methods used for formulating the recommendations are clearly described.

- The health benefits, side effects, and risks have been considered in formulating recommendations.
- There is an explicit link between the recommendations and the supporting evidence.
- The guideline has been externally reviewed by experts prior to publication.
- A procedure for updating the guideline is provided.
- Clarity and presentation
  - Recommendations are specific and unambiguous.
  - Different options for management of the condition or health issue are clearly presented.
  - Key recommendations are easily identifiable.
- Application
  - The guideline describes facilitators and barriers to its application.
  - The guideline provides advice and/or tools on how the recommendations can be put into practice.
  - The potential resource implications of applying the recommendations have been considered.
  - The guideline presents monitoring and/or auditing criteria.
- Editorial independence
  - The views of the funding body have not influenced the content of the guideline.
  - Competing interests of guideline development group members have been recorded and addressed (AGREE Next Steps Consortium, 2009, pp. 2–3).

The usefulness of a guideline depends on whether the actual recommendations in the guideline are meaningful and practical. Recommendations should be practical in relation to implementation, be as unambiguous as possible, address the frequency of screening and follow-up, and address clinically relevant actions. Other questions that the clinician must address in relation to guidelines include such factors as the setting of care, the patient population, and the strength of the recommendations (Beyea & Slattery, 2006).

Implementation Models for Evidence-Based Practice

Differences exist among evidence-based practice models, but most models do have common elements that include selection of a practice topic, critique and synthesis of evidence, implementation, evaluation of the impact on patient care and provider performance, and consideration of the context in which the practice is implemented (Titler, 2008). No one model of evidence-based practice is a perfect fit for every organization. Some models focus on the perspective of the individual clinician, or the researcher, whereas others focus on institutional efforts. Therefore, before embarking on this journey, the nurse or organization should consider several models and select or adapt one that fits the needs of the nurse or organization.

ACE Star Model of Knowledge Transformation

The Center for Advancing Clinical Evidence (ACE) Star Model of Knowledge Transformation, developed by Dr. Kathleen Stevens, is available at www.acestar .uthscsa.edu/acestar-model.asp. The model involves five steps: knowledge discovery, evidence summary, translation into practice recommendations, integration into practice, and evaluation. Discovery refers to the original research. During the second step, the task is to synthesize all the related research into a meaningful whole. It is during this step that information is reduced to a manageable form. During the step of translation, the scientific evidence is considered in the context of clinical expertise and values. This results in clinical practice guidelines, best practices, protocols, standards, or clinical pathways. During the stage of implementation, changes take place in practice. During evaluation, the impact of the change is measured. Variables such as specific health outcomes, length of stay, or patient satisfaction are examples of possible outcomes that might be examined.

The Iowa Model of Evidence-Based Practice

The Iowa Model of Evidence-Based Practice resembles a decision-making tree that identifies either problem-focused or knowledge-focused triggers that initiate the process in the organization. Problem-focused triggers within an organization can include risk management data, process improvement data, benchmarking data, financial data, or the identification of clinical problems. Knowledge-focused triggers within an organization can include the publication of new research or literature, a change in organizational standards and guidelines, changes in philosophies of care within the profession or organization, or questions from an institutional standards committee. Once there is either a problem-focused or a knowledge-focused trigger within the organization, a team must identify whether the topic is a priority for the organization. If the topic is indeed a priority, evidence is examined, and the change in practice can be piloted. This process is followed by monitoring and analysis of both the process and the outcome data and finally by dissemination of the results.

Agency for Healthcare Research and Quality Model

A model for maximizing and accelerating the transfer of research results from the AHRQ patient safety research portfolio to healthcare delivery includes three major stages of knowledge transfer: (1) knowledge creation and distillation, (2) diffusion and dissemination, and (3) organizational adoption and implementation. More specifically, knowledge creation and distillation refers to conducting research and then packaging relevant research findings into usable form such as practice recommendations. The diffusion and dissemination stage involves partnering with professional leaders, professional organizations, and healthcare organizations to disseminate knowledge to potential users such as nurses, physical therapists, or physicians. During the final stage of the process, the focus is on organizational adoption and implementation of evidence-based research findings and innovations in practice. In this model, the stages of knowledge transfer are viewed from the perspective of the researcher or the creator of new knowledge and begin with decisions about which research findings ought to be disseminated (Titler, 2008).

Johns Hopkins Nursing Evidence-Based Practice Model

The process used in the Johns Hopkins Nursing Evidence-Based Practice Model is known as PET, which refers to asking a practice question, finding the evidence, and translating the evidence to practice (Newhouse, Dearholt, Poe, Pugh, & White, 2007). In the model, questions are stated in the PICO format. Next, the research and nonresearch evidence undergoes appraisal. Nonresearch evidence includes not only expert opinion, patient experience data, and guidelines, but also evidence gathered from organizational experience such as quality improvement reports, program evaluations, and financial data analysis. The final step of the PET process is translation, assessing the evidence-based recommendations for transferability to the practice setting. During this process, practices are implemented, evaluated, and communicated, leading to a change in nursing processes and outcomes (p. 129).

Diffusion of Innovation Framework

Rogers's Diffusion of Innovation Framework (2003) posits that if a third of any group adopts a practice change based on new evidence, then the rest of the group will follow, considering the change in practice to be the norm. The key to using this framework to guide implementation is to work with people within the organization who are known to be innovators and early adopters

---

KEY COMPETENCY 10-4

Examples of Applicable
*Nurse of the Future: Nursing
Core Competencies*

Evidence-Based Practice:

Knowledge (K5) Explains the role of evidence in determining best clinical practice

Skills (S5) Facilitates integration of new evidence into standards of practice, policies, and nursing practice guidelines

Attitudes/Behaviors (A5a) Questions the rationale of supporting routine approaches to care processes and decisions

(A5b) Values the need for continuous improvement in clinical practice based on new knowledge

Source: Massachusetts Department of Higher Education. (2010). *Nurse of the future: Nursing core competencies* (p. 37).Retrieved from http://www.mass.edu/currentinit/documents/NursingCoreCompetencies.pdf

of change. There are five steps included in the framework: knowledge, persuasion, decision, implementation/trial, and confirmation. During the knowledge step, the innovation is described so that the decision-making unit develops an understanding of the suggested change. Next, the change agent works to develop favorable attitudes toward the innovation and subsequently a decision is made to adopt or reject the innovation. During the implementation or trial step, the innovation is in place and adjustments may occur. Finally, during the step of confirmation, the decision-making unit seeks reinforcement that the decision was correct, or they may choose to reverse the decision (Sellers & McCrea, 2014, p. 360).

Conclusion

Numerous models are available in the literature to guide nurses in the use of evidence-based practice. The models share similarities and differences but do have a common foundation because all use a planned action approach to moving knowledge to practice. The steps taken together provide a process for locating and synthesizing knowledge, and systematically using the change process for integrating and sustaining evidence-based changes in practice (Tracy & Barnsteiner, 2014).

Currently, the greatest challenge we face in fully implementing evidence-based practice in nursing as a profession is how to get the evidence to the practicing nurse. Nurses are very busy taking care of patients. From the perspective of the individual, it can indeed be daunting, especially when many practicing nurses are not knowledgeable about evidence-based nursing practice. Nevertheless, daunting or not, the impetus for evidence-based practice will continue to grow. As healthcare costs continue to climb, consistent, data-based answers to patient care problems are an expectation.

CASE STUDY 10-1 • MR. P.

Mr. P. is a 52-year-old, married, Hispanic male who is approximately 100 pounds overweight. Mr. P. has developed hypertension and adult-onset diabetes. He is currently being followed in a clinic setting. As a nurse working in the clinic setting, you have noticed that many of the patients you see in the clinic that are demographically similar to Mr. P. experience poorer health outcomes as compared with your patients who are members of different patient populations.

Case Study Questions

1. What PICO(T) questions can you ask to generate evidence for the patient population and patient problem(s) represented in the case study?
2. Based on a search of the literature, your expertise, and what you know about the preferences of this patient population, what are some evidence-based nursing interventions that you might want to translate into clinical practice in this clinic setting?

Classroom Activity 1

Have students create clinical questions in the PICO(T) format for a patient in a case study provided by the instructor or a patient recently cared for in the clinical setting.

Classroom Activity 2

Have students bring laptops to class or go to the computer lab as a class and access evidence from resources such as CINAHL, the National Guideline Clearinghouse, or the Cochrane Library to plan evidence-based care based on the questions created in Classroom Activity 1. If laptops or a computer lab is not available, then adapt this activity by having either students or the faculty access the sites via a computer projection system in the classroom and plan care as a group based on the search results. As an alternative, the students can do this activity outside of class and share their results during the following class.

Classroom Activity 3

Provide students with a clinical guideline (choose one that has recommendations students can audit for using the patient records provided), a clinical audit tool, and several example patient records. Have students perform an evidence-based clinical review (or audit) using the records provided to them. Have students summarize their findings for each recommendation and then suggest quality improvement actions to correct the identified problems.

Classroom Activity 4

Have students partner individually or as a group with a local clinical facility to work jointly on a project. Collaborate to identify PICO(T) questions, find evidence, and plan the process of translation of evidence into practice within the facility or on a nursing unit within the facility.

Classroom Activity 5

Numerous classroom and clinical activities related to evidence-based practice are available on the QSEN website at www .qsen.org/teaching-strategies/strategy-search/. Choose activities from the website for students to complete that meet specific course objectives.

References

Agency for Healthcare Research and Quality. (2002). *Systems to rate the strength of scientific evidence.* Evidence Report/Technology Assessment No. 47, AHRQ Publication No. 02-E016. Rockville, MD: Author.

AGREE Collaboration. (2003). Development and validation of an international appraisal instrument for assessing the quality of clinical practice guidelines: The AGREE project. *Quality and Safety in Health Care, 12,* 18–23.

AGREE Next Steps Consortium. (2009). *Appraisal of guidelines for research and evaluation.* Ottawa, Ontario: AGREE Research Trust.

American Association of Colleges of Nursing. (2008). *The essentials of baccalaureate nursing education for professional nursing practice.* Washington, DC: Author.

American Nurses Association. (2015). *Nursing: Scope and standards of practice* (3rd ed.). Silver Spring, MD: Author.

Beyea, S. C., & Slattery, M. J. (2006). *Evidence-based practice in nursing: A guide to successful implementation.* Marblehead, MA: Healthcare Compliance.

Critical Appraisal Skills Programme (CASP). (2010). Checklists. Retrieved from http://www.casp-uk.net/#!checklists/cb36

Cronenwett, L., Sherwood, G., Barnsteiner, J., Disch, J., Johnson, J., Mitchell, P., ... Warren, J. (2007). Quality and safety education for nurses. *Nursing Outlook, 55*(3), 122–131.

DelMonte, J., & Oman, K. S. (2011). Preparing and sustaining staff knowledge about EBP. In J. Houser & K. S. Oman (Eds.), *Evidence-based practice: An implementation guide for healthcare organizations* (pp. 55–71). Sudbury, MA: Jones & Bartlett Learning.

Houser, J. (2008). *Nursing research: Reading, using, and creating evidence.* Sudbury, MA: Jones and Bartlett.

Houser, J. (2011). Evidence-based practice in health care. In J. Houser & K. S. Oman (Eds.), *Evidence-based practice: An implementation guide for healthcare organizations* (pp. 1–19). Sudbury, MA: Jones & Bartlett Learning.

Institute of Medicine. (2008). *Evidence-based medicine and the changing nature of healthcare: 2007 IOM annual meeting summary.* Washington, DC: National Academies Press.

Institute of Medicine. (2011). *Clinical practice guidelines we can trust.* Washington, DC: National Academies Press. Retrieved from http://www.iom.edu/Reports/2011 /Clinical-Practice-Guidelines-We-Can-Trust.aspx

Levin, R. F. (2006a). Evidence-based practice in nursing: What is it? In R. F. Levin & H. R. Feldman (Eds.), *Teaching evidence-based practice in nursing: A guide for academic and clinical settings* (pp. 5–14). New York, NY: Springer.

Levin, R. F. (2006b). Teaching students to formulate clinical questions: Tell me your problems and then read my lips. In R. F. Levin & H. R. Feldman (Eds.), *Teaching evidence-based practice in nursing: A guide for academic and clinical settings* (pp. 27–36). New York, NY: Springer.

LoBiondo-Wood, G., & Haber, J. (2014). Integrating research, evidence-based practice, and quality improvement processes. In G. LoBiondo-Wood & B. Haber (Eds.), *Nursing research: Methods and critical appraisal for evidence-based practice* (8th ed., pp. 5–24). St. Louis, MO: Mosby.

Massachusetts Department of Higher Education. (2010). *Nurse of the future: Nursing core competencies.* Retrieved from http://www.mass.edu/currentinit/documents/NursingCoreCompetencies.pdf

Melnyk, B. M., & Fineout-Overholt, E. (2014). *Evidence-based practice in nursing and healthcare: A guide to best practice* (3rd ed.). Philadelphia, PA: Lippincott Williams & Wilkins.

Newhouse, R. P., Dearholt, S. L., Poe, S. S., Pugh, L. C., & White, K. M. (2007). *Johns Hopkins nursing evidence-based practice: Model and guidelines.* Indianapolis, IN: Sigma Theta Tau International.

Polit, D. F., & Beck, C. T. (2008). *Nursing research: Generating and assessing evidence for nursing practice* (8th ed.). Philadelphia, PA: Lippincott Williams & Wilkins.

Pugh, L. C. (2012). Evidence-based practice: Context, concerns, and challenges. In S. L. Dearholt & D. Dang (Eds.), *Johns Hopkins nursing evidence-based practice: Model and guidelines* (2nd ed., pp. 5–23). Indianapolis, IN: Sigma Theta Tau International.

Quality and Safety Education for Nurses. (2015). Evidence-based practice. Retrieved from http://qsen.org/competencies/pre-licensure-ksas/#evidence-based_practice

Revell, M. A. (2015). Role of research in best practices. *Nursing Clinics of North America, 50,* 19–32.

Rogers, E. M. (2003). *Diffusion of innovations* (5th ed.). New York, NY: Free Press.

Sellers, K. F., & McCrea, K. L. (2014). Evidence-based practice. In P. Kelly, B. A. Vottero, & C. A. Christie-McAuliffe (Eds.), *Introduction to quality and safety education for nurses* (pp. 339–370). New York, NY: Springer.

Spector, N. (2007). *Evidence-based health care in nursing regulation.* Chicago, IL: National Council of State Boards of Nursing.

Titler, M. G. (2008). The evidence for evidence-based practice implementation. In R. G. Hughes (Ed.), *Patient safety and quality: An evidence-based handbook for nurses* (pp. 1–49). Rockville, MD: Agency for Healthcare Research and Quality.

Tracy, M. F., & Barnsteiner, J. (2014). Evidence-based practice. In G. Sherwood & J. Barnsteiner (Eds.), *Quality and safety in nursing: A competency approach to improving outcomes* (pp. 133–148). West Sussex, UK: Wiley.

CHAPTER 11

Patient-Centered Care and Professional Nursing Practice

Kathleen Masters

Learning Objectives

After completing this chapter, the student should be able to:

1. Describe the characteristics of patient-centered care (PCC) and family-centered care (FCC).
2. Discuss the dimensions of PCC.
3. Discuss communication in the context of PCC and FCC.
4. Describe patient education in the context of PCC.
5. Describe the evaluation of PCC.

What exactly is **patient-centered care (PCC)**? As one of the six dimensions of quality identified by the Institute of Medicine (IOM), PCC is defined as "providing care that is respectful of and responsive to individual patient preferences, needs, and values and ensuring that patient values guide all clinical decisions" (2001, p. 40). The Quality and Safety Education for Nurses (QSEN) initiative refined this definition in the formation of the PCC competency. PCC is defined by QSEN in terms of the nurse recognizing "the patient or designee as the source of control and full partner in providing compassionate and coordinated care based on respect for the patient's preferences, values, and needs" (2012; Cronenwett et al., 2007). Another competency-based definition for PCC is that the nurse "will provide holistic care that recognizes an individual's preferences, values, and needs and respects the patient or designee as a full partner in providing compassionate, coordinated, age and culturally appropriate, safe and effective care" (Massachusetts Department of Higher Education, 2010, p. 9).

All three definitions share a common focus. The provision of care that is appropriate for each individual patient is based on the patient's preferences with the patient as a partner on the healthcare team. It is important to note that PCC is not the same as patient-focused care. In the patient-focused care

Key Terms and Concepts

» Patient-centered care (PCC)
» Family-centered care (FCC)
» Patient education
» Patient teaching
» Learning domains
» Andragogy
» Health Belief Model (HBM)
» Social learning theory
» Self-efficacy
» Readiness to learn
» Health literacy
» Age-related changes

scheme, the healthcare provider, rather than the patient, retains decision-making control (Walton & Barnsteiner, 2012). The remainder of this chapter will focus on the components of PCC and the nurse's role in the maintenance of a patient-centered environment.

Dimensions of Patient-Centered Care

Dimensions of PCC that are characteristic of a patient-centered environment include respect for patients' values, preferences, and expressed needs; coordination and integration of care; information, communication, and education; physical comfort; emotional support; involvement of family and friends; and transition and continuity (Gerteis, Edgman-Levitan, Daley, & Delbanco, 1993, pp. 5–11).

Nurses show respect for patients as individuals by sharing information with them and actively partnering to determine care priorities and the plan of care. In addition, tailoring the patient's level of involvement based on his or her preferences rather than the nurse's preferences and revising the plan as the situation changes also demonstrate respect for patients (Gerteis et al., 1993, pp. 5–6). For PCC to be a reality, clinicians must relinquish the role of expert, realizing that although they are technical experts, the patient and family are the experts regarding their own life experiences. The concept of compliance must be replaced by one of engagement and partnership, and clinicians must believe that the best decisions emerge through input from all who have knowledge relevant to a particular patient situation (Disch, 2012, p. 238).

Coordination and integration of care is evident as members of the healthcare team communicate effectively with one another and, in turn, deliver consistent messages to the patient and as nurses create smooth transitions across episodes of care. The role of nursing in the coordination and integration of care is increasingly important as care becomes more complex due to the simultaneous existence of multiple chronic conditions, increasing numbers of care providers involved in the episodes of care, numerous settings for care, and shorter episodes of care (Gerteis et al., 1993, pp. 6–7).

Adapting education and communication based on the patient's preference is a foundation of PCC. Information on clinical status, progress, and prognosis communicated to patients needs to make sense to patients and families and be at a level that they can understand. Education provided to patients to facilitate self-care and health promotion must also be at a level that the patient can understand (Gerteis et al., 1993, pp. 7–8).

Physical comfort should form the basis for the individualized plan of patient care. Assuring that the patient will be free of pain is an expectation of PCC, as are assistance with activities of daily living and a clean and private environment (Gerteis et al., 1993, p. 8). Periodic assessments of patient comfort are essential, as are the timely administration of medications and monitoring of the effects of medications and treatments (Walton & Barnsteiner, 2012).

In addition to physical discomfort, patients may experience anxiety and distress during their experience of care. Patients frequently experience anxiety over their clinical status, treatments, and prognosis as well as the impact of the illness on self and family and the financial impact of the illness. The nurse is in a position that allows for spiritual and emotional support of the patient and family during the care experience (Gerteis et al., 1993, p. 9).

Patient/family-centered care or **family-centered care (FCC)** is an extension of PCC that "widens the circle of concern to include those persons who are important to the patient's life" (Henneman & Cardin, 2002, p. 13), although it is important to note that FCC does not negate the patient's right to privacy and control. FCC requires the structuring of all aspects of the process of engaging the patient's family and friends around meeting the patient's needs rather than around the convenience of the organization. This includes accommodation for family and friends, inclusion of family in decision making (based on patient preference), recognizing the needs of the family, and providing support for the family in their caregiving role (Gerteis et al., 1993, pp. 9–10). It is important to view this aspect of PCC within the total context of the patient's care rather than based on a few policies because FCC "is a philosophy that considers the patient as the unit of attention in the context of his family (Walton & Barnsteiner, 2012); however, policies that promote the inclusion of the family may reflect the family-centered care philosophy of an organization. It is also important to note that in the context of PCC, *family* refers to those persons that the patient decides to call family rather than those defined by the provider (Walton & Barnsteiner, 2012).

Lastly, patients express anxiety about their ability to care for themselves once discharged from the healthcare setting. PCC includes support for patients as they transition to home including information related to medications, diet, and symptoms to report, provided in a manner that patients understand. PCC also provides for continuity of care and assures that patients understand the plan, how to obtain support services, and who to call for help once they are discharged from the acute care facility (Gerteis et al., 1993, pp. 10–11).

An eighth dimension, access to care, was added when these principles became known as the *Picker Principles of Patient-Centered Care* (Picker Institute, n.d.). This principle simply states that patients need to know that they can access care when it is needed and also deals with waits for admission and allocation of hospital beds.

In January 2010, the Joint Commission released a set of standards for patient-centered communication to advance effective communication, cultural competence, and PCC (p. 57). One of the new requirements specifically states that a family member, friend, or other individual will be allowed to be present with the patient to provide emotional support, comfort, and alleviate fear during the course of the hospital stay (2010, p. 61). This requirement is not meant to mandate visiting hours or other hospital policies; it is, however, intended to encourage patient-centered and FCC environments where policies allow for inclusion of those persons important to the patient.

One recent change on some nursing units has been the establishment of walking rounds to patient rooms during change of shift report. Using this model, the nurses, patient, and family members (if the patient wishes) are all involved in the exchange of information during the transition of care to the nurse coming on shift. Can you think of any other changes that you have observed in the healthcare setting that help to facilitate a PCC environment?*

Commonly cited components of PCC and FCC delivery models include many of the same types of strategies. Some of these components include:

- Coordination of care conference that includes the patient and/or family along with the interdisciplinary team to discuss goals of treatment and to initiate discharge planning
- Hourly rounding by the nurse to complete treatments that also includes assessment of pain, elimination, and positioning as well as other concerns of the patient and/or family members
- Bedside report with the patient at the center of the discussion, with family and friends present at the discretion of the patient or patient advocate
- Use of a patient care partner (may be a family member, friend, or volunteer) selected by the patient to participate at various times in educational, psychological, physical, and spiritual support
- Individualized care that is established on admission to include the patient's preferred name, the patient's priorities for care, the patient's learning style preference, and the patient's care partner selection
- Open medical record policy that allows patients to view their medical record and document their perspective if they choose
- Eliminating visiting restrictions in relation to family members because, in the context of FCC, family members are members of the healthcare team rather than visitors
- Allowing family presence with a chaperone during resuscitation and other invasive procedures, thus never separating them from the patient unless the patient requests it
- Silence and a healing environment where the patient is invited to report any discomfort with the noise level in their environment to the nurse, who will then intervene to decrease noise level as much as is possible (Flagg, 2015; Hunter & Carlson, 2014).

Communication as a Strategy to Support Patient-Centered Care

Effective communication between healthcare providers and the patient is an essential component of PCC (IOM, 2001). Communicating effectively in all areas of practice and with all members of the healthcare team, including the patient and the patient's support network, is an expectation of all registered nurses (American Nurses Association [ANA], 2015, p. 71), including entry-level nurses (American Association of Colleges of Nursing [AACN], 2008, p. 31; QSEN, 2012).

The nurse is responsible for assessment of his or her own communication skills, continuous improvement of communication skills, assessment of communication ability and preferences of patients, and communicating accurate information in a manner that demonstrates respect (ANA, 2015, p. 71).

In terms of a competency, communication is defined as the nurse interacting "effectively with patients, families, and colleagues, fostering mutual respect and shared decision making, to enhance patient satisfaction and health outcomes" (Massachusetts Department of Higher Education, 2010, p. 27). This definition not only includes the standards for communication and PCC, but also the desired outcomes of PCC.

The new standards published by the Joint Commission related to patient-centered communication were designed to improve the safety and quality of care for all patients and promote better communication and patient engagement (2010, p. 57). The standards include requirements that the hospital identifies the patient's oral and written communication needs, including the patient's preferred language, and that the hospital communicates in a manner that meets the patient's needs (p. 59).

Communication may be viewed from different vantage points and may be manifested in a variety of formats and styles. For example, communication may be oral or written, empathetic or nonempathetic, and verbal or nonverbal (Bankert, Lazarek-LaQuay, & Joseph, 2014).

Empathetic communication refers to communication with someone from the vantage point of the other person's feelings, values, and perspective. The nurse–patient relationship based on empathetic communication is characterized by a genuine respect for the patient's opinions and decisions. Empathetic communication is the foundation for establishing relationships that are consistent with PCC (Bankert et al., 2014, p. 164). Behaviors that facilitate empathetic communication include:

- Listens carefully and reflects back a summary of the patient's concerns
- Uses terms and vocabulary appropriate for the patient
- Calls the patient by his or her preferred name
- Uses respectful and professional language
- Asks the patient what he or she needs and responds promptly to those needs
- Provides helpful information
- Solicits feedback from the patient
- Uses self-disclosure appropriately
- Employs humor as appropriate
- Provides words of comfort when appropriate (Bankert et al., 2014, p. 165)

Behaviors can also hinder empathetic communication. Some of these behaviors may include:

- Interrupts the patient with irrelevant information
- Uses vocabulary that is either beneath the level of the patient or not understandable to the patient

- Uses language that may be perceived as patronizing or demeaning
- Uses nonprofessional language
- Reprimands or scolds the patient
- Preaches to the patient
- Provides the patient with inappropriate information
- Asks questions at inappropriate times or gives the patient advice inappropriately
- Self-discloses inappropriately (Bankert et al., 2014, p. 165)

Other elements to consider are verbal communication and nonverbal behaviors that, although discussed separately, take place simultaneously. The empathetic communicator will be attentive to conflicting messages related to verbal and nonverbal communication, paying particular attention to nonverbal messages because these provide the nurse with insight into the patient's inner feelings. Nonverbal behaviors that the nurse will want to observe include eye movement, body position and movement, facial expression, and tone of voice. To communicate effectively, the nurse must learn to attend to all of these elements of the communication process (Bankert et al., 2014, pp. 166–167).

Examples of specific questions, known as Kleinman's questions, that can help clinicians relate to a patient on his or her level to provide PCC are included here. The questions are designed to elicit the patient's perception of his or her illness. The wording of the questions can be revised based on the setting, illness, and characteristics of the patient.

- What do you think has caused your problem?
- Why do you think it started when it did?
- What do you think your problem does inside your body?
- How severe is your problem? Will it have a short or long course?
- What kind of treatment do you think you should receive?
- What are the most important results you hope to receive from this treatment?
- What are the chief problems your illness has caused you?
- What do you fear most about your illness/treatment? (Kleinman, 1980)

Patient Education as a Strategy to Support Patient-Centered Care

Patient education has formally been a part of nursing care since the time of Florence Nightingale (1860/1969). During the 1900s, patient education increasingly became identified as a role of the professional nurse; however, it was not until 1973 that the ANA (1973) defined patient education as a component of the practice of the registered nurse. Beginning in 1976, the Joint Commission on Accreditation of Healthcare Organizations (Joint

Commission, 1995) included patient and family education as a function critical to patient care. The AACN (1998, 2008) also recognized that the implementation of the professional nursing role requires that nurses are prepared to teach patients effectively. The standards of professional nursing practice Standard 5, states that the nurse is reponsible for implementation of an identified plan (ANA, 2015, p. 61). A subcategory of this standard entitled Health Teaching and Health Promotion indicates that the nurse employs strategies to promote health and a safe environment. Competencies under this standard include those related to the nurse providing health promotion education and health teaching (ANA, 2015, p. 65). Thus, in contemporary nursing practice, patient education is both a professional expectation and a legal obligation of the nurse.

"Patient education is any set of planned, educational activities designed to improve patients' health behaviors, health status, or both" (Lorig, 2001, p. xiii). There is nothing in this definition about improving knowledge, although a change in knowledge might be necessary to reach the goal of changing health status or health behaviors. In contrast, activities aimed at improving knowledge are known as **patient teaching** (Lorig, 2001, p. xiv). The point is that the purposes of patient education are more than a change in knowledge. The purposes of patient education are to maintain health, to improve health, or to slow deterioration of health. These purposes are met through changes in health-related behaviors and attitudes (Lorig, 2001), and these changes are not easily achieved. Effective patient education requires the nurse to have the ability to communicate effectively with patients to assess the individual needs, attitudes, and preferences of the patient that can affect health behaviors before any changes can be expected (Falvo, 2004, 2011).

Principles and Theories Related to Patient Education

In addition to communication and assessment skills, if the nurse is to be effective as a patient educator, then he or she must also have sufficient knowledge of the information that needs to be taught. If the knowledge base of the nurse is insufficient, the nurse risks providing inadequate or inaccurate information to the patient (Falvo, 2004, 2011). Finally, to be an effective patient educator, it is important that the nurse have an understanding of how to conduct patient education. Many educational theories and principles can be used to guide the patient education process. Some that are most commonly used in the healthcare setting are presented here.

Domains of Learning

First, we should examine the nature of learning in relationship to **learning domains**. Identification of the learning domain reflects the type of learning desired as a result of the patient education process. Learning occurs in three domains: the cognitive, the psychomotor, and the affective (Bloom, 1956). The framework includes categories or levels of learning that include knowledge, comprehension, application, analysis, synthesis, and evaluation. Each level builds on the previous one in a hierarchical fashion. In the cognitive and psychomotor domains, levels are arranged in order of increasing complexity. In the affective domain, levels are organized according to the degree of internalization of a value or attitude.

In the revised taxonomy (Anderson & Krathwohl, 2001), cognitive learning encompasses the intellectual skills of remembering, understanding, applying, analyzing, evaluating, and creating. The use of verbs rather than nouns to name the categories in the revised taxonomy underscores the dynamic nature of learning. Psychomotor learning refers to learning of motor skills and performance of behaviors or skills that require coordination. Affective learning requires a change in feelings, attitudes, or beliefs.

Understanding which domain is the target of learning helps guide the planning, implementation, and evaluation of learning. For example, if based on assessment you know that a patient is knowledgeable about insulin administration and is committed to administering the injection but has not yet been able to manipulate the syringe correctly to administer the injection, you know that your target domain for learning is the psychomotor domain. Thus, the focus of your objectives, planning, learning activities, and evaluation will be on the performance of the identified behaviors.

Andragogy

Andragogy, initially defined as "the art and science of helping adults learn" (Knowles, 1970), has taken on a broader meaning over the past 40 years and is currently used to refer to learner-focused education for people of all ages (Conner, 2004). The andragogic model asserts that the following four issues be considered and addressed in learning (Knowles, Swanson, & Holton, 1998, 2011):

- Letting learners know why something is important to learn
- Showing learners how to direct themselves through information
- Relating the topic to the learners' experiences
- Realizing that people will not learn until they are ready and motivated

Adults learn best when there is immediate opportunity for application. Adults in particular are motivated to learn when they recognize a gap between what they know and what they want to know or what they need to know (Knowles, 1970). Therefore, adult learners are rarely interested in learning detailed anatomy and physiology related to their chronic disease, but they are motivated to learn how to care for themselves after discharge from the hospital. Effective patient education will be based on principles that capitalize on these characteristics of the adult learner.

Health Belief Model

The **Health Belief Model (HBM)** is one of the most widely used frameworks in research and programs related to health promotion and patient education. This model was originally developed to predict the likelihood of a person following a recommended action and to understand the person's motivation and decision making regarding seeking health services (Hochbaum, 1958).

According to the HBM, the likelihood of a person acting in response to a health threat depends on six factors:

- The person's perception of the severity of the illness
- The person's perception of susceptibility to illness and its consequences
- The value of the treatment benefits (i.e., do the cost and side effects of treatment outweigh the consequences of the disease?)
- Barriers to treatment (i.e., expense, complexity of treatment)
- Costs of treatment in physical and emotional terms
- Cues that stimulate taking action toward treatment of illness (i.e., mass media campaigns, pamphlets, advice from family or friends, and postcard reminders from healthcare providers)

The HBM can provide a framework for assessing areas where patients have gaps in knowledge, such as severity of illness or susceptibility to illness, and then address those areas to increase the potential for compliance with the treatment regimen. Through use of the HBM, you can easily categorize and cover the essential components of your educational message, thus providing the patient with a basic understanding of the severity of the illness, the risk and consequences of the illness, the value of treatment, the barriers to treatment, and the costs of treatment.

Social Learning Theory

According to Bandura's **social learning theory**, if a person believes that he or she is capable of performing a behavior (**self-efficacy**) and also believes that the behavior will lead to a desirable outcome, the person will be more likely to perform the behavior (Bandura, 1997). In contrast, if a person does not believe that he or she is capable of performing a behavior, he or she will have no incentive to do so, even if the person is actually capable. Perceptions of self-efficacy are particularly important in relation to a patient's learning complex activities or long-term changes in behavior (Prohaska & Lorig, 2001).

There are four methods for developing or enhancing efficacy expectations if assessment reveals a need for such enhancement. These methods are as follows:

- Performance accomplishments
- Vicarious experience or modeling
- Verbal persuasion
- Interpretation of physiologic state

KEY COMPETENCY 11-2

Examples of Applicable *Nurse of the Future: Nursing Core Competencies*

Communication (Teaching/Learning):

Knowledge (K5d) Is aware of the three domains of learning: cognitive, affective, and psychomotor

Attitudes/Behaviors (A5c) Values the need for teaching in all three domains of learning

Source: Massachusetts Department of Higher Education. (2010). *Nurse of the future: Nursing core competencies* (p. 29). Retrieved from http://www.mass.edu/currentinit/documents/NursingCoreCompetencies.pdf

Performance accomplishment is the most direct and influential way to enhance self-efficacy. In this method, the patient first performs tasks that he or she can easily perform. By succeeding with these first tasks, the patient develops a sense of competence and enhancement of self-efficacy before proceeding to more difficult tasks. Along these same lines, it is also important to set short-term goals that are measurable so that patients can see their success and the impact of the change in their behavior. A patient who can see the benefits of a behavior change within a reasonable time is more likely to continue practicing the behavior.

The second method for enhancing self-efficacy is through modeling, where the patient observes others who appear to be similar and who are successfully performing behaviors. Modeling can also be achieved through the use of illustrations in pamphlets or in programming materials by using illustrations and models that are of various cultures, body shapes, and ages (Prohaska & Lorig, 2001).

Verbal persuasion can also be an effective method of enhancing self-efficacy expectations. The content of the message needs to include basic factual information that emphasizes the importance of performing the behavior. It is usually better to ask for incremental changes or ask the patient to do just slightly more than he or she is currently doing (Prohaska & Lorig, 2001). Encouragement and support not only from the nurse, but also from family and friends help the patient to be successful.

Most illnesses present with symptoms and most new behaviors cause some physiologic changes. Addressing the meaning of symptoms and physiologic states can influence self-efficacy. For example, a patient who is trying to quit smoking can expect withdrawal symptoms. If the patient understands the reasons for the symptoms and the limitation in the duration of the symptoms, the patient might decide that he or she has the ability to make the change. Without that knowledge, the patient might give up because he or she experiences physiologic changes that are not understood.

The Patient Education Process: Assessment

According to Redman (2001, 2006), the process of patient education can be viewed as parallel to the nursing process. Each of these processes begins with assessment, negotiation of goals and objectives, planning, intervention, and finally evaluation (Rankin, 2005; Rankin & Stallings, 2001; Rankin, Stallings, & London, 2005).

The goal of the nurse in the process of patient education is to assist the patient in obtaining the knowledge, skills, or attitude that will help the patient develop behaviors to meet needs and maximize the potential for positive health outcomes (Falvo, 2004, 2011). Because no patient or situation is exactly the same, an assessment is required.

Many available guides are helpful in assessing the learning needs of patients (Redman, 2003). Some nurses construct their own assessment tools to meet specific needs. Observation, interviews, open-ended questions, focus groups, and the patient's medical record are additional ways to gather information for the assessment of learning needs. Rankin and Stallings (2001, p. 200) suggest some specific questions that must be addressed in the assessment of learning needs. These questions are as follows:

- What information does the patient need?
- What attitudes should be explored?
- What skill does the patient need to be able to perform healthcare behaviors?
- What factors in the patient's environment may be barriers to the performance of desired behaviors?
- Is the patient likely to return home?
- Can the family or caregiver handle the care that will be required?
- Is the home situation adequate or appropriate for the type of care required?
- What kinds of assistance will be required?

Learning Styles

To provide the most effective patient teaching, the nurse must also assess patient learning style. Although most people learn best when multiple techniques are used in patient teaching, assessment of the patient's learning style is a fundamental step before beginning any learning activity. Learning styles are methods of interacting with, taking in, and processing information that allow individuals to learn. Learning styles are generally categorized as visual, auditory, or tactile/kinesthetic.

The patient who is a visual learner prefers written instructions rather than verbal instructions but prefers photographs and illustrations to written instructions. The nurse teaching the patient who is a visual learner should use a variety of interesting visual learning materials, including organized visual presentations, photographs, or computerized materials (Russell, 2006).

The patient who is an auditory learner remembers verbal instructions well and learns through discussion. The nurse teaching a patient who is an auditory learner will want to be sure the patient is positioned to be able to hear and will want to rephrase what is said several different ways to be sure the intended message is communicated. The nurse might also want to use multimedia that incorporates sound in patient teaching (Russell, 2006).

The patient who learns best through getting physically involved is the tactile or kinesthetic learner. The kinesthetic learner learns through doing or experiencing physically. The kinesthetic learner has difficulty staying in one place for very long and enjoys hands-on activities. The nurse teaching the kinesthetic learner should provide activities during the session and should provide samples or supplies for practicing or demonstrating skills (Russell, 2006).

Readiness to Learn

An important variable in the patient education process is **readiness to learn**. After a need to learn has been identified, a patient's readiness or evidence of motivation to receive information at that particular time must also be assessed (Falvo, 2004, 2011; Joint Commission, 2003; Redman, 2001). A variety of factors such as pain, anxiety, and emotional reactions can affect a patient's readiness to learn. Moderate to severe anxiety has been shown to interfere with a patient's ability to concentrate and understand new information (Stephenson, 2007). If a patient is distracted by physical or emotional pain, attempts at patient teaching will not be successful. The better choice is to wait until the pain has subsided or to address the anxiety that the patient is experiencing, and then when the patient is ready, proceed with patient education activities (Redman, 2001, 2006; Stephenson, 2007).

Health Literacy

Considering a patient's **health literacy** is an important component in PCC. Health literacy is generally defined as the ability to read, understand, and act on health information. The IOM (2004) consensus report on health literacy defined the concept as, "the degree to which individuals have the capacity to obtain, process, and understand basic health information and services they need to make appropriate health decisions" (p. 31).

Today there is more access to healthcare information than at any time in history. The low health literacy problem for most is not an issue of access to information, but rather is a crisis of not understanding medical information (Doak & Doak, 2002). Research studies have demonstrated that patients with low health literacy skills make more errors with their medications and treatments (Baker et al., 1996; Williams, Baker, Honig, Lee, & Nowlan, 1998) and are also at risk for experiencing preventable adverse events (Bartlett, Blais, Tamblyn, Clermont, & MacGibbon, 2008). They often fail to seek preventive care and are also at higher risk for hospitalization, which results in higher annual healthcare costs (Agency for Healthcare Research and Quality [AHRQ], 2011; Baker, Parker, Williams, & Clark, 1998; U.S. Department of Health and Human Services [USDHHS], 2012; Weiss, 1999).

In the United States, one in five adults and nearly two in five older adults and minorities read at the fifth-grade level or below. Only 12% of U.S. adults are considered to have proficient health literacy. The number of adults with only basic health literacy skills or below basic-level health literacy skills has reached 77 million. One-third of the U.S. adult population has difficulty with common health tasks such as following instructions on a medication label (USDHHS, 2012, p. 1). This is significant because persons with only basic health literacy skills or below basic-level health literacy skills have difficulty processing and understanding information and services and thus have difficulty making healthcare-related decisions (Miller & Stoeckel,

2011). Although health literacy is partially dependent on the patient's skill set, it is also dependent on the complexity of the information as well as how information is communicated (USDHHS, 2012).

The National Patient Safety Foundation (2015) has developed a program entitled Ask Me 3. According to the foundation, this program promotes improved health outcomes by encouraging patients to become active members of their healthcare team through improved communication between patients and their healthcare providers. The following are the three questions the program encourages patients to ask their healthcare provider:

- What is my main problem?
- What do I need to do?
- Why is it important for me to do this?

Another program that is used by nurses to become more effective patient educators is ACTS, an acronym for assess; compare; teach three, teach back; and survey. The best education strategies begin by asking the patient to identify his or her main concern. This simple question will shift the focus of the interaction from the nurse to a patient-centered encounter. Next, the nurse needs to discover the needs and preferences of the patient in order to individualize the teaching plan, as well as how the patient prefers to learn. Asking the patient or caregiver what they already know acknowledges his or her current level of expertise and supports the concepts of patient control and shared decision making. Finally, the nurse assesses patient core values and cultural, social, language, and physical influences. During the compare phase, the nurse compares the available resources to the needs and preferences of the patient to match relevant content to identified knowledge gaps. Teach three, teach back refers to the process in which patients are taught three or fewer key concepts or care skills in short segments and then the patient restates the concept in his or her own words or demonstrates the skill. If the patient has difficulty with restating or with skill demonstration, teaching should be repeated. Nurses should then close the loop by asking in an open ended manner if there are additional questions or learning needs (French, 2015, pp. 91–92).

When information is complex or time is limited, nurses frequently provide printed materials for patients to read or review at home. These materials are helpful when they provide patients who have adequate reading skills with a resource to remind them of the instructions given by the nurse, but for those patients with low health literacy skills, the printed materials might be of no use. The average American reads at the 8th- to 9th-grade level. Most materials used for patient education are written above the 10th-grade reading level (Doak & Doak, 2002; Doak, Doak, & Root, 1996). We know that when the reading level of printed materials is beyond the skill of the learner, comprehension is decreased, recall is sketchy and inaccurate, and motivation to learn is decreased (Redman, 2001, 2006).

KEY COMPETENCY 11-4

Examples of Applicable *Nurse of the Future: Nursing Core Competencies*

Communication (Teaching/Learning):

Knowledge (K5a) Understands the influences of different learning styles on the education of patients and families

Attitudes/Behaviors (A5a) Values different means of communication used by patients and families

Source: Massachusetts Department of Higher Education. (2010). *Nurse of the future: Nursing core competencies* (p. 29). Retrieved from http://www.mass.edu/currentinit/documents/NursingCoreCompetencies.pdf

KEY COMPETENCY 11-5

Examples of Applicable *Nurse of the Future: Nursing Core Competencies*

Communication (Teaching/ Learning):

Knowledge (K5e) Understands the concept of health literacy

Skills (S5a) Assesses factors that influence the patient's and family's ability to learn, including readiness to learn, preferences for learning style, and levels of health literacy

Source: Massachusetts Department of Higher Education. (2010). *Nurse of the future: Nursing core competencies* (p. 29). Retrieved from http://www.mass.edu/currentinit /documents/NursingCoreCompetencies.pdf

Patients with low health literacy skills are generally too embarrassed to reveal to the nurse that they cannot read or cannot read well enough to understand the written instructions. It is therefore important that the nurse take the initiative in assessing the literacy skills of patients before using written materials in the patient education process and to provide educational materials in various formats when possible.

Direct questioning of patients about reading ability is usually not effective. Thus, how can you determine the reading ability of the patient? One option is to use one of several instruments that have been developed to assess patient literacy quickly. Some of the literacy assessment instruments most commonly used in healthcare settings include the Rapid Estimate of Adult Literacy in Medicine (Davis et al., 1993) and the Wide Range Achievement Test (Jastak & Wilkinson, 1993).

One of the best ways to assess literacy is simply through careful observation of your patient. Clues that might be observed in a patient with low health literacy skills include forms that are filled out incompletely or incorrectly, written materials that are handed to a person accompanying the patient, and aloofness or withdrawal during provider explanations. Additional clues might include surveillance of the behavior of others in the same situation to copy their actions or a request for help from staff or other patients. Verbal responses such as "I will read this at home" or "I can't read this now because I forgot my glasses" are also common (Bastable, 2006; Doak & Doak, 2002).

Health literacy tools continue to focus primarily on reading ability, despite the IOM's recommendation that the focus change to skills-based health literacy tools that use a combination of skills that patients can use to manage health, such as verbal, computer, or other skills (AHRQ, 2011). Because reading ability continues to be the prevalent focus, we will consider assessment of readability of materials next.

Assessing the Readability of Patient Education Materials

Many health-related teaching materials are written on a level that is above the average patient's literacy level and contain too much medical jargon (National Center for Education Statistics, 2007). Written materials can still be useful supplements for patients with low health literacy skills if the written materials selected are appropriate to the reading level of the patient. Print materials for most patient populations should be written between the seventh- and eighth-grade reading levels. Print materials for patients with low health literacy skills should be written at or below the fifth-grade reading level (Doak & Doak, 2002).

Several readability formulas are available to determine the grade level of materials (Flesch, 1948; Fry, 1968; McLaughlin, 1969). One of the easiest formulas to use is the SMOG formula, which predicts the reading grade level of materials within 1.5 grades 68% of the time (McLaughlin, 1969). The procedure for using the SMOG readability formula for printed materials is outlined in **Box 11-1**.

CRITICAL THINKING QUESTIONS✱

Have you ever been assigned to read a book that had so many big words in it that you had to keep the dictionary by your side? If it was assigned for school, you probably struggled through it for the sake of not failing the test, but what about if you were not being graded? Would you bother to read it? If you did read it because you knew it would help you, would you have enough understanding to actually apply the information?✱

BOX 11-1 SMOG READABILITY FORMULA

1. Choose 10 consecutive sentences near the beginning, 10 consecutive sentences from the middle, and 10 consecutive sentences from the end of the material.
2. In these 30 sentences, count the number of words containing three or more syllables, including repetitions. Consider hyphenated words as one word. Proper nouns are also counted. Numerals and abbreviations should be counted as they would if the words were written out. When a colon divides words, each portion of the sentence is considered a separate sentence.
3. Estimate the square root of the number of polysyllabic words counted.
4. Add three to the square root. This gives the SMOG grading, which is the reading grade level that a person must have achieved to fully understand the material.
5. The quickest way to assess reading grade level is to use the SMOG conversion table. Simply compare the total number of words containing three or more syllables in the 30 sentences with the SMOG Conversion Table.

However, not all written patient education materials contain 30 sentences. To assess materials with fewer than 30 sentences:

1. Count all of the polysyllabic words.
2. Count the number of sentences.
3. Find the average number of polysyllabic words per sentence.

SMOG Conversion Table	
Word Count	Grade Level
0–2	4
3–6	5
7–12	6
13–20	7
21–30	8
31–42	9
43–56	10
57–72	11
73–90	12
91–110	13
111–132	14
133–156	15
157–182	16
183–210	17
211–240	18

Source: Developed by Harold C. McGraw, Office of Educational Research, Baltimore County Schools, Towson, Maryland.

(continued)

| BOX 11-1 SMOG READABILITY FORMULA (*continued*) |

4. Multiply that average by the number of sentences short of 30.
5. Add that figure to the total number of polysyllabic words.
6. Find the square root of the number you obtained in step 5 and add the constant of three. This procedure also gives you the SMOG grading.

Source: U.S. Department of Health and Human Services, National Institutes of Health, National Cancer Institute. (2004). Making health communication programs work: A planner's guide. Retrieved from http://www.cancer.gov/publications/health-communication /pink-book.pdf

Readability for materials available in an electronic format can be assessed using formulas embedded in word processing programs and also for free via several readability calculation websites on the Internet.

Low health literacy can be a barrier to effective patient education, but the patient with low health literacy skills is capable of learning if the nurse is willing to invest the extra time that is required. It is important for the nurse to take extra care to present information in terms that the patient is familiar with rather than using medical jargon, to use alternate formats such as pictographs when possible, to restate information using simple words, and to verify the patient's understanding by having him or her convey the information in his or her own words. The dividends for the extra effort include the patient who is able to manage his or her own illness, make informed health decisions, and make health-related behavior changes as a result of a patient education process that has accommodated for his or her weaknesses.

The Patient Education Process: Planning

The patient and the nurse share the planning process for patient education, but it is the responsibility of the nurse to guide the process using goals and objectives. Learning goals are derived from the learning assessment, and nursing diagnoses and objectives are developed based on goals in collaboration with the patient. The use of goals and objectives helps the nurse to focus on what is important for the patient to learn and keep patient education focused on outcomes (Rankin & Stallings, 2001; Rankin et al., 2005).

Patient education is directed toward behavioral change; therefore, the objectives for patient education are stated as behavioral objectives. There are three components of behavioral objectives: performance, conditions, and criteria (Mager, 1997). Performance refers to the activity that the patient will engage in and answers this question: What can the learner do? The condition refers to special circumstances of the patient's performance and answers this question: Under what conditions will the learner perform the behavior? The criteria or evaluation component refers to how long or how well the behavior must be performed to be acceptable and answers this question: What is the performance standard? (Rankin & Stallings, 2001; Rankin et al., 2005).

The learning objectives should be specific, measurable, and attainable (Rankin, 2005; Rankin & Stallings, 2001; Rankin et al., 2005). Learning objectives are also written in a manner that is learning-domain specific. Recognizing the targeted domain of learning as cognitive, psychomotor, or affective helps guide the process of writing behavioral learning objectives and thus guides the selection of learning activities.

The Patient Education Process: Implementation

The next stage of the process involves the actual intervention. Whether the teaching will occur in a group or with an individual patient, learning activities need to be consistent with learning objectives.

Using various learning activities can make learning more fun and more effective. Some common learning activities include lectures, demonstrations, practice, games, simulations, role playing, discussions, and self-directed learning through computer-assisted instruction or self-directed workbooks.

Patient education materials are frequently used in the implementation stage of the patient education process. Patient education materials can be designed to be used alone or to supplement other types of patient education activities but should be previewed before use and used only if consistent with learning objectives. There are many types of patient education materials currently on the market, or you might opt to produce your own materials.

Patient education materials generally include audiovisual materials, computer programs, Internet resources, posters, flip charts, charts, graphs, cartoons, slides, overhead transparencies, photographs, drawings, patient education newsletters, or written patient materials such as handouts, brochures, or pamphlets. These materials, even if designed to be used alone, should not be used without some verbal instruction as to why the patient is being instructed to view the video or read the brochure (Falvo, 2004, 2011). Additionally, the nurse should keep the door of communication open by inviting questions that the patient might have as a result of exposure to the teaching materials.

You must evaluate a variety of factors as you look at the appropriateness of patient education materials. Three important criteria for judging patient education materials are the following (Doak, Doak, Gordon, & Lorig, 2001, p. 184):

- The material contains the information the patient wants.
- The material contains the information the patient needs.
- The patient understands and uses the material as presented.

It is an expectation of the Joint Commission that the right educational materials are used in patient and family education and that the materials are accurate, age specific, easily accessible, and appropriate to patient needs (Joint Commission, 2003). To address all of these criteria, the nurse needs to conduct a needs assessment before preparing or choosing patient education materials.

Considerations: Patient Education with Older Adults

When caring for older adults, one of the primary considerations related to the patient education process is accommodation for age-related barriers to learning. The age-related barriers particularly important in the patient education process include **age-related changes** in cognition, vision, and hearing. Research has demonstrated that teaching is not as effective if it does not accommodate for age-related cognitive and sensory changes (Donlon, 1993; Masters, 2001; Weinrich, Weinrich, Boyd, Atwood, & Cervenka, 1994). Gerogogy in patient education has been defined as the transferring of essential information that has been designed, modified, and adapted to accommodate for the physiologic and psychologic changes in elderly persons by taking into account the person's disease process, age-related changes, educational level, and motivation (Pearson, 2012).

Age-related changes in cognitive function occur slowly and are thought to begin at approximately 60 years of age in healthy adults (Miller, 2004). Age-related visual changes are the most prevalent physical impairments affecting older adults. Hearing impairment ranks as one of the four most prevalent chronic conditions affecting the older population, occurring in one-third of the U.S. population between the ages of 65 and 74 years and in 47% of the population 75 years of age or older (National Institutes of Health, n.d.). Each of these age-related changes can have a profound effect on the teaching and learning process. Specific age-related changes in cognition, vision, and hearing are listed in **Box 11-2**.

BOX 11-2 AGE-RELATED BARRIERS TO LEARNING: COGNITIVE AND SENSORY CHANGES

Cognitive
  Changes in encoding and storage of information
  Changes in the retrieval of information
  Decreases in the speed of processing information*
Visual
  Smaller amount of light reaches the retina
  Reduced ability to focus on close objects
  Scattering of light resulting in glare
  Changes in color perception resulting in difficulty distinguishing colors such as dark green, blue, and violet
  Decrease in depth perception and peripheral vision[†]
Hearing
  Reduced ability to hear sounds as loudly
  Decrease in hearing acuity
  Decrease in ability to hear high-pitched sounds
  Decrease in the ability to filter background noise[†]

Sources: Data from *Merriam, S. B., & Caffarella, R. S. (1999). *Learning in adulthood: A comprehensive guide* (2nd ed.). San Francisco, CA: Jossey-Bass; *Merriam, S. B., Caffarella, R. S., & Baumgartner, L. M. (2007). *Learning in adulthood: A comprehensive guide* (3rd ed.). San Francisco, CA: Jossey-Bass; [†]Miller, C. A. (2004). *Nursing for wellness in older adults: Theory and practice* (4th ed.). Philadelphia, PA: Lippincott.

BOX 11-3 STRATEGIES TO ACCOMMODATE FOR AGE-RELATED BARRIERS TO LEARNING: COGNITIVE AND SENSORY CHANGES

Cognitive

Slow the pace of the presentation.

Give smaller amounts of information at a time.

Repeat information frequently.

Reinforce verbal teaching with audiovisuals, written materials, and practice.

Reduce distractions.

Allow more time for self-expression of learner.

Use analogies and examples from everyday experience to illustrate abstract information.

Increase the meaningfulness of content to the learner.

Teach mnemonic devices and imaging techniques.

Use printed materials and visual aids that are age specific*

Visual

Make sure patient's glasses are clean and in place.

Use printed materials with 14- to 16-point font and serif letters.

Use bold type on printed materials, and do not mix fonts.

Avoid the use of dark colors with dark backgrounds for teaching materials; instead use large, distinct configurations with high contrast to help with discrimination.

Avoid using blue, green, and violet to differentiate type, illustrations, or graphics.

Use line drawings with high contrast.

Use soft white light to decrease glare.

Light should shine from behind the learner.

Use color and touch to help differentiate depth.

Position materials directly in front of the learner.†

Hearing

Speak distinctly.

Do not shout.

Speak in a normal voice, or speak in a lower pitch.

Decrease extraneous noise.

Face the person directly while speaking at a distance of 3 to 6 feet.

Reinforce verbal teaching with visual aids or easy-to-read materials.†

Sources: Data from *Weinrich, S. P., Boyd, M., & Nussbaum, J. (1989). Continuing education: Adapting strategies to teach the elderly. *Journal of Gerontological Nursing, 15*(11), 17–21; †Oldaker, S. M. (1992). Live and learn: Patient education for the elderly orthopaedic client. *Orthopaedic Nursing, 11*(3), 51–56.

Specific strategies can be used during the patient education process to help overcome the age-related learning barriers in cognition, vision, and hearing. Some of these strategies are included in **Box 11-3**.

Cultural Considerations in Patient Education

Developing an educational program that is culturally appropriate is not much different from creating any other patient education program. You begin with a needs assessment; then, you write objectives and design the program. The difference is that you must be culturally sensitive and incorporate cultural information that you have learned about the target group into the patient education process (Bastable, 2006; Gonzalez & Lorig, 2001; Lengetti, Ordelt, & Pyle, 2007).

How important is it that you incorporate cultural information into the patient education process? Cultural awareness and sensitivity of nurses can influence the ability of patients to receive and apply information regarding their health care (Campinha-Bacote, Yahle, & Langenkamp, 1996). The way that information is communicated can influence a patient's perception of the healthcare system and affect adherence to prescribed treatments. In a recent study, patients who received care from nurses with cultural sensitivity training showed improvement not only in use of social resources, but also in overall functional capacity (Majumdar, Browne, Roberts, & Carpio, 2004).

In addition to the difference that it can make in relationship to patient outcomes, the standards of practice are clear that the nurse is responsible for using "health promotion and teaching methods in collaboration with the healthcare consumer's values, beliefs, health practices, developmental level, learning needs, readiness and ability to learn, language preference, spirituality, culture, and socioeconomic status" (ANA, 2015, p. 65). The Joint Commission standards also require not only that the patient's learning needs, abilities, and readiness to learn are assessed, but also that the patient's preferences are assessed. This assessment must consider cultural and religious practices as well as emotional and language barriers (Joint Commission, 2003).

How do you incorporate cultural information into the patient education process? Gonzalez and Lorig (2001, p. 172) suggest the following:

- Change the information into more specific or more relevant terminology.
- Create descriptions or explanations that fit with different people's understanding of key concepts.
- Incorporate a group's cultural beliefs and practices into the program content and process.

In addition, any visual aids that are used should reflect the target group or population. The use of culturally relevant analogies can also help people to understand complex, abstract, or foreign concepts (Gonzalez & Lorig, 2001).

The Patient Education Process: Evaluation

Evaluation determines worth by judging something against a standard. The standard used in the patient education process is the learning objective. Thus, the term *evaluation* as used here implies measuring the outcomes resulting from systematically planned activities implemented as a part of a patient education program or patient education process against the learning objectives to determine whether learning occurred.

KEY COMPETENCY 11-6

Examples of Applicable *Nurse of the Future: Nursing Core Competencies*

Patient-Centered Care:

Knowledge (K4) Describes how diverse cultural, ethnic, spiritual and socioeconomic backgrounds function as sources of patient, family, and community values

Attitudes/Behaviors (A4c) Supports patient-centered care for individuals and groups whose values differ from their own

Skills (S4a) Provides patient-centered care with sensitivity and respect for the diversity of human experience

Source: Massachusetts Department of Higher Education. (2010). *Nurse of the future: Nursing core competencies* (p. 10). Retrieved from http://www.mass.edu/currentinit/documents/NursingCoreCompetencies.pdf

Initiation of the patient education evaluation process is the responsibility of the nurse, and according to Rankin and Stallings (2001, p. 326), the evaluation process should include the following:

- Measuring the extent to which the patient has met the learning objectives
- Identifying when there is a need to clarify, correct, or review information
- Noting learning objectives that are unclear
- Pointing out shortcomings in patient teaching interventions
- Identifying barriers that prevented learning

Nurses commonly use several methods to evaluate patient learning. These methods include direct observation, the teach-back method or asking patients to explain something in their own words, situational feedback to determine if the patient selects the appropriate behavior, records of health-related behaviors that patients report, patient interviews and questionnaires, and critical incidents such as readmission, emergency department visits, and mortality (McNeill, 2012).

Evaluation of Patient-Centered Care

The National Strategy for Quality Improvement in Health Care was established by the secretary of the USDHHS to set priorities to guide the nation to increase access to high-quality health care. One of the priorities identified was the delivery of PCC and FCC (USDHHS, 2011). We know that there is a link between PCC and quality health care, but identifying specific measures of PCC is challenging.

The HCAHPS (pronounced H-CAPS) survey, also known as the Consumer Assessment of Healthcare Providers and Systems (CAHPS) Hospital Survey, was the first national, standardized, publically reported survey of patients' perspectives of hospital care. The intent of the survey is to provide a standard instrument to measure patient satisfaction with the hospital experience. The survey asks a core set of questions to assess patient satisfaction with the care provided by nurses, physicians, and other members of the healthcare team; the responsiveness of the hospital staff; pain management; communication about medications; and the cleanliness and quietness of the environment. The standardized questions allow for comparisons of patient care experiences.

A more recent addition to the CAHPS survey is the integration of a supplemental item set related to health literacy. The primary goal of the survey is to measure, from the patient's perspective, how well health-related information was communicated to them by health professionals during their care. This survey is available in English and Spanish. CAHPS supplemental item sets are also now available to assess cultural competence, to assess technology use, and for the patient-centered medical home (USDHHS, 2012).

Patient satisfaction with the care provided is recognized as a valid quality indicator (Bankert et al., 2014, p. 178). As consumers, patients provide their perspectives on the quality of care, delivery of care, outcomes of care, and the extent to which they were included as an active participant. PCC requires that evaluation of the care experience include the perspective of the patient (Walton & Barnsteiner, 2012).

Conclusion

The patient relationship with healthcare professionals has changed dramatically during the past few decades and continues to evolve. In just one generation, we have moved from a healthcare system in which the provider made all of the decisions for the passive patient, to a system where our goal is full partnership with the patient. This shift requires nurses to actively engage patients in all dimensions of their care while communicating in a manner that conveys empathy and respect for patient preferences.

CASE STUDY 11-1 ▪ MR. MARTIN

Mr. Martin, an 82-year-old African American patient, is ready for discharge from the medical unit after a 3-day hospitalization resulting from exacerbation of heart failure. Before discharge from the hospital, the student nurse reviews the medication orders and provides Mr. Martin with standard patient education materials related to control of heart failure symptoms.

Case Study Questions

1. What else could the student nurse in the case study do to enhance the effectiveness of the patient education process for Mr. Martin?

2. Do you have any suggestions for the student nurse related to accommodating for age-related changes of this patient?

3. Do you have any suggestions for the student nurse related to cultural considerations as she educates this patient?

Classroom Activity 1

Provide students with a copy of printed patient education materials. These can be obtained from a local healthcare organization or from online sources such as the American Heart Association. Ask students to evaluate the materials for readability using the SMOG formula in Box 11-1. Next, ask students to evaluate the materials for use with older adults using the information presented in Box 11-2 and Box 11-3. Finally, have students evaluate the materials for use with a population of a different culture. Ask students to share findings during informal presentations to classmates.

Classroom Activity 2

Divide the class into small groups and ask students to create a patient education brochure that conforms to recommended reading levels, considers age-related learning barriers, and accommodates cultural differences. The group may choose a fictitious case scenario or an actual scenario from a recent clinical experience. For this activity, several students will need to bring laptops to class or the class will need to have access to a computer lab. Alternately, this activity could be assigned to students to complete outside of class to be shared with the class or submitted for a grade.

Classroom Activity 3

Share highlights of the story of Lia Lee from Anne Fadiman's book, *When the Spirit Catches You and You Fall Down*. Next share the responses of Lia's mother to Dr. Arthur Kleinman's questions, available at http://www.donnathomson.com/2012/11/eight-questions-that-can-heal.html. Discuss the differing perspective of the issues once someone asks the patient and/or family what they think.

Classroom Activity 4

Numerous classroom and clinical activities related to PCC are available on the QSEN website at http://qsen.org/teaching-strategies/strategy-search/. Choose activities from the website for students to complete that meet objectives specific to your course.

References

Agency for Healthcare Research and Quality. (2011). *Health literacy interventions and outcomes: An updated systematic review*. Publication No. 11E-006. Rockville, MD: U.S. Department of Health and Human Services.

American Association of Colleges of Nursing. (1998). *The essentials of baccalaureate education for professional nursing practice*. Washington, DC: Author.

American Association of Colleges of Nursing. (2008). *The essentials of baccalaureate education for professional nursing practice.* Washington, DC: Author.

American Nurses Association. (1973). *Standards of nursing practice.* Kansas City, MO: Author.

American Nurses Association. (2015). *Nursing: Scope and standards of practice* (3rd ed.). Silver Spring, MD: Author.

Anderson, L. W., & Krathwohl, D. R. (Eds.). (2001). *A taxonomy for learning, teaching and assessing: A revision of Bloom's taxonomy of educational objectives.* New York, NY: Addison-Wesley.

Baker, D. W., Parker, R. M., Williams, M. V., & Clark, W. S. (1998). Health literacy and the risk of hospital admission. *Journal of General Internal Medicine, 13,* 791–798.

Baker, D. W., Parker, R. M., Williams, M. V., Pitkin, K., Parikh, N. S., Coates, W., & Imara, M. (1996). The health care experience of patients with low literacy. *Archives of Family Medicine, 5,* 329–334.

Bandura, A. (1997). *Self-efficacy: The exercise of control.* New York, NY: W. H. Freeman.

Bankert, E., Lazarek-LaQuay, A., & Joseph, J. M. (2014). Patient-centered care. In P. Kelly, B. A. Vottero, & C. A. Christie-McAuliffe (Eds.), *Introduction to quality and safety education for nurses* (pp. 161–189). New York, NY: Springer.

Bartlett, G., Blais, R., Tamblyn, R., Clermont, R. J., & MacGibbon, B. (2008). Impact of patient communication problems on the risk of preventable adverse events in acute care settings. *Canadian Medical Association Journal, 178*(12), 1555–1562.

Bastable, S. B. (2006). *Essentials of patient education.* Sudbury, MA: Jones and Bartlett.

Bloom, B. (1956). *Taxonomy of educational objectives.* New York, NY: Addison-Wesley.

Campinha-Bacote, J., Yahle, T., & Langenkamp, M. (1996). The challenge of cultural diversity for nurse educators. *Journal of Continuing Education in Nursing, 27*(2), 59–64.

Conner, M. (2004). *Introduction to andragogy and pedagogy.* Retrieved from http://www.agelesslearner.com/intros/andragogy.html

Cronenwett, L., Sherwood, G., Barnsteiner, J., Disch, J., Johnson, J., Mitchell, P., … Warren, J. (2007). Quality and safety education for nurses. *Nursing Outlook, 55*(3), 122–131.

Davis, T. C., Long, S. W., Jackson, R. H., Mayeaux, E. J., George, R. B., & Murphy, P. W. (1993). Rapid estimate of adult literacy in medicine: A shortened screening instrument. *Family Medicine, 25,* 391.

Disch, J. (2012). Are we really ready for patient-centered care? *Nursing Outlook, 60*(5), 237–239.

Doak, C., Doak, L., Gordon, L., & Lorig, K. (2001). Selecting, preparing, and using materials. In K. Lorig (Ed.), *Patient education: A practical approach* (3rd ed., pp. 183–197). Thousand Oaks, CA: Sage.

Doak, C. C., Doak, L. G., & Root, J. H. (1996). *Teaching patients with low literacy skills.* Philadelphia, PA: Lippincott.

Doak, L. G., & Doak, C. C. (Eds.). (2002). Pfizer health literacy principles. Retrieved from http://www.pfizerhealthliteracy.com

Donlon, B. C. (1993). *The effect of practical education programming for the elderly (PEPE) on the rehospitalization rate of older congestive heart failure patients:*

A quasi-experimental study. Unpublished doctoral dissertation. University of Southern Mississippi.

Falvo, D. (2004). *Effective patient education: A guide to increased compliance* (3rd ed.). Sudbury, MA: Jones and Bartlett.

Falvo, D. R. (2011). *Effective patient education: A guide to increased adherence* (4th ed.). Sudbury, MA: Jones & Bartlett Learning.

Flagg, A. J. (2015). The role of patient-centered care in nursing. *Nursing Clinics of North America, 50,* 75–86.

Flesch, R. (1948). A new readability yardstick. *Journal of Applied Psychology, 32*(3), 221–233.

French, K. (2015). Transforming nursing care through health literacy ACTS. *Nursing Clinics of North America, 50,* 87–98.

Fry, E. (1968). A readability formula that saves time. *Journal of Reading, 11,* 513–577.

Gerteis, M., Edgman-Levitan, S., Daley, J., & Delbanco, T. L. (1993). *Through the patient's eyes: Understanding and promoting patient-centered care.* San Francisco, CA: Jossey-Bass.

Gonzalez, V. M., & Lorig, K. (2001). Working cross-culturally. In K. Lorig (Ed.), *Patient education: A practical approach* (3rd ed., pp. 163–182). Thousand Oaks, CA: Sage.

Henneman, E. A., & Cardin, S. (2002). Family-centered critical care: A practical approach to making it happen. *Critical Care Nurse, 22*(6), 12–19.

Hochbaum, G. M. (1958). *Public participation in medical screening programs: A socio-psychological study.* Public Health Service Publication No. 572. Washington, DC: U.S. Government Printing Office.

Hunter, R., & Carlson, E. (2014). Finding the fit: Patient-centered care. *Nursing Management, 45,* 39–43.

Institute of Medicine. (2001). *Crossing the quality chasm: A new health system for the 21st century.* Washington, DC: National Academies Press.

Institute of Medicine. (2004). *Health literacy: A prescription to end confusion.* Washington, DC: National Academies Press.

Jastak, S., & Wilkinson, G. S. (1993). *Wide range achievement test: Review 3.* Wilmington, DE: Jastak Associates.

Joint Commission. (1995). *Comprehensive accreditation manual for hospitals* (Vols. 1 and 2). Oakbrook Terrace, IL: Author.

Joint Commission. (2003). *Joint Commission guide to patient and family education.* Oakbrook Terrace, IL: Author.

Joint Commission. (2010). *Advancing effective communication, cultural competence, and patient- and family-centered care: A roadmap for hospitals.* Oakbrook Terrace, IL: Author.

Kleinman, A. (1980). *Patients and healers in the context of culture: An exploration of the borderland between anthropology, medicine, and psychiatry.* Berkeley, CA: University of California Press.

Knowles, M. (1970). *The modern practice of adult education: Andragogy versus pedagogy.* New York, NY: Association Press.

Knowles, M., Swanson, R., & Holton, E. (1998). *The adult learner: The definitive classic in adult education and human resource development.* Houston, TX: Gulf.

Knowles, M., Swanson, R., & Holton, E. (2011). *The adult learner: The definitive classic in adult education and human resource development* (7th ed.). New York, NY: Elsevier.

Lengetti, E., Ordelt, K., & Pyle, N. (2007, November). Patient teaching competency for staff. *Patient Education Management*, 123–124.

Lorig, K. (2001). *Patient education: A practical approach* (3rd ed.). Thousand Oaks, CA: Sage.

Mager, R. (1997). *Preparing instructional objectives* (3rd ed.). Atlanta, GA: Center for Effective Performance.

Majumdar, B., Browne, G., Roberts, J., & Carpio, B. (2004). Effects of cultural sensitivity training on health care provider attitudes and patient outcomes. *Journal of Nursing Scholarship, 36*(2), 161–166.

Massachusetts Department of Higher Education. (2010). *Nurse of the future: Nursing core competencies*. Retrieved from http://www.mass.edu/currentinit/documents/NursingCoreCompetencies.pdf

Masters, K. (2001). *The effect of education that is modified to accommodate for age-related barriers to learning in older adult home health patients with congestive heart failure*. Unpublished doctoral dissertation. Louisiana State University Health Sciences Center.

McLaughlin, G. H. (1969). SMOG grading—a new readability formula. *Journal of Reading, 12,* 639–646.

McNeill, B. E. (2012, January–March). You "teach" but does your patient really learn?: Basic principles to promote safer outcomes. *Tar Heel Nurse*, 9–16.

Merriam, S. B., & Caffarella, R. S. (1999). *Learning in adulthood: A comprehensive guide* (2nd ed.). San Francisco, CA: Jossey-Bass.

Merriam, S. B., Caffarella, R. S., & Baumgartner, L. M. (2007). *Learning in adulthood: A comprehensive guide* (3rd ed.). San Francisco, CA: Jossey-Bass.

Miller, C. A. (2004). *Nursing for wellness in older adults: Theory and practice* (4th ed.). Philadelphia, PA: Lippincott.

Miller, M. A., & Stoeckel, P. R. (2011). *Client education: Theory and practice*. Sudbury, MA: Jones & Bartlett Learning.

National Cancer Institute, Office of Cancer Communications. (1989). *Making health communications work*. Rockville, MD: Author.

National Center for Education Statistics. (2007). Literacy in everyday life: Results from the 2003 National Assessment of Adult Literacy. Retrieved from http://nces.ed.gov/pubsearch/pubsinfo.asp?pubid=2007480

National Institutes of Health. (n.d.). NIHSeniorHealth: Hearing loss. Retrieved from http://nihseniorhealth.gov/hearingloss/hearinglossdefined/01.html

National Patient Safety Foundation. (2015). Ask Me 3. Retrieved from http://www.npsf.org/?page=askme3

Nightingale, F. (1969). *Notes on nursing: What it is and what it is not*. New York, NY: Dover. (Original work published 1860)

Oldaker, S. M. (1992). Live and learn: Patient education for the elderly orthopaedic client. *Orthopaedic Nursing, 11*(3), 51–56.

Pearson, M. (2012, June–August). Gerogogy in patient education—revisited. *Oklahoma Nurse*, 12–17.

Picker Institute. (n.d.). Picker principles of patient-centered care. Retrieved from http://cgp.pickerinstitute.org/?page_id=1319

Prohaska, T. R., & Lorig, K. (2001). What do we know about what works: The role of theory in patient education. In K. Lorig (Ed.), *Patient education: A practical approach* (3rd ed., pp. 21–55). Thousand Oaks, CA: Sage.

Quality and Safety Education for Nurses. (2012). Competencies: Prelicensure KSAS. Retrieved from http://qsen.org/competencies/pre-licensure-ksas/

Rankin, S. H. (2005). *Patient education in health and illness*. Philadelphia, PA: Lippincott.

Rankin, S. H., & Stallings, K. D. (2001). *Patient education: Principles and practice* (4th ed.). Philadelphia, PA: Lippincott.

Rankin, S. H., Stallings, K. D., & London, F. (2005). *Patient education in health and illness* (5th ed.). Philadelphia, PA: Lippincott.

Redman, B. K. (2001). *The practice of patient education* (9th ed.). St. Louis, MO: Mosby.

Redman, B. K. (2003). *Measurement tools in patient education* (2nd cd.). New York, NY: Springer.

Redman, B. K. (2006). *The practice of patient education: A case study approach* (10th ed.). St. Louis, MO: Mosby.

Russell, S. S. (2006). An overview of adult-learning processes. *Urologic Nursing, 26*(5), 349–352, 370.

Stephenson, P. L. (2007). Before teaching begins: Managing patient anxiety prior to providing education. *Clinical Journal of Oncology Nursing, 10*(2), 241–246.

U.S. Department of Health and Human Services, National Institutes of Health, National Cancer Institute. (2004). Making health communication programs work: A planner's guide. Retrieved from http://www.cancer.gov/publications/health-communication/pink-book.pdf

U.S. Department of Health and Human Services. (2011). *National strategy for quality improvement in health care*. Washington, DC: Author.

U.S. Department of Health and Human Services. (2012). CAHPS item set for assessing health literacy. Retrieved from https://cahps.ahrq.gov/surveys-guidance/item-sets/literacy/index.html

Walton, M. K., & Barnsteiner, J. (2012). Patient-centered care. In G. Sherwood & J. Barnsteiner (Eds.), *Quality and safety in nursing: A competency approach to improving outcomes* (pp. 67–89). West Sussex, UK: Wiley.

Weinrich, S. P., Boyd, M., & Nussbaum, J. (1989). Continuing education: Adapting strategies to teach the elderly. *Journal of Gerontological Nursing, 15*(11), 17–21.

Weinrich, S. P., Weinrich, M. C., Boyd, M. D., Atwood, J., & Cervenka, B. (1994). Teaching older adults by adapting for aging changes. *Cancer Nursing, 17*(6), 494–500.

Weiss, B. D. (1999). *Twenty common problems in primary care*. New York, NY: McGraw-Hill.

Williams, M. V., Baker, D. W., Honig, E. G., Lee, T. M., & Nowlan, A. (1998). Inadequate literacy is a barrier to asthma knowledge and self-care. *Chest, 114*, 1008–1015.

CHAPTER 12

Informatics in Professional Nursing Practice

Kathleen Masters and Cathy K. Hughes

Learning Objectives

After completing this chapter, the student should be able to:

1. Consider the role of informatics in nursing practice.
2. Discuss various informatics competencies for professional nursing practice.
3. Consider security and privacy issues related to electronic health records (EHRs).
4. Discuss basic computer competencies required for nursing practice.
5. Discuss information literacy skills needed to practice nursing.
6. Examine the role of information management nursing practice.
7. Envision the future of healthcare information systems based on current influences.

Healthcare delivery depends on information for effective decision making. Having entered the era of the electronic health records (EHRs) and telecommunication systems, informatics has become an indispensable element in the practice of nursing. All professional nurses now utilize informatics skills in their practice.

Key Terms and Concepts

» Nursing informatics (NI)
» Electronic health record (EHR)
» Search engines
» Database
» Email
» Listservs
» Social media
» Telehealth
» EBSCO Publishing
» Cumulative Index to Nursing and Allied Health Literature (CINAHL)
» Cochrane Library

Informatics: What Is It?

Nursing informatics (NI) is both a field of study and an area of specialization. In the mid-1900s, NI was first identified as the use of information technology in nursing practice (Hannah, 1985). In 1992, the American Nurses Association (ANA) first recognized NI as a nursing specialty. The original ANA *Scope and Standards of Nursing Informatics Practice* was published in 2001 and then revised in 2008 and 2014. Key components of the definition include that nursing informatics is a specialty within the profession of nursing that "integrates nursing science, computer science, and information science" for the purpose of managing and communicating data, information, and knowledge (ANA, 2008, p. 92). Nursing informatics is useful in supporting decision making through "information structures, information processes, and information technology" (ANA, 2008, p. 92).

Thus, the specialty of NI focuses on developing and implementing solutions for the management and communication of health information pertinent to providing better quality patient care (Zykowski, 2003).

Clinical informatics is a broader term that includes nursing as well as other medical and health specialties and addresses the use of information systems in patient care. The domains of clinical informatics include the three areas of health systems, clinical care, and information and communication technologies and may include issues ranging from decision support to EHR documentation to electronic order entry (Alexander, 2015b, pp. 7–8). Health informatics is an even broader term that encompasses the "interdisciplinary study of the design, development, adoption, and application of IT-based innovations in healthcare services delivery, management and planning" (Procter, 2009).

Informatics, the broadest of the terms, is the science of collecting, managing, and retrieving information. The informatics discipline began decades ago, but an Institute of Medicine (IOM) report published in 1991 brought national attention to the lack of use of information technology in the healthcare industry as compared to other industries (IOM, 1997). That report, along with subsequent IOM reports, became the impetus for the transition to information systems to support the provision of health care (Silsbee & Reed, 2014). In today's healthcare systems, information and computer technologies are major infrastructure components of patient safety and integral tools used by healthcare providers (Walton, 2012).

The Impact of Legislation on Health Informatics

Several IOM (1997, 1999, 2001) reports informed Congress about legislation needed to bring about change in health care related to informatics that resulted in the passage of several laws that have expedited the health informatics agenda. There are three primary laws that have affected health information management. The Health Insurance Portability and Accountability Act (HIPAA) of 1996 contains provisions for privacy and security of health information. The Health Information Technology for Economic and Clinical Health (HITECH) Act of 2009 provided federal money in the form of grants to advance use of health information technology (HIT). The Patient Protection and Affordable Care Act of 2010 also provides for funding of HIT (Silsbee & Reed, 2014).

HIPAA and Health Information Privacy

Movement toward electronic information management in health care was slow, in part due to concern over the lack of privacy of patient health records in an electronic system. In 1996, Congress passed HIPAA to improve the efficiency and effectiveness of the healthcare system by encouraging the development of a health information system. Some areas addressed by the act include simplifying healthcare claims, developing standards for data transmission, and implementing privacy regulations. The privacy regulations protect clients by limiting the ways that health plans, pharmacies, hospitals, and other entities can use clients' personal medical information. The regulations protect medical records and other individually identifiable health information, whether communicated orally, on paper, or electronically. Accompanying the privacy regulations are specific security rules that protect health information in electronic form. To be in compliance, agencies must ensure the confidentiality and integrity of all electronic health information that is created, received, transmitted, or stored; protect against threats to security; protect against disclosures of information; and ensure compliance of their employees (Garner, 2003).

Protecting an individual's personal and private information has historically been a significant issue for nursing. Healthcare information is a collection of data relating to personal aspects of an individual's life. Improper disclosure can cause devastating consequences. Patients assume that information provided to a healthcare provider will not be disclosed. It is not only possible, but probable that patients will not disclose certain types of information essential to their care if they believe the information is not confidential. The introduction of electronic documentation and communication has increased the difficulty of maintaining privacy. Improved access to healthcare information can and does increase efficiency and improve patient care, but accompanying the benefits are greater difficulties in maintaining privacy and confidentiality. Preserving the security of the health information system is critical because unauthorized access to the computerized health information system compromises the privacy and confidentiality of patient health records. Protection against unauthorized access can be achieved by implementing a login process that verifies that the user has permission to use the system. The majority of systems rely on a user ID and password for verification. Passwords must be changed

CRITICAL THINKING QUESTION✳

What is your role as a nurse in protecting patient healthcare information?✳

KEY COMPETENCY 12-1

Examples of Applicable
*Nurse of the Future: Nursing
Core Competencies*

Informatics and Technology:

Skills (S6b) Maintains privacy
and confidentiality of patient
information

Source: Massachusetts Department of Higher
Education. (2010). *Nurse of the future:
Nursing core competencies* (p. 24). Retrieved
from http://www.mass.edu/currentinit
/documents/NursingCoreCompetencies.pdf

frequently to protect against breach of security. Users should never divulge or share passwords. Healthcare agencies have written policies regarding the penalties of misuse of the system. Consequences are usually severe, with many including termination of employment.

HITECH

The HITECH Act provided money to providers and organizations to encourage use of the **electronic health record (EHR)**. As an incentive to move healthcare systems to the use of EHRs within a short time, under the Centers for Medicare and Medicaid Services (CMS) Incentive Program, healthcare providers and organizations can receive financial incentives for meaningful use of certified EHRs through 2016. However, by 2015 a provider that had not shown meaningful use of a certified EHR received less reimbursement. A certified EHR is one that meets requirements of interoperability and formatting standards.

Meaningful use criteria and objectives have evolved each year. Stage one involved data capture and sharing such as using information captured in a standardized format to track clinical conditions or coordinate care. Stage two involved advanced clinical processes such as electronic transmission of patient care summaries across multiple settings. Stage three involves improved outcomes such as improving quality, safety, and efficiency, leading to improved health outcomes and improving population health (Alexander, 2015a; Silsbee & Reed, 2014).

Nursing Informatics Competencies

The current expectation is that all nurses demonstrate proficiency in the use of information and patient care technology; therefore, many of the national nursing organizations have promulgated lists of expectations for either nursing students or nurses related to informatics skills. Defined levels of informatics competencies vary depending on the experience and specialty of the nurse. For example, differing levels of expertise in informatics are expected from the beginning nurse, experienced nurse, informatics specialist, and informatics innovator (Hebda & Czar, 2009; McGonigle & Mastrian, 2009; Staggers, Gassert, & Curran, 2001).

The entry-level professional nurse is expected to have computer literacy and basic information management skills. Important technology skills of the entry-level nurse include knowing how to use nursing-specific software such as computerized documentation; use of patient care technologies such as monitors, pumps, and medication dispensing; and information management for patient safety (American Association of Colleges of Nursing [AACN], 2008, pp. 19–20). In our world of electronic communication and data management, maintaining privacy, security, and confidentiality of patient information as mandated by HIPAA is an expectation of all nurses, including nursing students.

Experienced nurses should be skilled in information management and computer technology to sustain their specific area of practice. These skills include making judgments based on trends of data in addition to collaboration with informatics nurses in the development of nursing systems. An informatics nurse specialist has graduate-level informatics preparation and is prepared to assist the practicing nurse in meeting his or her needs for information (ANA, 2008). The informatics innovator also has graduate-level informatics preparation and possesses skills for developing theory and conducting informatics research (Thede, 2003). The focus of this chapter is on the generalist nurse rather than the informatics specialist or informatics innovator.

AACN Information Management and Application of Patient Care Technology

The AACN (2008) includes information management and application of patient care technology as an essential component of a baccalaureate education in nursing in order to prepare the graduate to deliver safe and effective care. The AACN names informatics and technology-related outcomes for baccalaureate nursing graduates that include the following:

- Demonstrate skills in using patient care technologies, information systems, and communication devices that support safe nursing practice.
- Use telecommunication technologies to assist in effective communication in a variety of healthcare settings.
- Apply safeguards and decision-making support tools embedded in patient care technologies and information systems to support a safe practice environment for both patients and healthcare workers.
- Understand the issues of clinical information systems to document interventions related to achieving nurse-sensitive outcomes.
- Use standardized terminology in a care environment that reflects nursing's unique contribution to patient outcomes.
- Uphold ethical standards related to data security, regulatory requirements, confidentiality, and clients' right to privacy.
- Recognize that redesign of workflow and care processes should precede implementation of care technology to facilitate nursing practice (AACN, 2008, pp. 18–19).

Quality and Safety Education for Nurses Informatics Competencies

Sponsored by the Robert Wood Johnson Foundation, Quality and Safety Education for Nurses (QSEN) has the overall goal of "preparing future nurses who will have the knowledge, skills and attitudes (KSAs) necessary to continuously improve the quality and safety of the healthcare systems within which they work" (QSEN, n.d.). The purpose of this initiative is to develop competencies of future nursing graduates in six key areas: patient-centered care, evidence-based practice, quality improvement, teamwork and collaboration, safety, and informatics. The application of informatics in nursing practice is also a vital component in the mastery of the other defined KSAs.

Informatics is defined in the QSEN (n.d.) initiative as the use of information and technology to communicate, manage knowledge, mitigate error, and support decision making. The entry-level informatics skill domain competencies identified by QSEN include:

- Seek information about how information is managed in care settings before providing care.
- Apply technology and information management tools to support safe processes of care.
- Navigate the EHR.
- Document and plan patient care in an EHR.
- Employ communication technologies to coordinate care for patients.
- Respond appropriately to clinical decision-making supports and alerts.
- Use information management tools to monitor outcomes of care processes.
- Use high-quality electronic sources of healthcare information (QSEN, n.d.).

Nurse of the Future Core Competencies: Informatics and Technology

The Nurse of the Future Core Competencies for informatics uses the definition from QSEN and incorporates the informatics knowledge, skills, and attitudes from multiple sources to provide a document that synthesizes all of the competency recommendations into a succinct format (Massachusetts Department of Higher Education, 2010, pp. 22–26).

Technology Informatics Guiding Education Reform Initiative

In 2004, the Technology Informatics Guiding Education Reform (TIGER) initiative was formed to bring together various nursing stakeholders in order to develop a shared vision, strategies, and specific actions for improving nursing practice, education, and patient care delivery through the use of information technology (Technology Informatics Guiding Education Reform, 2008, p. 2). The TIGER Informatics Competencies Collaborative Team was formed to develop competencies for all practicing nurses and graduating nursing students. The resultant TIGER Informatics Competency Model has three components: basic computer competencies, information literacy, and information management (p. 3).

Basic computer competencies include understanding the concepts of information and communication technology, possessing skill in the use of a computer and managing files, word processing, spreadsheets, using databases, presentations, Web browsing, and communication (p. 7). Information literacy builds on computer competencies and includes skills such as being able to identify information needed for a specific purpose, locate pertinent information, evaluate the information, and correctly apply the information. Information literacy skills are prerequisites for the practice of evidence-based nursing (p. 9). The information management process consists of collecting data, processing the data, and presenting and communicating the processed data as information or knowledge. A foundational concept in information management is what is known as the data–information–knowledge continuum. Data are symbols, such as a numeric value of 1.5. Information is data that are organized or processed in a way that gives them meaning, such as 1.5 ng/ml. Knowledge is information that is transformed or combined in a way that is useful in making judgments and decisions. An example of knowledge is a combination of information such as that a digoxin level of 1.5 ng/ml is a therapeutic level for an adult patient (p. 11). The organization of the remainder of this chapter reflects the three components of the TIGER Competency Model.

Basic Computer Competencies

Basic computer competencies include understanding the concepts of information and communication technology, possessing skill in the use of a computer and managing files, word processing, spreadsheets, using databases, presentations, Web browsing, and communication (TIGER, 2008, p. 7). An overview of some of those skills is presented in the following sections of the chapter.

Web Browsing

Not since the invention of the printing press has the speed with which new information can be accessed changed so much as with the development of the Internet. Search tools and **search engines** assist users in finding specific topics on the Web by compiling a **database** of Internet sites. Popular search engines include AltaVista, InfoSeek, WebCrawler, Yahoo!, Northernlight, and Hotbot. All have different search features and produce somewhat differing results. In addition to search engines, there are metasearch engines. A metasearch engine conducts a search of a variety of search engines. Metacrawler (www.metacrawler.com), Google (www.google.com), and Dogpile (www.dogpile.com) are examples of metasearch engines. Each search engine queries different databases using different search techniques (Bliss & DeYoung, 2002) and uses a range of engines for retrieval of information.

Communication: Email

Email (electronic mail) can be sent to anyone in the world who has an email address. In moments, messages can be sent across time zones, allowing instant communication. For several reasons, attention must be paid to the content of messages sent by email. Someone other than the intended recipient can access a message while it is transmitted over the Internet. In addition, messages containing sensitive information can accidentally or purposefully be forwarded. Although email can be a way of facilitating direct communication between consumers of health care and healthcare providers, precautions must be taken to ensure that only the intended recipient receives health-related email messages.

To send and receive email, a person must have an individual address that consists of two main parts separated by an @ sign. The first part is called a login name or a user ID. The part after the @ is the name of the network or service provider used to access the Internet. The characters after the last dot in an email address indicate the domain or main subdivision of the Internet to which the computer belongs. Addresses must be accurate for the intended recipient to receive the message. Appropriateness must be considered when selecting your login name. Professionals should not use suggestive or insensitive wording for their login names.

Email is a special form of communication and carries its own form of etiquette. Pagana (2007) suggests nurses follow these guidelines when sending a business or professional message:

- Do not use all uppercase letters. Typing in all caps is deemed shouting.
- Include a specific subject line.
- Sign your messages with text that includes your email address and contact information.
- Use the "reply to all" function appropriately. Not everyone is interested in receiving your comments.
- Avoid forwarding chain letters, and delete all unnecessary information from forwarded messages.
- Do not send confidential information, and check for correct recipients before sending.
- Use the spell-check and grammar functions.
- Do not use email for thank-you correspondence.

Communication: Listserv Groups and Mailing Lists

Mailing lists and **listservs** are forms of group email that provide an opportunity for people with similar interests to share information. Subscribing to a list is usually free. Once subscribed, you can send and receive messages to and from the list. The communication is asynchronous, meaning it does not occur in real time. Someone posts a question or comment to the list, and other members reply in time. List groups are usually either layperson oriented or professional oriented. There are numerous groups devoted to the topic of nursing. To find a list, ask friends and colleagues or visit CataList, an official catalog of listservs that includes a searchable database. You can access CataList at www.lsoft.com/catalist.html.

Most listservs provide specific instructions on subscribing. Every listserv has two addresses. One address is used to join, and the second is used to send messages that can be read by the group. Listserv groups can be open to anyone, or you might have to have permission to join. It is important to remember that messages sent to the listserv are read by everyone subscribed to the listserv. Posting a personal message to an individual on a listserv is considered inappropriate. Do not send attachments to the list. The list might have hundreds of members, and some will not have computers that support sophisticated graphics or large files. Additionally, viruses can be transmitted in attachments.

Communication: Social Media

Social media are "Internet-based applications that enable people to communicate and share resources and information" (Lindsay, 2011). Examples of social media are YouTube, Facebook, LinkedIn, and Twitter, as well as blogs, wikis, and chat rooms. The many choices of how users can share information can be found on the ANA website (www .nursingworld.com). The drop-down menu on the Share button lists the various options available for users.

Growing participation in social networking sites poses challenges for nursing. Although social networking aids with personal and professional knowledge exchange and prompts interaction with others, it comes with risks. Personal and patient privacy issues can be raised and some networking discussions might be viewed as "fact" and not validated. The ANA has adopted the Principles for Social Networking, which include the following:

- Nurses must not transmit or place online individually identifiable patient information.
- Nurses must observe ethically prescribed professional patient–nurse boundaries.
- Nurses should understand that patients, colleagues, institutions, and employers might view postings.
- Nurses should take advantage of privacy settings and seek to separate personal and professional information online.
- Nurses should bring content that could harm a patient's privacy, rights, or welfare to the attention of appropriate authorities.
- Nurses should participate in developing institutional policies governing online contact (ANA, 2011a, 2011b).

The National Council of State Boards of Nursing (NCSBN) has also adopted guidelines related to the responsible use of social media and has endorsed the principles adopted by the ANA. The guidelines from the NCSBN (2011) are available at www.ncsbn.org/Social_Media.pdf and address issues of confidentiality and privacy, common myths and misunderstandings related to social media, possible consequences in the use of social media including consequences with board of nursing implications, and how to avoid problems. The guidelines also include seven scenarios related to social media use by nurses with board of nursing implications.

According to the NCSBN (2011) white paper, depending on the jurisdiction, the board of nursing might investigate reports of inappropriate disclosures related to the use of social media on the grounds of the following: unprofessional conduct, unethical conduct, moral turpitude, mismanagement of patient records, revealing a privileged communication, and breach of confidentiality. If allegations are found to be true, the nurse could face disciplinary action by the board of nursing that can include a reprimand, a sanction, an assessment of a fine, or the temporary or permanent loss of licensure. In addition, improper use of social media might violate state and federal laws, resulting in civil or criminal penalties that carry with them fines or jail time.

Social networking can have both positive and negative consequences. Negative consequences can affect not only nurses' personal reputations, but also their professional standing. Nurses should consider that current or future employers might view their personal social media pages.

On the other hand, social media can be used in disasters as a means of disseminating information and as an emergency management tool. Social media can be a source of information in a crisis as well as part of a plan to mobilize responders. In disaster preparation, social media sites can be used to publicize training events and dates (Lindsay, 2011).

Future challenges of social media include the use of the technology for the delivery of accurate and pertinent information by experts and healthcare providers and by peers and the lay public. Healthcare providers' uses of social media technology may include public education related to sources of information and monitoring the impact of social media on health outcomes.

Communication: Telehealth

Telehealth is the use of electronic information and telecommunications technologies to support long-distance clinical health care, patient and professional health-related education, public health, and health administration (U.S. Department of Health and Human Services [USDHHS], n.d.b). The use of this technology has many implications in the provision of health care in the context of both access and quality. For example, healthcare providers can monitor patients in their homes for changes in health status. Images and other data can be transmitted for consultation with other healthcare providers. Practitioners in geographically remote areas or in a prison setting can connect to a large hospital for consultations and second opinions without transporting the patient to that site. From a motor vehicle crash site, the emergency medical system response field team can transmit information and documentation to the emergency department for direction on care of the patient.

> **CRITICAL THINKING QUESTIONS**✳
>
> What needs of populations in your region or state could be addressed with the use of telehealth? What ideas can you envision to assist in the access to and delivery of healthcare services where you live or work?✳

Information Literacy

Information literacy builds on basic computer competencies and includes skills such as being able to identify information needed for specific purposes, locating pertinent information, evaluating the information, and correctly applying the information. The following section will discuss information location and evaluation specific to nursing and health care.

Electronic Databases

An increasing number of databases are available on the Internet and can be accessed through local libraries or by subscription from a vendor such as **EBSCO Publishing**, which provides access to online databases and e-journals. Most of the databases allow keyword searches and are capable of advanced searching. Many full text resources are available via databases making information available very quickly. Some of the most beneficial databases to nursing include the following:

- The **Cumulative Index to Nursing and Allied Health Literature (CINAHL)** is a resource for nursing and allied health professionals, students, educators, and researchers. This database provides indexing and abstracting for more than 1,700 current nursing and allied health journals and publications dating back to 1982, totaling more than 880,000 records. The **Cochrane Library** is an online collection of six databases with "independent high-quality evidence for healthcare decision making" (Cochrane Collaboration, n.d.). This is available at academic institutions and is funded for free access in many countries and regions of the world.
- The **Educational Resource Information Center (ERIC)** is a national information system supported by the U.S. Department of Education, the National Library of Education, and the Office of Educational Research and Improvement. It provides access to information from journals included in the Current Index of Journals in Education and Resources in Education Index. ERIC provides full text of more than 2,200 digests along with references for additional information, citations, and abstracts from more than 1,000 educational and education-related journals.

> **KEY COMPETENCY 12-2**
>
> Examples of Applicable *Nurse of the Future: Nursing Core Competencies*
>
> Informatics and Technology:
>
> Knowledge (K9) Describes general applications available for research
>
> Skills (S9a) Conducts on-line literature searches
>
> Attitudes/Behaviors (A9) Values technology as a tool for generating knowledge
>
> *Source:* Massachusetts Department of Higher Education. (2010). *Nurse of the future: Nursing core competencies* (p. 25). Retrieved from http://www.mass.edu/currentinit/documents/NursingCoreCompetencies.pdf

CRITICAL THINKING QUESTION *

How can you locate online sources for more information on a new treatment or medications for a health condition you discussed in a nursing class or clinical this week? *

- Google Scholar (googlescholar.com), launched in 2004, contains some full-text peer-reviewed journals, abstracts, links to subscription journals, and articles for purchase as well as technical reports, theses, and books.
- **Health Source**, the Nursing Academic Edition, provides more than 550 scholarly full-text journals, including more than 450 peer-reviewed journals focusing on many medical disciplines including nursing and allied health.
- **MEDLINE**, created by the National Library of Medicine, is the largest biomedical literature database and provides authoritative medical information on medicine, nursing, dentistry, veterinary medicine, the healthcare system, and preclinical sciences. In MEDLINE, users can search abstracts from more than 4,600 current biomedical journals. Included are citations from Index Medicus, International Nursing Index, Index to Dental Literature, PREMEDLINE, AIDSLINE, BIOETHICSLINE, and HealthSTAR.
- **PsycINFO** contains nearly 2 million citations and summaries of journal articles, book chapters, books, dissertations, and technical reports, all in the field of psychology. It also includes information about the psychological aspects of related disciplines such as medicine, psychiatry, nursing, sociology, education, pharmacology, physiology, linguistics, anthropology, business, and law.

Internet access to government organizations and nonprofit organizations is also available. The U.S. National Library of Medicine (www.nlm.nih.gov /hinfo.html) offers access to a myriad of health information websites. PubMed and MedlinePlus permit searches of multiple retrieval systems and provide excellent information. The evaluation guidelines discussed in the following section should be applied to all Internet sites before using the information in patient teaching (Thede & Sewell, 2010).

KEY COMPETENCY 12-3

Examples of Applicable *Nurse of the Future: Nursing Core Competencies*

Informatics and Technology:

Skills (S2b) Evaluates information and its sources critically and incorporates selected information into his or her own professional knowledge base

(S5f) Assesses the accuracy of health information on the Internet

Source: Massachusetts Department of Higher Education. (2010). *Nurse of the future: Nursing core competencies* (pp. 22–23). Retrieved from http://www.mass.edu/currentinit /documents/NursingCoreCompetencies.pdf

Website Evaluation

The Internet has grown rapidly since its beginning, and information can be published easily and inexpensively. An Internet website can be created by anyone with the ability to create a webpage, and many webpage templates are available for little or no cost, making this very easy. Many sites are for commercial purposes; others simply publish the opinions of the website owner. Websites are under no guidelines or standards. Additionally, no official organization is responsible for site evaluation. As a result, a vast amount of information is available on the Internet, but not all information is reliable. Applying the following guidelines can assist you in evaluating resources on the Internet so that the information you obtain is reliable:

- *Accuracy*: Is the information accurate, reliable, and free from error? Spelling and punctuation errors can indicate an untrustworthy site.

- *Authority or source*: Look for the credentials of the author or the reputation of the hosting organization. A good indication of authority is peer review.
- *Objectivity*: What are the goals and objectives of the site? What biases are present? Is the site trying to present a specific or neutral point of view?
- *Currency or timeliness*: Look for publication and updated dates to determine if the information is current. Dead links can indicate old information.
- *Coverage or quality*: Is the subject matter presented on the site of appropriate quality for the intended audience?
- *Intended purpose*: Does the site have choices for users such as the public, healthcare providers, students, or educators?
- *Usability*: Is the site designed for easy navigation? Are there excessive graphics that require long download times? Are all links current and do they load easily? (Hebda & Czar, 2009; Thede & Sewell, 2010)

CRITICAL THINKING QUESTION ✳

What is your role as a nurse in the evaluation of information on the Internet? ✳

Health Information Online

The number of people accessing health information online continues to grow. This increase in numbers demonstrates how critically important it is that healthcare websites provide reliable and credible information. Nurses are responsible for assisting the public in evaluating health information available on the Internet.

Whether nurses are developing online materials or using existing online information, it is important for them to understand what makes the information accessible to all people and to be able to make informed recommendations about websites to individuals with disabilities (Carmona, 2005; Smeltzer, Zimmerman, Frain, DeSilets, & Duffin, 2003). Some websites that feature webinars and online programs have closed captioning and copies of the scripts available on demand for these programs. Language options are available on some websites for print and audible programs (Thede & Sewell, 2010). Contents of sites should be presented in a way that people with disabilities and with low-end technology are able to navigate and use.

Vulnerable populations and underserved populations, which include persons with lower socioeconomic status, with lower reading levels, in rural areas, or with disabilities, have issues with access to care and access to information about health care. For persons in these populations, the term *digital divide* has typically been used to describe decreased access to information technologies, particularly via the Internet (Chang et al., 2004, p. 449).

More people are using the Internet for finding health information. Knowledgeable nurses need to assist patients and their families in evaluating the quality of Internet resources. The Health on the Net Foundation (HON), founded in 1995, is a nonprofit organization dedicated to assisting people in obtaining reliable health information on the Internet (HON, n.d.). To obtain certification, a website applies for registration. The site is evaluated and, if approved, is qualified to display the HONcode seal. The site is randomly checked for compliance. From the HON website, Internet users can download the HON toolbar, which will be added to their Web browser. When a certified site is accessed, the seal will be illuminated on the user's toolbar. The HONcode criteria in brief include:

- *Authoritative*: Indicate the qualifications of the authors.
- *Complementarity*: Information should support, not replace, the doctor–patient relationship.
- *Privacy*: Respect the privacy and confidentiality of personal data submitted to the site by the visitor.
- *Attribution*: Cite the source(s) of published information; date medical and health pages.
- *Justifiability*: Back up claims relating to benefits and performance.
- *Transparency*: Accessible presentation, accurate email contact.
- *Financial disclosure*: Identify funding sources.
- *Advertising policy*: Clearly distinguish advertising from editorial content.

Several sites from the Office of the National Coordinator (ONC) for Health Information Technology (ONC HIT, n.d.a), such as HealthIT.gov, have information on e-health tools for the public to review and use that focus on health and wellness. Sites such as Health 2.0 Developer Challenge (n.d.) hold innovation competitions and community action programs to address solutions for key challenges in HIT.

Information Management

Information management consists of collecting data, processing the data, and presenting and communicating the processed data as information or knowledge. Data sets that are very large and can be analyzed to reveal patterns, trends, and associations are known in informatics as "big data." Examples of healthcare databases with big data are those run by the CMS and National Institutes of Health (NIH) Library of Medicine. Health Service Research Information Central is the arm of the NIH Library of Medicine that serves as the data repository.

One of the current issues in nursing that prevents use of data sets to their full potential is a lack of standardized nomenclature. A lack of standardization inhibits the exchange of information, quality measurement, and analysis of data to identify patterns and associations related to nursing interventions on performance measures such as clinical outcomes.

Even within one organization using similar nomenclature, after years of using the EHR, nurses still have difficulty using collected data to report on safety and quality issues. Nurses are, however, becoming increasingly skillful in the use of the EHR for tasks related to documentation and tasks associated with the routine care of patients such as medication administration.

The primary information management system used by nurses is the EHR, so this section will begin with an overview of information management and then specifically address the EHR in more detail.

Due to a concern over patient privacy and lack of funding for information systems, the process of implementing health records was slow after the 1991 IOM report (IOM, 1997). In 1997, a revised report was published, again calling for progress in the use of information systems in health care. Subsequently the IOM published two landmark reports (1999, 2001) that called attention to human error in health care, called for system solutions to make it more difficult to make human errors, and called for the use of computer systems as tools to assist with order entry, including links with clinical practice guidelines, clinical decision support systems, and patient management systems.

Electronic Health Records

As part of the National Health Information Infrastructure, President George W. Bush established a technology agenda authorizing the development of an EHR for all Americans by 2014 (Healthcare IT, 2004). Information on this agenda is available via the USDHHS website (White House Archives, 2004).

The EHR as envisioned is to be a longitudinal record of the patient's healthcare record across the life span and to include input from different healthcare facilities and practitioners. Although the record is actually located in various locations and on various computers, the record appears as one record to the EHR user as data are imported from multiple computer systems as needed. This is in contrast to the electronic medical record, which allows information to be created, gathered, managed, and consulted but can only be used within one healthcare organization. For access across institutions to occur, there must be agreed-upon standards of operability between hardware and software companies that allow for the exchange of information across health information systems. Many standards do exist and more continue to be developed. The process of developing standards for health information systems is coordinated by the Healthcare Information Technology Standards Panel of the American National Standards Institute (Silsbee & Reed, 2014).

Another IOM report (2011) identified characteristics for software designers to consider in the creation of electronic information systems for use by health professionals. These characteristics included that data should be accurate, timely, reliable, and entered directly into the system; easy to navigate; simple to use; and intuitive to the user, with evidence available at point of care to aid in decision making. The characteristics should also enhance and streamline workflow and automate mundane tasks, have minimal time required for upgrades, and allow data to be easily imported and exchanged between systems.

EHRs also include an integrated database of clinical information known as a clinical decision support system. The purpose of the clinical decision support system is to aid the nurse or other provider by leading the user through a decision-making process based on a set of data in the system. The clinical decision support system uses a decision tree model, so during this process, the EHR user is guided through a series of questions to narrow down the options for a correct diagnosis or most effective treatment plan (Silsbee & Reed, 2014). In addition, EHRs include pharmacological and lab value databases and clinical guidelines, resources that are all available to the nurse at the patient's bedside. The EHR clinical decision support system can also provide clinical alerts and reminders, identify abnormal parameters of laboratory and assessment data, and prompt clinicians on important tasks and protocols (Hebda & Czar, 2009). Thus, the electronic information system can maximize the time nurses spend with the patient at the bedside, improve the accuracy of documentation, and decrease medication errors, thus supporting patient quality and safety initiatives.

Many other information systems can be imported into the EHR. Two of the most common are the computerized provider order entry (CPOE) and bar code medication administration (BCMA). The CPOE feature of the EHR allows the provider to enter patient care orders directly into a computer system. The orders can be entered from any location, which not only eliminates the issue of order legibility, but also eliminates the need for verbal or telephone orders. CPOE also decreases delays in care; for example, with use of the CPOE, orders for lab tests are transmitted to the lab and medication orders are transmitted to the pharmacy. The BCMA is a system that receives orders from the CPOE system and prints bar-coded labels that contain a patient-specific identification number. The bar-coded label is attached to the medication sent from the pharmacy, and before the nurse administers the medication, both the bar code on the patient's bracelet and the bar code on the medication are scanned. This feature of the EHR checks for the right medication and right patient as well as the right time and frequency, right dose, and right route for the medication (McGonigle & Mastrian, 2012), thus reducing the potential for medication error.

In the healthcare setting today, information systems are interwoven into almost every process. Admission/discharge/transfer systems interact with outpatient registration systems to collect and track patient information, such as demographics, hospital number, relatives, and primary physician. All patient encounters are connected to these interacting systems. Information systems within healthcare organizations organize data and track fiscal operations of an organization including reporting, scheduling, payroll, and billing. Ancillary applications permit sharing of information among multiple systems and specialty areas such as those of radiology, laboratory, physical therapy, and pharmacy. Acuity applications attempt to predict the resources necessary for patient care and are integrated with other systems such as staffing to create adequate patient unit staffing. Systems are found in specialized units within

---

KEY COMPETENCY 12-4

Examples of Applicable *Nurse of the Future: Nursing Core Competencies*

Informatics and Technology:

Knowledge (K5) Describes the computerized systems presently utilized to facilitate patient care

Skills (S5a) Applies technology and information management tools to support safe processes of care and evaluate impact on patient outcomes

(S5b) Accesses, enters, retrieves data used locally for patient care

Attitudes/Behaviors (A5) Values the importance of technology on patient care

Source: Massachusetts Department of Higher Education. (2010). *Nurse of the future: Nursing core competencies* (p. 23). Retrieved from http://www.mass.edu/currentinit /documents/NursingCoreCompetencies.pdf

the healthcare setting that include monitoring equipment in intensive care units that automatically measure and record physiologic data, generate trends, sound alarms for abnormalities, and interact with other information systems within the patient environment including physician notification of abnormal patient data and trends. Critical pathways, generated by information systems, identify specific patient outcomes and make integrated documentation by different disciplines possible that, in turn, promotes cost-effective care through effective communication. **Table 12-1** shows expected EHR roles in relation to key tasks.

TABLE 12-1   Expected Electronic Health Record Tasks

| Key Tasks | Electronic Health Record Role | | | |
	Memory	Computation	Decision Support	Collaboration
Review patient history	Display available history and demographics	Provide contextual view of overall patient health	Recommend care based on patient characteristics	Incorporate information from outside sources
Conduct patient assessment	Prompt for required information	Compute statistics (body mass index, etc.)	Provide action-oriented clinical reminders	Coordinate across multiple providers
Determine clinical decision	Relate assessment to patient history	Display trends, reference ranges	Support based on outside research/ recommendations	Staff views/ instructions
Develop treatment plan	Standards of care, care plans, evidence-based guidelines	Apply standards of care based on patient characteristics	Evidence-based care adjusted by patient characteristics	Patient summary, educational tools
Order additional services	Review previous services/results	Determine appropriate provider/location	Alignment with insurance requirements	Create referrals, facilitate provider communication
Prescribe medications	Medication history, allergies, formulary	Dose calculation	Interactions, contraindications, effectiveness	Patient instructions, side effects and warnings
Document visit	Diagnosis and treatment codes	Prompts/ automatic population	Insurance guidelines	Patient education, coordination with multiple providers

Source: Armijo, D., McDonnell, C., & Werner, K. (2009). *Electronic health record usability: Evaluation and use case framework.* Publication No. 09(10)-0091-1-EF. Rockville, MD: U.S. Department of Health and Human Services, Agency for Healthcare Research and Quality.

Sensmeier (2008) offers ways to improve nursing practice with technology, including seeking nursing input related to workflow, investing in informatics training, promoting informatics excellence, and working for a staged approach to adopting a paperless EHR. Thede (2008) suggests that nursing professionals must engage in discussion to decide how data will be used, consider which data are to be included in the EHR, and the acceptable terminology to be used when recording the data. Work must be done to refine and implement standardized nursing terminologies that better express nursing care. As standardized nursing terminologies become unique to nursing, some benefits will include better communication, improved patient care, and a uniform style for nursing data collection that will aid in evaluation of nursing care outcomes (Thede & Schwiran, 2011). A "cardinal rule in informatics is one entry of a piece of data, many uses" (Thede, 2012, p. 2). The same data can be used in a variety of reports leading to decreased redundancy of charting, and clinical documentation systems have the advantage of easily collecting data for use in planning and evaluation, particularly if the data are in a standardized format and use standardized terminology.

Handheld Devices

Personal digital assistants (PDAs) are handheld devices that have wireless connectivity and can synchronize data and information between the PDA and a computer. Use of the PDA has become popular in health care and nursing. The devices can be used as a digital reference for obtaining drug information, dosage calculations, and diagnostic test results, as well as decision protocols for administration. They are useful tools for data collection and management of patient outcomes. Some PDAs can be interfaced with the EHR to obtain and update vital patient information. Immediate access to the Internet allows the healthcare provider to obtain valuable information through national and international resources.

Hybrid devices have a combination of capabilities, such as a cell phone that is also an Internet-enabled PDA with an MP3 player and camera that includes text messaging capabilities, maps and direction assistance, and inter-active voice assistance. Available options can vary with different service plans, coverage areas, and memory size. Upon employment and when there are any policy changes, nurses must review the healthcare facility policies on the use of handheld devices while at work.

HIPAA regulations must be strictly followed when using PDAs and other wireless technology (Thompson, 2005). The use of PDAs in the clinical setting must be compliant with HIPAA rules and regulations; PDAs are not allowed by many facilities due to concerns about patient privacy (Mastrian, McGonigle, Mahan, & Bixler, 2011).

Personal Health Record

In addition to electronic health information for professional use, patients also have access to an electronic record of health-related information through what is known as a **personal health record**. The personal health record conforms to interoperability standards and is available via a patient portal. The patient manages, shares, and controls the information in the personal health record (Johnson, 2010). The patient portal can also be used to provide discharge or medication teaching, health promotion, and prevention education, and engage the patient as a partner in care through use of software programs and patient pathways.

In addition, patients have access to a myriad of health-related technology in the form of wellness applications (apps), personal wellness devices, and wellness tracking sites. From coordination of chronic disease using implantable devises for glucose monitoring to wearable activity monitors, calorie monitors, and sleep monitors to enhance wellness, the future of both caring for the sick and personal wellness are increasingly joined to the use of technology.

Current and Future Trends

Clearly, computerized technology will shape the future of health care for individuals, populations, and organizations. Recognizing this fact, the Healthy People 2010 objectives (USDHHS, 2000) called for increasing the number of households with access to the Internet. Health communication and HIT are also objectives of Healthy People 2020, with the goal to improve healthcare quality and safety (USDHHS, n.d.a). Many healthcare organizations and public service agencies use the Internet as the main avenue for information delivery; thus, having access to the Internet will be essential to acquiring health information and services.

Beginning in 2012, an initiative of the CMS, the Hospital Value Based Purchasing (VBP) Program, was introduced to gather data related to performance and quality of care and uses the data to determine how much the hospital is paid for services. Several specific patient care measures related to nursing are reported. Some process measures include discharge instructions, serum glucose levels for postoperative cardiac patients, and several other specific measures for the patient undergoing surgery. Some measures of patient experiences include communication with nurses, communication about medicines, responsiveness of the hospital staff, and discharge information (CMS, n.d.). Education, surveillance, reporting, and communication

---

KEY COMPETENCY 12-6

Examples of Applicable *Nurse of the Future: Nursing Core Competencies*

Informatics and Technology:

Knowledge (K6) Describes patients' rights as they pertain to computerized information management

Skills (S6a) Discusses the principles of data integrity, professional ethics, and legal requirements

Skills (S6c) Describes ways to protect data

Attitudes/Behaviors (A6) Values the privacy and confidentiality of protected health information in electronic health records

Source: Massachusetts Department of Higher Education. (2010). *Nurse of the future: Nursing core competencies* (p. 24). Retrieved from http://www.mass.edu/currentinit/documents/NursingCoreCompetencies.pdf

---

CRITICAL THINKING QUESTION *

Discuss issues of the digital divide. Explore resources in your city and county for the general public to have free Internet access and assistance. What other technology-type resources are available for underserved populations? *

of VBP measures for the nursing and hospital staff will be a priority for healthcare organizations because the impact is fiscal.

Just as the VBP program has a fiscal impact, so do the Medicare and Medicaid EHR Incentive Programs have the focus of the "meaningful use" of certified EHR information systems that were discussed earlier in this chapter. Financial incentives are attached to the health-related goals (ONC HIT, n.d.b); thus, nurses will play an essential role in aiding organizations to meet meaningful use criteria of EHR systems (Alexander, 2015a). The use of health information systems is currently vital and will continue to be so in healthcare programs and delivery systems. It will be imperative to the financial viability of healthcare organizations to have a qualified workforce with the competencies to function in this increasingly complex environment. Nursing has positioned itself well to meet this challenge.

Conclusion

Informatics provides the solution to many of the challenges that health care is facing—from easing the strain of the nursing shortage to improving patient safety. Nurses must embrace technology and integrate it into their nursing practice. Technology will not go away. It will continue to transform healthcare delivery systems. Because of technology, individuals and groups communicate in new ways, the methods with which we teach and learn have changed, and the way health care is delivered has changed. Nursing must continue to take a leadership role in the incorporation of technology into health care, and each professional nurse should strive to fully incorporate informatics competencies into his or her own practice to improve healthcare quality and patient safety.

Classroom Activity 1

Explore possible online sources to locate support groups available for individuals needing services in your area, county or parish, region, and state.

Classroom Activity 2

View the NCSBN Social Media Guidelines video during class and then allow discussion related to the guidelines, behaviors, and consequences of behaviors related to the inappropriate use of social media. The video is available at https://www.ncsbn.org/347.htm.

Classroom Activity 3

Numerous classroom and clinical activities related to informatics are available on the QSEN website at http:// qsen.org/teaching-strategies/strategy-search/. Choose activities from the website for students to complete that meet specific course objectives.

References

Alexander, S. (2015a). The electronic health record. In S. Alexander, K. H. Frith, & H. Joy (Eds.), *Applied clinical informatics for nurses* (pp. 200–221). Burlington, MA: Jones & Bartlett Learning.

Alexander, S. (2015b). Overview of informatics in health care. In S. Alexander, K. H. Frith, & H. Joy (Eds.), *Applied clinical informatics for nurses* (pp. 3–15). Burlington, MA: Jones & Bartlett Learning.

American Association of Colleges of Nursing. (2008). The essentials of baccalaureate education for professional nursing practice. Retrieved from http://www.aacn.nche .edu/education-resources/BaccEssentials08.pdf

American Nurses Association. (2001). *Scope and standards of nursing informatics practice*. Washington, DC: Author.

American Nurses Association. (2008). *Scope and standards of nursing informatics practice*. Washington, DC: Author.

American Nurses Association. (2011a). *Fact sheet. Navigating the world of social media*. Silver Spring, MD: Author.

American Nurses Association. (2011b). *6 tips for nurses using social media*. Silver Spring, MD: Author.

American Nurses Association. (2014). *Nursing informatics: Scope and standards of practice* (2nd ed.). Washington, DC: Author.

Armijo, D., McDonnell, C., & Werner, K. (2009). *Electronic health record usability: Evaluation and use case framework*. Publication No. 09(10)-0091-1-EF. Rockville, MD: U.S. Department of Health and Human Services, Agency for Healthcare Research and Quality.

Bliss, J. B., & DeYoung, S. (2002). *Working the Web: A guide for nurses*. Upper Saddle River, NJ: Prentice Hall.

Carmona, R. H. (2005, July 26). A call to caring: Remarks at press conference to launch "The Surgeon General's Call to Action to Improve the Health and Wellness of Persons with Disabilities." Retrieved from http://www.surgeongeneral.gov/news /speeches/07262005.html

Centers for Medicare and Medicaid Services. (n.d.). Hospital value-based purchasing. Retrieved from http://www.cms.gov/Medicare/Quality-Initiatives-Patient -Assessment-Instruments/hospital-value-based-purchasing/index.html?redirect =/Hospital-Value-Based-Purchasing/

Chang, B. L., Bakken, S., Brown, S. S., Houston, T. K., Kreps, G. L., Kukafka, R., ... Stavri, P. Z. (2004). Bridging the digital divide: Reaching vulnerable populations. *Journal of the American Medical Informatics Association, 11*(6), 448–457.

Cochrane Collaboration. (n.d.). The Cochrane Library. Retrieved from http://www .thecochranelibrary.com/view/0/index.html

Garner, J. C. (2003). Final HIPAA security regulations: A review. *Managed Care Quarterly, 3*(11), 15–27.

Hannah, K. (1985). Current trends in nursing informatics: Implications for curriculum planning. In K. Hannah, E. J. Builenmin, & D. N. Corkin (Eds.), *Nursing uses of computer and information science* (pp. 181–187). Amsterdam, Netherlands: North-Holland.

Health on the Net Foundation. (n.d.). HON code of conduct. Retrieved from http:// www.hon.ch/HONcode/Pro/intro.html

Health 2.0 Developer Challenge. (n.d.). Developer challenge. Retrieved from http:// www.health2con.com/devchallenge/

Healthcare IT. (2004). President Bush continues EHR push, sets national goals. Retrieved from http://www.healthcareitnews.com/news/president-bush-continues -ehr-push-sets-national-goals

Hebda, T., & Czar, P. (2009). *Handbook of informatics for nurses and healthcare professionals* (4th ed.). Upper Saddle River, NJ: Pearson Prentice Hall.

Institute of Medicine. (1997).The computer-based patient record: An essential technology for health care. Retrieved from https://www.iom.edu/Reports/1997 /The-Computer-Based-Patient-Record-An-Essential-Technology-for-Health-Care -Revised-Edition.aspx

Institute of Medicine. (1999). *To err is human: Building a safer health care system.* Washington DC: National Academies Press.

Institute of Medicine. (2001). *Crossing the quality chasm: A new health system for the 21st century*. Washington DC: National Academies Press.

Institute of Medicine. (2011). Health IT and patient safety: Building safer systems for better care. Retrieved from https://www.iom.edu/Reports/2011/Health-IT-and -Patient-Safety-Building-Safer-Systems-for-Better-Care.aspx

Johnson, J. K. (2010). Health informatics competency resource paper. Retrieved from http://qsen.org/faculty-resources/

Lindsay, R. (2011). *Social media and disasters: Current uses, future options, and policy considerations*. Congressional Research Service, 7-5700. CRS Report R41987. Retrieved from http://www.crs.gov

Massachusetts Department of Higher Education. (2010). *Nurse of the future: Nursing core competencies*. Retrieved from http://www.mass.edu/currentinit/documents /NursingCoreCompetencies.pdf

Mastrian, K. G., McGonigle, D., Mahan, W. L., & Bixler, B. (2011). *Integrating technology in nursing education. Tools for the knowledge era.* Sudbury, MA: Jones & Bartlett Learning.

McGonigle, D., & Mastrian, K. (2009). *Nursing informatics and the foundation of knowledge*. Sudbury, MA: Jones and Bartlett.

McGonigle, D., & Mastrian, K. (2012). Introduction to cognitive science and cognitive informatics. In D. McGonigle & K. G. Mastrian (Eds.), *Nursing informatics and the foundation of knowledge* (2nd ed., pp. 121–145). Burlington, MA: Jones & Bartlett Learning.

National Council of State Boards of Nursing. (2011). White paper: A nurse's guide to the use of social media. Retrieved from https://www.ncsbn.org/Social_Media.pdf

Office of the National Coordinator for Health Information Technology. (n.d.a). Health IT. Retrieved from http://www.healthit.gov

Office of the National Coordinator for Health Information Technology. (n.d.b). How to implement EHRs. Retrieved from http://www.healthit.gov/providers-professionals /ehr-implementation-steps/step-5-achieve-meaningful-use

Pagana, K. D. (2007). E-mail etiquette. *American Nurse Today, 2*(7), 45.

Procter, R. (2009). *Health informatics.* Retrieved from http://www.nlm.nih.gov /hsrinfo/informatics.html

Quality and Safety Education for Nurses. (n.d.). About QSEN. Retrieved from http:// qsen.org/about-qsen/

Sensmeier, J. (2008, September). Deep impact: Informatics and nursing practice. *Nursing Management, 2,* 4, 6. Retrieved from http://journals.lww.com /nursingmanagement/Fulltext/2008/09001/Deep_impact__Informatics_and _nursing_practice.1.aspx?WT.mc_id=HPxADx20100319xMP. doi:10.1097/01 .NUMA.0000357564.51644.42

Silsbee, D., & Reed, F. I. (2014). Informatics. In P. Kelly, B. A. Vottero, & C. A. Christie-McAuliffe (Eds.), *Introduction to quality and safety education for nurses* (pp. 270–308). New York, NY: Springer.

Smeltzer, S., Zimmerman, V., Frain, M., DeSilets, L., & Duffin, J. (2003). Accessible online health promotion information for persons with disabilities. *OJIN: The Online Journal of Issues in Nursing.* Retrieved from http://nursingworld.org /MainMenuCategories/ANAMarketplace/ANAPeriodicals/OJIN/TableofContents /Volume92004/No1Jan04/ArticlePreviousTopic/AccessibleInformation.html

Staggers, N., Gassert, C. A., & Curran, C. (2001). Informatics competencies for nurses at four levels of practice. *Journal of Nursing Education, 40*(7), 303–316.

Technology Informatics Guiding Education Reform. (2008). *The TIGER initiative. Collaborating to integrate evidence and informatics into nursing practice and education: An executive summary.* Retrieved from http://www.thetigerinitiative .org/docs/TIGERCollaborativeExecSummary_20090405_002.pdf

Thede, L. (2008, August 18). The electronic health record: Will nursing be on board when the ship leaves? *OJIN: The Online Journal of Issues in Nursing, 13*(3). doi:10.3912/OJIN.Vol13No03InfoCol01

Thede, L. (2012, January 23). Informatics: Where is it? *OJIN: The Online Journal of Issues in Nursing, 17*(1). doi:10.3612/OJIN.Vol17No1InfoCol01

Thede, L., & Schwiran, P. (2011, February 25). Informatics: The standardized nursing terminologies: A national survey of nurses' experiences and attitudes—survey I. *OJIN: The Online Journal of Issues in Nursing, 16*(2). doi:10.3912/OJIN .Vol16No02InfoCol01

Thede, L. Q. (2003). *Informatics and nursing: Opportunities and challenges* (2nd ed.). Philadelphia, PA: Lippincott Williams & Wilkins.

Thede, L. Q., & Sewell, J. P. (2010). *Informatics and nursing competencies and applications.* Philadelphia, PA: Wolters Kluwer/Lippincott Williams & Wilkins.

Thompson, B. W. (2005). HIPAA guideline for using PDAs. *Nursing, 99*(35), 24.

U.S. Department of Health and Human Services. (2000, November). *Healthy People 2010: Understanding and improving health and objectives for improving health* (2nd ed., 2 vols.). Washington, DC: U.S. Government Printing Office.

U.S. Department of Health and Human Services. (n.d.a). Healthy People 2020. Retrieved from http://healthypeople.gov/2020/topicsobjectives2020/overview.aspx?topicid=18

U.S. Department of Health and Human Services. (n.d.b). Telehealth. Retrieved from http://www.hrsa.gov/ruralhealth/about/telehealth/

Walton, J. J. (2012). Informatics. In G. Sherwood & J. Barnsteiner (Eds.), *Quality and safety in nursing: A competency approach to improving outcomes* (pp. 171–187). West Sussex, UK: Wiley.

White House Archives. (2004). Fact sheet: Transforming health care for all Americans. Retrieved from http://georgewbush-whitehouse.archives.gov/news/releases/2004/05/20040527-2.html

Zykowski, M. E. (2003). Nursing informatics: The key to unlocking contemporary nursing practice. *AACN Clinical Issues, 14*(3), 271–281.

CHAPTER 13

Teamwork and Collaboration in Professional Nursing Practice

Sharon Vincent and Kathleen Masters

Learning Objectives

After completing this chapter, the student should be able to:

1. Discuss how patient care is delivered in a complex healthcare system.
2. Describe nursing care delivery models.
3. Explore the roles of the professional nurse.
4. Discuss teamwork and collaboration In the context of quality and safety.
5. Explore communication strategies for effective interprofessional teams.
6. Examine barriers to the effective functioning of interprofessional teams.

Perhaps you wonder why hospitals are called healthcare delivery systems and not just hospitals, or why nurses are referred to as professional nurses and not just nurses. This chapter explores what the healthcare delivery system means to us and some of the roles nurses play that define what it means to be a professional nurse. In addition, various models of nursing care delivery are discussed so that the graduate nurse possesses a greater understanding of the healthcare delivery environment. The method used to assign staff nurses and technicians might seem like a distant concept at this moment, but as a baccalaureate entry-level nurse, you could be making assignments soon after graduation.

All nurses today are managers. Registered nurses (RNs) manage the care of specific groups of patients, perform care themselves, direct others to provide care, and collaborate with other healthcare providers. Nurses must know how to delegate, supervise, evaluate, motivate, and communicate with other disciplines, nurses, and unlicensed personnel. Nurses must also lead teams. In the management of care, each nurse directs the nursing care within a delivery setting to protect the patients, significant others, and healthcare personnel.

Key Terms and Concepts

» Complex adaptive systems (CASs)
» Models of patient care delivery
» Team nursing
» Total patient care
» Case management
» Collaborative critical pathway
» Delegation
» Interprofessional healthcare team
» Teamwork and collaboration

The professional nurse assesses patients and evaluates the expertise of nursing staff when making assignments. The nurse's role encompasses both interprofessional and intraprofessional collaboration in the continuity of care from admission to discharge and through rehabilitation. This chapter clearly defines some of the concepts that are needed for the entry-level nurse to maintain safe and competent entry-level practice.

Healthcare Delivery System

The healthcare delivery system has changed profoundly over the past several decades for many reasons. Population shifts (demographic changes), cultural diversity, the patterns of diseases, advances in technology, and economic changes have all affected the practice of nursing. Population changes affect delivery of health care. Health care is needed now more than in the past because the population is growing, the composition of the population is changing, birth rates are decreasing, and the life span is lengthening. People older than 85 years of age, who often require health care for chronic conditions, make up one of the fastest-growing segments of the population. More senior citizens, many of whom are women, are a factor in health care because of the healthcare resources they consume.

A significant portion of the population also now resides in urban areas, with a steady influx of ethnic minorities. Homeless persons, including homeless families, are on the rise. Cultural diversity increases as people from different nationalities enter the country. The professional nurse must know how to provide for the diverse needs of people from varied cultural backgrounds. Being culturally aware within the healthcare delivery system helps the nurse avoid imposing personal value systems when the patient has a different point of view.

In the last 50 years, evolving patterns of diseases have brought significant changes to the healthcare delivery system. Infectious diseases that were once isolated are spread across the globe quickly in our increasingly mobile society. Because of the widespread inappropriate use of antibiotics, an increasing number of infectious agents are becoming resistant to antibiotic therapy. Obesity is now a major health challenge as are its comorbidities—hypertension, coronary heart disease, diabetes mellitus, and cancer.

In addition, the improvement in techniques for trauma and acute care means that more people are surviving catastrophic events and living decades longer with disability and chronic conditions. Technology has boosted surgical and diagnostic service areas so that patients can receive sophisticated treatment on an outpatient basis. Communication techniques provide a means to train providers and deliver health care to remote countries or islands by satellite. The Veterans Administration has a program of post-traumatic stress disorder and telemental health for veterans in tribal reservations and on remote islands.

In the past, the healthcare delivery system was mainly hospital based with an acute care focus. Currently, many patients stay in the hospital for only a very short time Other facets of current healthcare delivery include hospital testing and precertification, telecommunications, home health, mobile vans, and mall clinics. Historically, as healthcare costs became alarmingly high, cost containment mandated by Congress initiated the beginning of diagnosis-related groups (DRGs), a plan to cut costs related to Medicare reimbursement. Treatment became focused on cost and profit, and the quality of nursing care declined. Nurses experienced work-related stress and burnout, and many left nursing as hospitals operated with fewer resources. Because of cost constraints and a shortage of available nurses, cross-training became a common practice. For example, one nurse could be cross-trained to work in the operating room and the postanesthesia care unit and thus possess the specialized skills to work in either unit when the need arose (Blais, Hayes, Kozier, & Erb, 2006). Nurses are trained to fill two departments or more because fewer nurses are being hired because of cost constraints. Nurses are challenged more than ever to provide quality care with fewer resources.

The chain of command refers to the hierarchy of authority and responsibility in an organization. Line authority is a type of authority in traditional healthcare delivery systems in which the supervisor directs activities of employees he or she supervises. A chain of command allows employees to understand their tasks and to manage supervisory relationships within the organization. This structure provides an avenue for reporting issues that need management's attention. Organizational charts with chain of command illustrate flow of responsibility from staff nurse to nurse managers and on up to the chief nursing officer. This model is reflective of the traditional centralized/decentralized approach commonly observed in a hospital setting.

Other models of healthcare delivery are emerging as organizations face increasing unpredictability and the need for change. Healthcare organizations (HCOs) are examples of complex systems. The term **complex adaptive systems (CASs)** refers to a collection of individual agents who are free to act in ways not totally predictable and whose actions are interconnected so that one action changes the context for other agents or units (Wilson & Holt, 2001). A CAS is highly adaptive and is characterized by self-organization, emergence of new patterns or behaviors, and distributed rather than centralized control. Patterns and behaviors enable understanding of CASs. Plsek and Wilson (2001) advocate applying CAS concepts to organizational structure. Such application to HCOs would describe a zone of complexity in which CASs have the ability to adapt to different conditions (Engebretson & Hickey, 2011). One unit or agent can change the order of behavior, and this change does not necessarily follow a linear hierarchy structure.

In HCOs, the CAS implications are that hospitals are examples of high-order complex systems, and they typically contain systems embedded within systems. New models of organizational development are needed to understand the dynamic and fast-paced unpredictability of healthcare delivery. These new models must replace outdated ones, including models of organizational development and change based on linearity, vertical organization, hierarchical decision making, and controlled change strategies, which are outmoded and no longer work for contemporary HCOs.

Complexity science offers new mental models. Complexity science is a vehicle for change and creates a lens through which we can understand organizations and change. Mental models are generalizations we make about reality that form patterns that organize how we understand the world. Healthcare professionals must begin to abandon linear models, accept unpredictability and creativity, and respond to emerging opportunities (Plsek & Wilson, 2001). For example, nurses can adopt a new paradigm of complexity of human physiology and can then provide more individualized care that augments adaptive components of the human body. As organizations struggle to be more responsive to issues, the ability to be flexible, adaptive, and innovative becomes essential for survival. Nurses must understand the framework of CASs if they are to sustain a dynamic organization ready for innovation and change in the complex health environment (Engebretson & Hickey, 2011).

Newer healthcare delivery systems also use interprofessional teams, collaboration techniques, and case management, whereas in previous eras, the physician directed all patient care, and everyone else followed the physician's lead. The care of patients has shifted from care of the sick to health promotion and prevention programs, continuity of care, and complementary health alternatives. The focus on billing with cost containment has shifted to a focus on accountability of caregivers, continuous quality improvement (CQI), and care maps or critical pathways (Blais et al., 2006).

Nursing Models of Patient Care

The healthcare delivery system is continuously changing and evolving. Within the healthcare delivery system, there are several **models of patient care delivery**. Nurses are leaders and managers within various models of patient care delivery. The methods of care delivery might differ significantly from one organization to another. The purpose of a care delivery model is to provide a framework for nurses to deliver care to a specific group of patients. The delivery of care includes use of the nursing process and includes assessing and triaging patients so that the order of care can be prioritized, a care plan formulated, and patient responses to nursing interventions evaluated in collaboration with other health team members (National Council of State Boards of Nursing, 2012).

The methods and models of nursing care have evolved over the years and have included functional nursing (task nursing), team nursing, total patient care, primary nursing, and case management. The continual evaluation of nursing models of care has been prompted by changes in nursing staff availability, reduction in hospital revenue and reimbursement, changes in acuity levels, shorter stays in the hospital, consumer demands for quality care, consumer demands for value, and demands by healthcare workers for improvements.

Team Nursing

The **team nursing** model of care is used in the United States most frequently in hospitals and in long-term and extended care facilities. This arrangement evolved after the functional nursing of the 1940s. With this approach, the nursing staff is divided into teams, and total patient care is provided to a group of patients who might be grouped according to their diagnoses. A team might consist of an RN, a licensed practical nurse (LPN), and two unlicensed assistive personnel (UAPs). The RN is the team leader responsible for making assignments and has overall responsibility for patient care by team members. The team works collaboratively, with each member performing activities he or she is best trained to do. The team communicates patient care needs and possible changes in the care plan to the team leader. The team acts as a whole with a holistic perspective of the personal needs of each patient. The team leader takes the lead to resolve problems that the team encounters by updating care plans and communicating with physicians and other members of the interprofessional healthcare team. Often the team leader makes rounds with physicians. The nursing reports communicated at the beginning of each shift are a key feature to high-quality team nursing.

Team nursing has several advantages. One is that UAPs can carry out some of the functions that do not require an RN's expertise. Team nursing also allows tasks to be carried out that require several persons because an assigned team is readily available. Several disadvantages can surface with a team. If communication skills are not adequate, the holistic view of the patient might be fragmented. In addition, UAPs and LPNs might feel resentment if they perceive the RN to be focused totally on paperwork and documentation and less on the physical needs of the patient. For a team leader to be effective, delegation, communication, and problem-solving skills are essential.

Total Patient Care

Appearing as early as the 1920s, the first model of patient care delivery was **total patient care** (Sullivan & Decker, 2005). In this model, the RN has responsibility for all aspects of care of the patient or patients. The RN works directly with the patient, other nursing staff, and physicians in implementing a plan of care. The objective of total patient care is to have one nurse provide all care to the same patient or patients for the entire shift. Currently, this model is practiced in areas such as critical care units or postanesthesia recovery units

KEY COMPETENCY 13-1

Examples of Applicable
*Nurse of the Future: Nursing
Core Competencies*

Systems-Based Practice:

Knowledge (K3a) Understands
the concept of patient care
delivery models

Skills (S3a) Considers
resources available on the
work unit when contributing
to the plan of care for a
patient or group of patients

Attitudes/Behaviors (A3a)
Acknowledges the tension
that may exist between a
goal-driven and a resource-
driven patient care delivery
model

Source: Massachusetts Department of Higher
Education. (2010). *Nurse of the future:
Nursing core competencies* (p. 20). Retrieved
from http://www.mass.edu/currentinit
/documents/NursingCoreCompetencies.pdf

where a high level of expertise is required. This system's advantages are that nurses provide holistic continuous care, there is continuity of communication from patients to interprofessional team members, and the nurse has total accountability for that shift. The disadvantage to this model is that it is more expensive than other models because nurses are providing patient care that lesser-skilled persons are able to perform.

Case Management

A current nursing model of nursing care delivery is **case management**, which relies on clinical pathways to evaluate care. The clinical pathway refers to expected outcomes and interventions established by the collaborative practice team (Sullivan & Decker, 2005). The professional nurse is responsible for initiating and updating the plan of care, care map, or clinical pathway that is used to guide and evaluate patient care. The clinical pathway provides a timeframe for expected outcomes of care and involves an interdisciplinary team of caregivers who use the pathway to provide consistent care.

Nursing case management focuses on managing a group (caseload) of patients and the members of the interprofessional healthcare team caring for those patients. The case manager organizes patient care by major diagnoses or DRGs and focuses on specific timeframes to achieve predetermined patient outcomes and contain costs. The case manager makes referrals to other healthcare providers and manages the quality of care. Important characteristics to the role of nursing case managers are collaboration, identification of patient outcomes with timeframes, and the use of CQI analysis. The case manager does not usually provide direct patient care but supervises the provision of care by UAPs and licensed personnel.

A case manager's role in an acute care setting involves the management of a caseload of 10 to 15 patients. Case managers follow patient progression from admission through discharge and solve problems of variances from the expected outcomes. A variance would be, for example, that a total hip surgery patient was not discharged on day 6 (expected outcome by timeframe) as planned. Instead, that person was hospitalized for 10 days. The case manager intervenes and communicates with the healthcare team to analyze specific patient progression and outcomes and determine why the patient was not discharged. Usually, case managers have considerable nursing experience and an advanced degree.

To manage the cases of a group of patients, a team is selected that includes clinical experts from the disciplines needed such as nursing, medicine, or physical therapy. The key features of case management are support by administration and physicians, a qualified case manager, collaboration of the teams, a CQI system, and critical pathways. All members of the team must agree on the critical pathways and accept responsibility and accountability for interventions and patient outcomes. Case management contributes to the reduction of complications that arise during hospitalization.

The caseload selected for case management includes high-volume, high-cost, and high-risk cases. One such example is the total hip replacement population in orthopedics. The number of hip replacement surgeries performed is higher than the number of many other procedures; they cost more and include higher risks such as pulmonary emboli and surgical site infections. The total cost to the patient and related departments is higher, so careful monitoring is necessary. Other high-risk patients are those in critical condition, in the intensive care unit (ICU) for more than 2 days, or on a ventilator. Baseline data such as length of stay, cost of care, and complications are collected on these groups and analyzed.

The critical path quickly orients the staff to the expected outcomes that should be achieved for that day. Nursing diagnoses identify the outcomes needed. If these are not achieved, the case manager is notified and the situation analyzed. An example of a **collaborative critical pathway** for a patient having a total hip replacement is described here. A critical path for a total hip replacement patient on days 1 and 3 postoperatively might include the following:

- Day 1 Operating Room and Postoperative Care
  Activity: Bed rest, turn/cough/deep breath q 2 hrs
  NSG: VS q h × 4, then q 4 hrs, circulation/neuro checks q h × 4, then q 4 hrs
  Hemovac: Check q hr × 4, then q 4 hrs, I & O
  Medications: Antibiotics, pain control
  Nutrition: NPO to clear liquids as tolerated
  Teaching: Pain control, assist devices, incentive spirometry, mobility plan, D/C plan, home health evaluation
- Day 3 Postoperatively
  Activity: Continue mobility plan, turn/cough/deep breath q 2 hrs, skin protocols
  NSG: VS q 8 hrs, D/C assessment, D/C hemovac, ck drainage, I & O q 8 hrs, D/C Foley, continue elastic hose
  Medications: Antibiotics, p.o. pain control, continue stool softeners, IV to heplock, continue Coumadin
  Nutrition: Diet as tolerated, repeat teaching as needed
  D/C plans: Review transfer orders, D/C needs

Normally, a total hip replacement patient would be expected to be discharged on the sixth day after surgery. The critical path continues all 6 days, with potential nursing diagnoses attached, such as pain control deficit or impaired mobility. The critical path is also given to the patient's family so that they know what to expect during an uncomplicated total hip surgery hospitalization.

Critical pathways are implemented through collaboration with input from various departments. Critical pathways are also called interdisciplinary or interprofessional plans, or action plans. The interprofessional teams deal

KEY COMPETENCY 13-2

Examples of Applicable
*Nurse of the Future: Nursing
Core Competencies*

Systems-Based Practice:

Knowledge (K3b) Understands
role and responsibilities
as a member of the health
care team in planning and
using work unit resources
to achieve quality patient
outcomes

Skills (S3b) Collaborates with
members of the health care
team to prioritize resources,
including one's own work
time and activities delegated
to others, for the purposes
of achieving quality patient
outcomes

Attitudes/Behaviors (A3b)
Values the contributions of
each member of the health
care team to the work unit

Source: Massachusetts Department of Higher
Education. (2010). *Nurse of the future:
Nursing core competencies* (p. 20). Retrieved
from http://www.mass.edu/currentinit
/documents/NursingCoreCompetencies.pdf

with patient-related problems and help the patient progress through the clinic and hospital efficiently. The physician or nurse practitioner sees the patient and recommends consultations as needed. The nurse's role is to assess the need for consultations and identify expected outcomes of consultation, along with the need for revising care, as patient needs change. For example, nurse–nurse (interprofessional) consulting might occur between a staff nurse and an enterostomal therapist related to the care of a patient's excoriated ostomy site secondary to radiation and chemotherapy. This type of consultation is documented in the patient record after obtaining a physician's order for an enterostomal therapist consult; then, the enterostomal nurse intervenes and documents the care rendered. The primary nurse revises the plan of care with continuous reassessment and evaluation of outcomes. The following sections further define some of the many roles that nurses assume.

Roles of the Professional Nurse

The role of the professional nurse is one of the most exciting areas to discuss for entry-level nurses. Think about it. You go from high school student to professional in zero to 4 years or so! The role of the professional nurse has expanded in response to changing populations and the philosophical shift toward health promotion rather than illness cure. Several roles of nurses include caregiver, advocate, educator, leader, manager, collaborator, and researcher. Placing *RN* after your name means that you are committed to the legal, ethical, and moral responsibilities that define the professional roles of the nurse. These responsibilities are based on the American Nurses Association's (ANA's) *Nursing: Scope and Standards of Practice* (2015b), *Code of Ethics for Nurses with Interpretive Statements* (2015a), and *Nursing's Social Policy Statement* (2010). You are the fulcrum of patient care and the patients' safety net as well as their advocate. The following sections examine some important aspects of a few of the roles of the entry-level nurse.

Caregiver

The role of the nurse as caregiver has changed tremendously during the past century. The role as a dependent person to the physician who only provided personal care has evolved to that of the educated nurse who is an autonomous and informed professional. As a caregiver, the nurse practices nursing as both an art and a science. The nurse provides interventions to meet physical, psychosocial, spiritual, and environmental needs of patients and families using the nursing process and skills of clinical judgment. Holistic care is a philosophical approach that emphasizes the uniqueness of the individual and in which interacting wholes are more important than the sum of each part;

that is, the whole person is greater than merely each component part of the patient—biophysical, psychological, social, and spiritual parts. The science (knowledge base) of nursing becomes the art of nursing through caring, where the nurse demonstrates concern for the patient. The nurse and patient are connected. The nurse as a caregiver is skilled and empathetic, knowledgeable and caring.

Advocate

As the nurse–patient relationship develops, the nurse uses professional knowledge to assist patients in their decision making. The nurse assumes the role of patient advocate in healthcare delivery, intervening during times of crises whether the situation be related to the diagnosis of acquired immune deficiency syndrome, homelessness, drug and alcohol abuse, teenage pregnancy, child and spouse abuse, or increasing healthcare costs. A patient advocate is a person who pleads the cause for patients' rights. The purpose of this nursing role is to respect patient decisions and support patient autonomy. Patient advocacy includes developing a therapeutic nurse–patient relationship to secure patient self-determination, protecting patients' rights, and acting as an intermediary among patients and their significant others and healthcare providers (Blais et al., 2006). A patient advocate is concerned with empowering the patient. The nurse represents the interests of the patient, who has needs that are unmet and are likely to remain unmet without the nurse's intervention. Examples of situations where the nurse must speak up for the patient might relate to pain control, the patient's refusal of treatment, or issues of resuscitation status.

Ethical challenges may face the nurse in the role of patient advocate, but the nurse has an obligation to advocate for high-quality and safe patient care as a member of the interprofessional team (American Association of Colleges of Nursing, 2008, p. 23; ANA, 2015a). To be an effective patient advocate, the nurse must do the following:

- Be assertive, knowing that the nurse's primary responsibility is to the patient.
- Recognize the patient's values and preferences as more important than the healthcare providers' values and preferences.
- Ensure adequate information is provided so that patients and families can make informed decisions.
- Be aware that moral or ethical conflicts can arise that require consultation or negotiation among healthcare providers.

Nurses may need to assist patients in the clarification of their values as they relate to a particular health problem or end-of-life issue. End-of-life issues such as advance directives should be addressed early in the course of patient hospitalizations while the patient is capable of making personal choices.

KEY COMPETENCY 13-3

Examples of Applicable *Nurse of the Future: Nursing Core Competencies*

Systems-Based Practice:

Knowledge (K4) Understands role and responsibilities as patient advocate, assisting patient in navigating through the health care system

Skills (S4a) Serves as a patient advocate

Attitudes/Behaviors (A4a) Values role and responsibilities as patient advocate

Source: Massachusetts Department of Higher Education. (2010). *Nurse of the future: Nursing core competencies* (p. 20). Retrieved from http://www.mass.edu/currentinit /documents/NursingCoreCompetencies.pdf

Manager

In exploring the concept of management in practice, all nurses are managers. They direct the work of professionals and nonprofessionals to achieve expected outcomes of care. All nurses need to learn management and leadership skills to be efficient and effective in their respective fields. In the healthcare setting, a manager is an individual who is employed by an organization and is responsible and accountable for the goals of that organization (Sullivan & Decker, 2005). In practice, nurses are expected to manage the care of each patient assigned to them for that shift. So, imagine you have just received a report on your patients. Where do you begin? Assessments and medicines are due. Patients need to go to surgery and radiology. Breakfast trays are being distributed. Insulin is past due. Charting is needed. Student nurses want report. So much to do, and so little time! How can you get everything done, provide quality care, and still be standing at the end of your shift? These are all reasons that delegation is a terrific concept!

It is easy to say "delegate," but delegation is a difficult leadership role for nurses to adopt and one that is not readily learned during nursing education. Both experienced nurses and entry-level nurses struggle to develop delegation and prioritization skills. Nurse managers must continually expand delegation skills to survive. With cost containment, it is necessary now more than ever to delegate effectively. **Delegation** is defined as the process by which responsibility and authority for performing a certain task are transferred from one individual to another while retaining accountability for the outcome (ANA, 2015b). To delegate, the person delegating (delegator) must be the one who is responsible for the task.

It is important to understand the acceptance of delegation. The one to whom a task is being delegated (delegatee) must realistically decide whether he or she has the skills and abilities for the task being assigned and the time to do it. If not, the individual must inform the person delegating that he or she does not have the skills. The delegator has the option to delegate parts of a task, but the one delegated to also has the option to negotiate for the parts of the task that can be accomplished. After the participants agree on the responsibilities to be assumed, they must clarify the timeframe and other expectations. The delegatee must communicate with the delegator effectively throughout the completion of the task.

The nurse is responsible for using informed judgment and basing the decision to delegate on the person's competencies and qualifications. The procedure should be communicated with clear instructions that allow opportunity for clarification and questions. If the outcome does not meet expectations, the nurse should lead a discussion to identify reasons for the unexpected outcome and determine what can be learned from the experience

---

KEY COMPETENCY 13-4

Examples of Applicable *Nurse of the Future: Nursing Core Competencies*

Leadership:

Knowledge (K6) Understands the principles of accountability and delegation

Skills (S6b) Assigns, directs, and supervises ancillary personnel and support staff in carrying out particular roles/functions aimed at achieving patient care goals

Attitudes/Behaviors (A6a) Recognizes the value of delegation

Attitudes/Behaviors (A6b) Accepts accountability for nursing care given by self and delegated to others

Source: Massachusetts Department of Higher Education. (2010). *Nurse of the future: Nursing core competencies* (p. 18). Retrieved from http://www.mass.edu/currentinit/documents/NursingCoreCompetencies.pdf

to improve care in the future (Altmiller, 2014). Delegation is a skill that can be learned, but practice is required. Successful nurses learn the process of delegation. Nurses accomplish more by delegating than if they try to do everything themselves.

Interprofessional Teams and Healthcare Quality and Safety

Health care has become so complex today that it takes several professional providers delivering care in a collaborative environment to provide patient-centered care with high-quality patient outcomes. We know that teamwork among healthcare professionals is associated with the provision of safe, high-quality patient care (Barnsteiner, Disch, Hall, Mayer, & Moore, 2007). Thus, all members of the **interprofessional healthcare team** must combine their skills, knowledge, and resources to improve outcomes, and nurses and physicians must modify their traditional roles and work more collaboratively as colleagues.

One of the many roles of the professional nurse is participation in collaboration as a member of interprofessional and intraprofessional teams. The interprofessional team consists of members of more than one discipline and may be composed of those who provide direct care to patients such as physicians, nurses, and family members, as well as those who provide support services such as social workers, dieticians, pharmacists, physical therapists, transport services, and housekeeping (Altmiller, 2014, p. 133). Interprofessional teams provide a full range of expertise through each of the team members, and thus all contribute to patient outcomes.

One of the 10 rules for redesign of the healthcare system recommended by the Institute of Medicine (IOM) in the 2001 *Crossing the Quality Chasm* report was making cooperation among clinicians a priority to ensure appropriate exchange of information and coordination of care. The IOM report that followed, *Health Professions Education: A Bridge to Quality* (2003), included the recommendation that health professions work in interdisciplinary teams cooperating, collaborating, communicating, and integrating care to ensure that care is continuous and reliable.

Interprofessional Teamwork and Collaboration

Teamwork and collaboration are competencies expected of health professionals and refer to functioning effectively within nursing and interprofessional teams, fostering open communication, mutual respect, and shared decision making to achieve quality patient care (Quality and Safety Education for Nurses [QSEN],

KEY COMPETENCY 13-5

Examples of Applicable
*Nurse of the Future: Nursing
Core Competencies*

Teamwork and Collaboration
(Self):

Knowledge (K1) Identifies
own strengths, limitations,
and values in functioning as
a member of a team

Skills (S1a) Demonstrates
self-awareness of strengths
and limitations as a team
member

Attitudes/Behaviors (A1a)
Recognizes responsibility
for contributing to effective
team functioning

(A1b) Appreciates the importance of collaboration

Source: Massachusetts Department of Higher
Education. (2010). *Nurse of the future:
Nursing core competencies* (p. 31). Retrieved
from http://www.mass.edu/currentinit
/documents/NursingCoreCompetencies.pdf

2007; Massachusetts Department of Higher Education, 2010). The ultimate purpose of teamwork and collaboration is to achieve high-quality patient care. Providing collaborative care requires that each professional coordinate care with other professionals on the healthcare team so that redundancies, deficits, and errors are prevented (Lomax & White, 2015, p. 61). Other goals of collaborative care include the following:

- Enhance continuity across the continuum of care from wellness and prevention, through acute episodes of illness, to discharge or transfer and rehabilitation.
- Provide research-based, high-quality, cost-effective care that is driven by expected outcomes.
- Promote mutual respect and communication among the patient, nurse, and caregiver to form a coalition.
- Provide opportunities to solve issues and problems.

Interprofessional teams may come together for provision of patient care or to focus on specific problems in order to identify possible solutions on a patient care unit or as a part of a healthcare system. A common example of an interprofessional team in the acute care setting is the code or resuscitation team whose members respond to situations involving cardiac or respiratory arrest. Another interprofessional team developed in Australia (Berwick, 2014) and found in acute care facilities is the rapid response team (RRT). An RRT is a group of specific professionals with specialized skills who can mobilize and deliver immediate intervention to the patient at the bedside at the first signs of deterioration in a patient's health status. The RRT differs from the code team and is minimally composed of a physician, a critical care nurse, and a respiratory therapist. The RRT can be called to the patient's bedside by anyone, including family members (Altmiller, 2014, p. 133). This single intervention resulted in a 27% decline in mortality after its implementation in Australia (Berwick, 2014).

The ability to collaborate is particularly important for staff nurses. Collaboration is one of the key skills required in nursing; but what exactly is collaboration? According to the ANA (2015b), collaboration is a professional healthcare relationship that is grounded in a reciprocal and respectful recognition and acceptance of each partner's unique expertise, power, and sphere of influence and responsibilities. Also included in the definition is the concept of commonality of goals and the mutual safeguarding of the legitimate interest of each party.

The advent of group practice, managed care, and practice standards has driven the need for collaboration. On a continuum, collaboration at the lowest level begins with communication among all involved disciplines and the patient, with everyone asking similar questions (Blais et al., 2006). Each professional has separate interventions with a separate plan of care, and decision making is independent. Coordination and consultation represent a middle-range level of collaboration, where the professionals seek to make best use of the resources. Comanagement and referral represent the highest level of collaboration, in which providers are responsible and accountable for their own aspects of care, and then patients are directed to other providers when the problem is beyond a particular provider's expertise. The main levels on the continuum of collaboration are represented in **Figure 13-1**.

Nurses collaborate with patients, peers, and other professionals in the healthcare delivery system. Specifically, the nurse's role as a collaborator with the patient includes acknowledging and supporting the patient in healthcare decisions, encouraging patient autonomy, helping patients set goals for care, and providing patient consultation in a collaborative fashion. With other healthcare professionals, the nurse's role is to recognize the contribution and expertise of each member of the interdisciplinary team, listen, share responsibilities in exploring options and setting goals, and participate in collaborative interprofessional research to increase knowledge of a particular clinical problem. A nurse can also collaborate within professional organizations by serving on committees at the local, state, national, or international level to create solutions for professional and healthcare concerns.

When one team member is confident in the actions of another, trust occurs. HCOs have not always fostered mutual caring and respect among professionals, so nurses must strive to promote positive relationships with team members despite lingering negative attitudes from the past. When professionals work closely together on a team, giving and receiving timely and relevant feedback are some of the most difficult challenges but are important to the team process. Type of feedback given can be affected by a person's perceptions, roles, confidence, beliefs, and environment. Helpful feedback is characterized by warm, caring, and respectful communication. Opportunities to practice listening and giving and receiving feedback can enhance professional communication skills. Giving and receiving feedback helps the professional collaborative team develop an understanding and effective working relationship.

KEY COMPETENCY 13-6

Examples of Applicable *Nurse of the Future: Nursing Core Competencies*

Teamwork and Collaboration (Team):

Knowledge (K2) Describes scope of practice and roles of interdisciplinary and nursing health care team members

Skills (S2) Functions competently within own scope of practice as a member of the health care team

Attitudes/Behaviors (A2) Values the perspectives and expertise of all health care team members

Source: Massachusetts Department of Higher Education. (2010). *Nurse of the future: Nursing core competencies* (p. 31). Retrieved from http://www.mass.edu/currentinit /documents/NursingCoreCompetencies.pdf

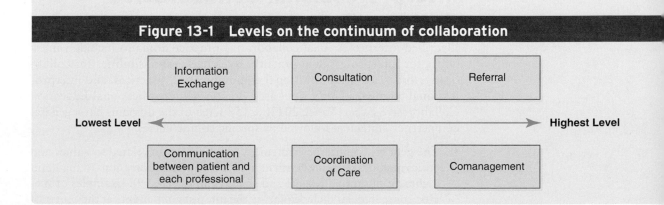

Figure 13-1   Levels on the continuum of collaboration

One of the most difficult challenges in promoting collaboration among professionals is giving and receiving feedback. What is your experience in giving and receiving timely and helpful feedback with a team? Think of an example of receiving both negative and positive feedback. Compare the effect of the negative and positive feedback. Compare the experiences. *

Another key element of collaboration by the interdisciplinary team involves responsibility for the expected outcome. To achieve a solution, team decision making should begin with a clear definition of the problem and be directed at the objectives of the specific effort. By focusing on the patient's priority needs first, organization of interventions can be planned accordingly. The discipline best able to address the patient's highest needs at the moment is given priority in planning and is responsible for providing its interventions in a timely manner. In order to make these determinations, it is necessary to understand the scope of practice of the individual team members.

Often, nurses take the lead to help the team identify priorities and focus on areas that require further referral or attention. Take, for example, a terminal oncology patient who requires care post abdominal surgery to correct a bowel obstruction caused by an invasive tumor. Cancer has affected the patient's spine, causing neurologic deficits of the extremities. The patient has an implanted port for chemotherapy, parenteral nutrition, and requires multiple antibiotic infusions. Several decubiti have developed. The primary nurse ensures patient-centered care by communicating with the patient and significant others. The nurse then collaborates with the physician for pain control and postoperative care. The nurse ensures expert intravenous lines for chemotherapy and multiple antibiotic infusions, collaborating with peers if necessary. The nurse consults per physician orders with the enterostomal therapist for wound care of the decubiti and consults with the dietician for hyperalimentation (total parenteral nutrition) needs. The nurse collaborates with physical therapy for resumption of activity for neurologic deficits. Each member of the interprofessional team contributes his or her own expertise to common goals of care to ensure quality care for the patient.

Interprofessional Collaborative Practice Domains

Identified interprofessional collaborative practice domains include values/ethics for interprofessional practice, roles and responsibilities for collaborative practice, interprofessional communication practices, and interprofessional teamwork and team-based practice (Interprofessional Education Collaborative Expert Panel, 2011, p. 15). Each of the domains has a general competency statement followed by specific competencies.

- The general competency statement for the domain related to values and ethics includes working "with individuals of other professions to maintain a climate of mutual respect and shared values" (p. 19). Examples of specific competencies include placing the interests of patients at the center of interprofessional care delivery and respecting the dignity and privacy of patients while maintaining confidentiality in the delivery of team-based care (p. 19).

- The general competency statement related to roles and responsibilities states that one "uses the knowledge of their own role and those of other professions to appropriately assess and address the healthcare needs of the patients and populations served" (p. 21). Examples of specific competencies include communicating one's roles and responsibilities clearly to patients, families, and other professionals and recognizing one's limitations in relation to skills, knowledge, and abilities (p. 21).

- The general competency statement related to interprofessional communication states that one "communicates with patients, families, communities, and other health professionals in a responsive and responsible manner that supports a team approach to the maintenance of health and treatment of disease" (p. 23). Examples of specific competencies include organizing and communicating information to patients, families, and healthcare team members in a form that is understandable, avoiding discipline-specific terminology and using respectful language appropriate for a given difficult situation, crucial conversation, or interprofessional conflict (p. 23).

- The general competency statement related to teamwork and team-based practice includes applying "relationship-building values and the principles of team dynamics to perform effectively in different team roles to plan and deliver patient-/population-centered care that is safe, timely, efficient, effective, and equitable" (p. 25). Examples of specific competencies include engaging other health professionals, as appropriate to the specific situation, in shared patient-centered problem solving and reflecting on individual and team performance (p. 25).

The full document with all of the specific competencies for each of the domains is available online.

Interprofessional Team Performance and Communication

Effective interprofessional healthcare teams function in an environment where all members can voice concerns and opinions and all members contribute and share in decision making. Clear and focused communication with respectful negotiation promotes camaraderie among team members and reduces the potential for human error in judgment (Altmiller, 2014). The complexity of the healthcare environment, coupled with the limitations of human performance, make it critically important for clinicians to work in environments where they are empowered to express concerns and have standardized tools to communicate (O'Daniel & Rosenstein, 2008, p. 275).

In addition, poor communication is associated with patient error; the Joint Commission indicated that communication failure was the most frequently identified root cause of sentinel events reported between 1995 and 2008 (Disch, 2012, p. 94). The reporting of sentinel events to the Joint Commission is voluntary and therefore represents a small proportion of actual events; however, it is worth noting that 532 out of 901 sentinel events in 2012, 563 out of 887 sentinel events in 2013, and 248 out of 394 sentinel events in 2014 were identified as having a root cause related to communication issues (Joint Commission, n.d.).

Interprofessional Communication Techniques

Several initiatives have been developed to provide mechanisms for effective communication techniques among members of the interprofessional healthcare team. For example, TeamSTEPPS is an evidence-based teamwork system that was developed by the Agency for Healthcare Research and Quality (AHRQ, n.d.) to optimize patient outcomes through the provision of training in effective communication and teamwork skills. TeamSTEPPS includes ready-to-use materials and a training curriculum to facilitate integration into any healthcare system.

Another communication framework, more familiar to most nurses, is SBAR. Developed by the military, this is an acronym for the words *situation, background, assessment*, and *recommendation*. Using SBAR, the situation describes what is happening with the patient; the background includes a brief backdrop of the patient's circumstances that provide context; the assessment identifies what data the provider has regarding the situation; and the recommendations identify what the provider thinks needs to be done to correct the situation. The idea behind the use of SBAR is that significant information regarding a patient's status or care is communicated from one provider to another using a standardized format (Altmiller, 2014, p. 140).

Cross-monitoring is a process of monitoring the actions of other team members that can be used to share workload and avoid errors. This requires that team members listen carefully to the details communicated and provide correction for the team if needed. An example of this technique might include a situation where interventions agreed upon during grand rounds with the interprofessional team are not those included in the written orders. A nurse asking for clarification of the orders because she recalls something different from grand rounds is an example of cross-monitoring (Altmiller, 2014, p. 141).

Another technique is CUS, an acronym for *concerned, uncomfortable*, and *safety*. CUS is a standardized tool that nurses and other team members can use to take an assertive stance in advocating for patients. For example, using the CUS tool, the nurse who is concerned about a larger than recommended medication dose may approach the ordering provider and state, "I am concerned about the medication dose that has been ordered. I am uncomfortable giving the dose to this patient because of her renal status. I don't think it is safe" (Altmiller, 2014, p. 141).

A call out is used to bring attention to the entire team at one time regarding a patient situation. Using a call out, a team member calls out to others for assistance. The call out is followed by a check back that verifies the receipt of the call out information and provided feedback and an appropriate response. Requiring the check back means that the call out message is acknowledged and there is opportunity for correction if necessary. The two-challenge rule refers to the obligation of the team member to make a second attempt to make the patient's problem known to others on the team if he or she believes that the first attempt was not successful. This rule, designed for when the team member's input is purposefully ignored, stipulates that the team member is still obligated to make a second attempt. For example, when a nurse communicates to the physician a concern about a change in the level of consciousness of a patient and the physician does not address the concern, the nurse is obligated to bring the concern to the physician a second time (Altmiller, 2014, p. 141).

Interprofessional Team Performance and Communication Issues

Factors that enhance the performance of teams include open communication, nonpunitive environment, clear direction and roles for team members, respectful atmosphere, clear decision-making procedures, routine communication and information sharing, appropriate balance of team member participation for the task, clear specifications about authority and accountability, and shared responsibility for team success (Disch, 2012, pp. 95–96). Several factors have been identified that can compromise team effectiveness.

Groupthink is the mode of thinking that persons engage in when concurrence seeking becomes dominant and tends to override realistic appraisal of alternative courses of action, or when the flow of information to the group is controlled such that it restricts the decision making of a group by limiting the ability to explore all options in a particular situation. Symptoms of groupthink may also be observed when members of decision-making groups become motivated to avoid being too harsh in their judgments of their leaders' or their colleagues' ideas (Janis, 2007). Considering the factors that contribute to effective interprofessional team performance, it is clear that groupthink can potentially limit team performance and therefore healthcare quality.

Excessive authority gradients and excessive courtesy may also impede effective team performance. If deference is given to the senior leader on the team or to the physician to make decisions for the team in all situations, then the team performance is compromised. These behaviors may be related to a hierarchal organizational structure or to the perceived abilities of team members. In addition, performance-shaping behaviors that may include high

KEY COMPETENCY 13-7

Examples of Applicable *Nurse of the Future: Nursing Core Competencies*

Teamwork and Collaboration (Team Communication):

Knowledge (K5) Understands the principles of effective collegial communication

Skills (S5a) Adapts own communication style to meet the needs of the team and situation

(S5b) Demonstrates commitment to team goals

(S5c) Solicits input from other team members to improve individual and team performance

Attitudes/Behaviors (A5) Values teamwork and the relationships upon which it is based

Source: Massachusetts Department of Higher Education. (2010). *Nurse of the future: Nursing core competencies* (p. 32). Retrieved from http://www.mass.edu/currentinit/documents/NursingCoreCompetencies.pdf

stress, excessive fatigue, deficiencies in skill, or the work environment may affect the abilities of teams to function effectively (Sasou & Reason, 1999).

Barriers to interprofessional communication and collaboration may include issues such as cultural differences, gender differences, generational differences, personality differences, hierarchy, organizational culture, differences in schedules and routines, differences in jargon, professional rivalry, disruptive behavior, differing values and expectations, varying qualifications and status, and complexity of care requiring rapid decision making (O'Daniel & Rosenstein, 2008). Some of these barriers may actually manifest as conflict.

One barrier related to interprofessional communication and collaboration that has gotten attention in the recent past is disruptive behavior. This behavior may be manifested verbally with outbursts of anger or profanity or may be manifested by physical acts such as throwing objects. According to the Joint Commission (2008), disruptive behavior is a behavior that undermines a culture of safety. Intimidating and disruptive behaviors foster medical errors, contribute to poor patient satisfaction, contribute to preventable adverse outcomes, increase the cost of care, and cause qualified clinicians, administrators, and managers to seek new positions in more professional environments. Therefore, the Joint Commission has embedded in its leadership accreditation requirements two elements that address disruptive behavior.

- *EP 4:* The hospital/organization has a code of conduct that defines acceptable and disruptive and inappropriate behaviors.
- *EP 5:* Leaders create and implement a process for managing disruptive and inappropriate behaviors.

In addition, suggestions from the Joint Commission included the implementation of training programs to foster professional interactions and the development and implementation of organizational policies with "zero tolerance" for intimidating and/or disruptive behaviors, protection for those who report disruptive behaviors, and responding to patients and their families who witness disruptive behaviors.

Interpersonal conflict might occur when individuals are working together on teams and their expectations are incompatible. Conflicts between people can affect interprofessional collaboration. To reduce conflict, team members can conduct interprofessional conferences, take part in interprofessional educational programs, and recognize and accept personal responsibility for teamwork. Sometimes the failure of professionals to collaborate is because they lack the skills necessary to contribute to effective teamwork. In the past, nursing has been interested in emphasizing nursing research and nursing practice. Attention is now shifting to focus on interprofessional collaboration and the recognition of different points of view. Collaboration among disciplines requires that nurses have the ability to articulate their own theories while considering different perspectives, to determine the best approach to specific problems. The key to effective collaboration among an interprofessional team is the building of relationships among all members that reflect trust and respect.

Conclusion

This chapter has introduced healthcare delivery systems and the role of the professional nurse. It explored various models of nursing care delivery. All nurses are managers of the care of a specific group of patients and collaborate with other healthcare providers in the delivery of patient-centered and safety-focused care. Nurses must possess the skills of clinical judgment, delegation, supervision, collaboration, evaluation, motivation, and communication to function effectively as a member of the interprofessional team. This chapter introduced some of the concepts necessary for the entry-level nurse to function competently in the roles required in professional nursing practice, including as a member of the interprofessional healthcare team.

Classroom Activity 1

The nurse is planning the discharge of an 82-year-old man who has heart failure and chronic obstructive pulmonary disease. Divide the class into small groups of students to discuss how the case manager would intervene for the patient and family and provide continuity of care from ICU to home. Have a spokesperson for each group briefly present each group's plan, or include an interprofessional team perspective on care and have each student in the group present from the perspective of a different team member (for example, nursing, social work, dietetics, physician, physical therapy), being sure to address competencies in each of the interprofessional domains in the discussion.

Classroom Activity 2

Numerous classroom and clinical activities related to teamwork and collaboration are available on the QSEN website at: http://qsen.org/teaching-strategies/strategy-search/. Choose activities from the website for students to complete that meet specific course objectives.

References

Agency for Healthcare Research and Quality. (n.d.). TeamSTEPPS ®: Strategies and tools to enhance performance and patient safety. Retrieved from http://www.ahrq.gov /professionals/education/curriculum-tools/teamstepps/index.html

Altmiller, G. (2014). Interprofessional teamwork and collaboration. In P. Kelly, B. A. Vottero, & C. A. Christie-McAuliffe (Eds.), *Introduction to quality and safety education for nurses* (pp. 131–160). New York, NY: Springer.

American Association of Colleges of Nursing. (2008). *The essentials of baccalaureate education for professional nursing practice.* Washington, DC: Author.

American Nurses Association. (2010). *Nursing's social policy statement: The essence of the profession.* Silver Spring, MD: Author.

American Nurses Association. (2015a). *Code of ethics for nurses with interpretive statements.* Silver Spring, MD: Author.

American Nurses Association. (2015b). *Nursing: Scope and standards of practice* (3rd ed.). Silver Spring, MD: Author.

Barnsteiner, J., Disch, J. M., Hall, L., Mayer, D., & Moore, S. M. (2007). Promoting interprofessional education. *Nursing Outlook, 55*(3), 144–150.

Berwick, D. M. (2014). *Promising care: How we can rescue health care by improving it.* San Francisco, CA: Jossey-Bass.

Blais, K. K., Hayes, J. S., Kozier, B., & Erb, G. (2006). *Professional nursing practice concepts and perspectives* (5th ed.). Upper Saddle River, NJ: Pearson Prentice Hall.

Disch, J. (2012). Teamwork and collaboration. In G. Sherwood & J. Barnsteiner (Eds.), *Quality and safety in nursing: A competency approach to improving outcomes* (pp. 91–112). West Sussex, UK: Wiley.

Engebretson, J. C., & Hickey, J. V. (2011). Introduction to complexity science. In J. Butts & K. Rich (Eds.), *Philosophies and theories for advanced nursing practice* (pp. 115–141). Sudbury, MA: Jones & Bartlett Learning.

Institute of Medicine. (2001). *Crossing the quality chasm: A new health system for the 21st century.* Washington, DC: National Academies Press.

Institute of Medicine. (2003). *Health professions education: A bridge to quality.* Washington, DC: National Academies Press.

Interprofessional Education Collaborative Expert Panel. (2011). *Core competencies for interprofessional collaborative practice: Report of an expert panel.* Washington, DC: Interprofessional Education Collaborative. Retrieved from https://ipecollaborative .org/Resources.html

Janis, I. L. (2007). Groupthink. In R. P. Vecchio (Ed.), *Leadership: Understanding the dynamics of power and influence in organizations* (2nd ed., pp. 157–169). Notre Dame, IN: University of Notre Dame Press.

Joint Commission. (2008). Behaviors that undermine a culture of safety. Retrieved from http://www.jointcommission.org/sentinel_event_alert_issue_40_behaviors _that_undermine_a_culture_of_safety/

Joint Commission. (n.d.). Sentinel event data: Root causes by event type. Retrieved from http://www.jointcommission.org/sentinel_event.aspx

Lomax, S. W., & White, D. (2015). Interprofessional collaborative care skills for the frontline nurse. *Nursing Clinics of North America, 50*, 59–73.

Massachusetts Department of Higher Education. (2010). *Nurse of the future: Nursing core competencies*. Retrieved from http://www.mass.edu/currentinit/documents/NursingCoreCompetencies.pdf

National Council of State Boards of Nursing. (2012). *2013 NCLEX-RN detailed test plan: Candidate version*. Chicago, IL: Author. Retrieved from https://www.ncsbn.org/1287.htm

O'Daniel, M., & Rosenstein, A. H. (2008). Professional communication and team communication. In R. G. Hughes (Ed.), *Patient safety and quality: An evidence-based handbook for nurses* (Vol. 2, pp. 2-271–2-283). Publication No. 08-0043. Rockville, MD: Agency for Healthcare Research and Quality (AHRQ).

Plsek, P. E., & Wilson, T. (2001). Complexity, leadership and management in healthcare organisations. *British Medical Journal, 323*, 746–749.

Quality and Safety Education for Nurses. (2007). Competencies: Prelicensure KSAS. Retrieved from http://qsen.org/competencies/pre-licensure-ksas/

Sasou, K., & Reason, J. (1999). Team errors: Definition and taxonomy. *Reliability Engineering and System Safety, 65*, 1–9.

Sullivan, E. J., & Decker, P. J. (2005). *Effective leadership and management in nursing* (6th ed.). Upper Saddle River, NJ: Pearson Prentice Hall.

Wilson, T., & Holt, T. (2001, September). Complexity and clinical care. *British Medical Journal, 323*, 685–688.

CHAPTER 14

Ethical Issues in Professional Nursing Practice

Janie B. Butts and Karen L. Rich

Learning Objectives

After completing this chapter, the student should be able to:

1. Explain important ethical issues related to nurses' relationships with patients, families, and colleagues.
2. Examine key ethical concepts involved in nurses' work, such as professional boundaries, dignity, and patient advocacy.
3. Discuss the concept of patient rights in health care.
4. Contrast the meaning and details of end-of-life advance directives—living will and durable power of attorney for designation of health care.
5. Identify complex problems in determining healthcare allocation and explore standards of distributive justice.
6. Analyze three major ethical issues surrounding organ transplantation.
7. Explore the Organ Procurement and Transplantation Network's (OPTN's) strategies for ensuring a fair and balanced allocation decision.
8. Differentiate among active, passive, voluntary, and nonvoluntary euthanasia.
9. Define key concepts related to end-of-life care, such as withdrawing and withholding life support and medical futility.
10. Identify appropriate decision-making standards when patients have lost decision-making capacity.
11. Distinguish between the meaning of brain death and persistent vegetative state.
12. Contrast the terms *terminal sedation (TS)*, *rational suicide*, and *physician-assisted suicide (PAS)*.
13. Explain the relationship between rule of double effect and palliative care.
14. Summarize the American Nurses Association's (ANA's) opinions in the *Code of Ethics for Nurses with Interpretive Statements* on palliative care, the alleviation of pain and suffering, and a nurse's ethical obligation to provide care.
15. Identify moral dilemmas that occur during end-of-life care and decision making.

Medical ethics, which later became known as bioethics, stemmed from rapid medical, ethical, and technological advances and increasing concern about the mistreatment of human beings in research and other experiments. The inhumane treatment of persons and violations of human rights during the era of World War II, which came to light during the Nuremberg Trials of 1947, as well

Note: Fourth edition chapter revised by Janie B. Butts.

© robertiez/iStock/Getty Images Plus/Getty

Key Terms and Concepts

» Unavoidable trust
» Professional boundaries
» Dignity
» Patient advocacy
» Moral right

as other atrocities around the world initiated the birth of bioethics. The term *bioethics* came into existence in the late 1970s. Technological progress came with a human price. New and intriguing moral dilemmas continue to surface as technological advances evolve in professional healthcare practice and patient care situations emphasizing the need for nurses in every venue to have the skills of ethical reflection and moral reasoning—a "good grasp of everyday ethical comportment" (Benner, Sutphen, Leonard, & Day, 2010, p. 28).

Relationships in Professional Practice

Professional healthcare practices gained credibility because of formal expert knowledge. Healthcare relationships originated from natural human conditions, such as illness, and became the foundation for healthcare practices (Sokolowski, 1991). If nurses follow the guidance of the ANA's *Code of Ethics for Nurses with Interpretive Statements* (2015), patients will remain the central focus of nursing care and nursing relationships. The quality of patient care depends on harmonious relationships between nurses and physicians, other nurses, and other healthcare workers. Nurses who are concerned about providing compassionate patient care and developing harmonious relationships with patients also must be concerned about their relationships with colleagues. The quality of a nurse's relationships and the moral climate surrounding those relationships can affect the well-being of patients.

Nurse–Physician Relationships

In 1967, Stein, a physician, wrote an article characterizing a type of relationship between medical doctors and nurses, which he labeled "the doctor–nurse game" (Stein, Watts, & Howell, 1990). This hierarchical relationship, with doctors in the position of the superior, formed the basis for the game. Avoidance of open disagreement between physicians and nurses was the game's hallmark. Experienced nurses had the ability to avert conflict by cautiously suggesting thoughts so the physician did not directly perceive consultative advice as coming from a nurse. In the past, student nurses were educated about the rules of "the game" while attending nursing school. Over the years, other people have given credence to the historical accuracy of Stein's characterization of doctor–nurse relationships (Fry & Johnstone, 2002; Jameton, 1984; Kelly, 2000).

Stein, along with two other physicians, wrote an article in 1990 revisiting the doctor–nurse game, 23 years after he coined the phrase (Stein et al., 1990). They discovered that nurses unilaterally had stopped playing the game. This behavior evolved gradually as nurses increased their use of dialogue rather than gamesmanship and began viewing the nursing profession as having an equal partnership status with other healthcare professions. Other factors at work included an alignment of nurses with the civil rights and women's movements, an increase in nurses receiving higher education, and a more collaborative approach between nurses and physicians. The dismantling of the doctor–nurse game encouraged nurses to establish nursing as an autonomous profession by continuing the fight for freedom from physician domination. Physicians and nurses must pursue a common goal between care and cure while steadfastly following the moral traditions that are so noticeable in the healthcare professions. The two professions must work together cohesively for the well-being of individual patients, groups, and communities. When overt or covert battles arise between nurses and physicians, so do ethical issues, and patients could be the losers.

Nurse-Patient-Family Relationships

Unavoidable Trust

When patients enter the healthcare system, they are usually entering an environment that they perceive as foreign and threatening (Chambliss, 1996; Zaner, 1991). When patients are in need of help from nurses and access health care, they frequently feel a sense of vulnerability and heightened tension. Personal interactions and intimate activities, such as touching and probing, which generally do not occur between strangers, are commonplace between patients and healthcare professionals. Patients are frequently stripped of their clothes, subjected to sitting alone in cold and uninviting rooms, and made to wait anxiously for frightening news regarding the continuation of their very being. In most cases, patients at the point of needing care have no option but to trust nurses and other healthcare professionals, a phenomenon Zaner (1991) recognized as **unavoidable trust**.

At the beginning of the point-of-care encounter, an asymmetrical and uneven power structure exists, which pushes patients and families into an unavoidable trust situation with nurses or other healthcare professionals. Because of this unavoidable trust, nurses must commit to the highest possible quality of care and promise "not only to take care of, but to care for, the patient and family—to be candid, sensitive, attentive, and never to abandon them" (Zaner, 1991, p. 54). Oddly enough, patients must trust healthcare professionals before they ever receive any care, but whether trust was warranted can only be determined by patients once the care is delivered to them. That type of structure results in a significant degree of implied nursing power over the patient; therefore, nurses must never take for granted the fragility of patients' trust and the permission patients give so unquestioningly, or even questioningly.

Professional Boundaries

In Provision 2.4 of the *Code of Ethics for Nurses with Interpretive Statements* (ANA, 2015), the ANA made a significant case for respecting professional boundaries in nursing. Nurses must sustain the integrity of the professional boundaries and recognize the risks for violating those professional lines. Butts (2016c) defined **professional boundaries** as "limits that protect the space between the nurse's professional power and the patient's vulnerabilities. Boundaries facilitate a safe connection because they give each person in the relationship a sense of legitimate control, whether the relationships are between a nurse and a patient, a nurse and a physician, a nurse and an administrator, or a nurse and a nurse" (p. 78). In addition to the issues of trust discussed in the previous section, staying within the boundaries of practice also will increase the trust between patients and the nurse.

The nature of the profession of nursing has a personal element, which increases the risks for departing from a boundary. According to Butts (2016c), two types of departures from professional boundaries occur.

> The first type of departure is boundary violations, which are actions that do not promote the best interest of another person in a relationship and pose a potential risk, harm, or exploitation to another person in the relationship. Boundary violations widely vary, from misuse of power, betrayal of trust, disrespect, and personal disclosure to more severe forms, such as sexual misconduct and exploitation. The second type of departure, boundary crossings, is a lesser and more short-lived type that accidentally or intentionally occurs during normal nursing interventions and will not necessarily happen again. (p. 79)

Potential violations of nurse–patient boundaries can involve gifts, intimacy, limits, neglect, abuse, and restraints (Maes, 2003). The gifts patients give to nurses must be considered in terms of the implication of why the gift was given, its value, and whether the gift might provide therapeutic value for the patient but not influence the level of care provided by the nurse. Gifts generally lead to boundary violations and need to be discouraged most of the time. In addition to an obvious violation of intimacy through inappropriate sexual relationships, a violation of intimacy might occur if a nurse inappropriately shares information with other people in ways that violate patients' privacy. Nurses and patients need to observe limits to prevent either person from becoming uncomfortable in the relationship. Nurses must take care to provide reasonable care to all patients according to the *Code* (ANA, 2015) and the particular state's nurse practice acts rules and regulations so as not to be neglectful in the provision of nursing care, and they must do everything possible to prevent or intervene to stop patient abuse in whatever form it occurs. Restraining patients, whether the restraint is physical, chemical, or environmental, will increase nurses' risks for violating or crossing a boundary. The policies of employers as well as the standards set by accrediting agencies to safeguard patients will serve as legal guidelines for nurses.

CRITICAL THINKING QUESTIONS

New nurses have not necessarily developed their own professional boundaries when they begin practice. They may violate a boundary without even knowing they crossed it (Maes, 2003).

What do you think? What signs might alert you to a potential professional boundary violation or crossing?

Dignity

In the first provision of the *Code of Ethics for Nurses with Interpretive Statements*, the ANA (2015) included the standard that a nurse must have "respect for human dignity" (p. 17). Shotton and Seedhouse (1998) propose the term **dignity** has been used in vague ways. They characterize dignity as being related to persons in a position to use their capabilities. In general terms, a person has dignity "if he or she is in a situation where his or her capabilities can be effectively applied" (p. 249). For example, nurses will enhance the dignity of elders by assessing their priorities and determining what the person has been capable of in the past and what the person is capable of in the present.

A lack of or loss of capability is frequently an issue when caring for patients such as children, elders, and people who are physically and mentally disabled. Having absent or diminished capabilities is consistent with what MacIntyre (1999) refers to in his discussion of human vulnerability. People generally progress from a point of vulnerability in infancy to achieving varying levels of independent practical reasoning as they mature (MacIntyre, 1999). All people, including nurses, would do well to realize that persons have been or will be vulnerable at some point in their lives. Taking a "there but for the grace of God go I" stance can prompt nurses to develop what MacIntyre calls the virtues of acknowledged dependence. Those virtues are just generosity, *misericordia*, and truthfulness and are exercised in communities of giving and receiving. Just generosity is a form of giving generously without "keeping score" of who gives or receives the most; *misericordia* is a Latin word to signify giving without prejudice when an urgent need occurs; and truthfulness means to give information needed by patients for their own good and not withholding the information. Nurses who cultivate these three virtues can move toward preserving patient dignity and the common good of the community.

Patient Advocacy

Nurses acting as patient advocates try to identify unmet patient needs and then follow up to address the needs appropriately (Jameton, 1984). **Patient advocacy**, as opposed to patient advice, involves the nurse's moving from the patient's values to the healthcare system rather than moving from the nurse's values to the patient. The concept of advocacy has been a part of the International Council of Nurses' *Code of Ethics* (2012) and the ANA's *Code* since the 1970s. In the *Code of Ethics for Nurses with Interpretive Statements*, the ANA (2015) supports patient advocacy in terms of nurses providing social justice and requiring nurses to work collaboratively with others to attain the goal of addressing the healthcare needs of patients and the public. Nurses commonly act to ensure that all appropriate parties are involved in patient care decisions, patients are provided with the information needed to make informed decisions, and collaboration is used to increase the accessibility and availability of health care to all patients who need it. The International Council of Nurses (2012), in the *Code of Ethics for Nurses*, affirmed:

- The nurse shares with society the responsibility for initiating and supporting action to meet the health and social needs of the public, in particular those of vulnerable populations. (p. 2)
- The nurse advocates for equity and social justice in resource allocation, access to health care and other social and economic services. (p. 2)

Nurse–Nurse Relationships

As in the case of nurse–physician relationships, nurse–nurse relationships can be thought of as relationships within a community. Nurses in a nursing community might be what Engelhardt (1996) calls moral friends. According to Wildes (2000), moral friends exist together within communities and use similar moral language. They "share a moral narrative and commitments [and] common understandings of the foundations of morality, moral reason, and justification" (p. 137). Communities are strongest when moral friends share "common moral traditions, practices, and [a] vision of the good life" (p. 137). In putting patients first in nurses' priorities, nurses in a community work together for a common good, using professional traditions to guide the communal narrative of nursing.

Unfortunately, nurses often treat other nurses in hurtful ways through what some people have called lateral or horizontal violence (Kelly, 2000; McKenna, Smith, Poole, & Coverdale, 2003). Lateral or horizontal violence, currently known as workplace bullying, involves interpersonal conflict, harassment, intimidation, harsh criticism, sabotage, and abuse among nurses. Some people believe oppression among nurses occurs because nurses feel oppressed by other dominant groups such as physicians or institutional administrators. Some nurses have characterized the violence perpetrated against nurses who excel and succeed as the "tall poppy syndrome," which is a phrase that traces back to the Greek and Roman philosophers, but more recently, the term was repopularized in Australia and New Zealand. Nurses who succeed are ostracized, thereby creating a culture to discourage success among nurses.

Lateral violence in nursing is counterproductive for the profession. A more productive path for nurses might be to cultivate the virtue of sympathetic joy. *Sympathetic joy* refers to experiencing happiness in terms of the good things experienced by others. The nursing community does not benefit from lateral violence, but nurses who cultivate the virtue of sympathetic joy can strengthen the sense of community among nurses. Nurses must support other nurses' success rather than treat colleagues as tall poppies that must be cut down.

However, there are occasions when unpleasant action must be taken in regard to nursing colleagues. In addition to advocating directly for patients' unmet needs, nurses are advocates when they take appropriate action to protect patients from the unethical, incompetent, or impaired practice of other nurses (ANA, 2015). When nurses are aware of these situations, they must deal compassionately with the offending coworkers while assuring that patients are receiving safe, quality care. Concerns must be expressed to the offending nurse when personal safety and patient safety are not jeopardized, and appropriate guidance must be obtained from supervisory personnel and institutional policies. Although action must be taken to safeguard patients' care, the manner in which a nurse handles situations involving unethical, incompetent, or impaired colleagues must not involve gossip, condescension, or unproductive derogatory talk.

Moral Rights and Autonomy

In a perfectly just society, moral rights and legal rights would overlap, but the two types of rights are not the same in our society. A **moral right** is a person's right

> [T]o perform certain activities (a) because they conform to the accepted standards or ideas of a community (or of a law, or of God, or of conscience), or (b) because they will not harm, coerce, restrain, or infringe on the interests of others, or (c) because there are good rational arguments in support of the value of such activities. (Angeles, 1992, p. 264)

Generally, moral rights are separated into welfare rights and liberty rights. Welfare rights allow persons to pursue their legitimate interests or those personal interests that do not interfere with the other persons' interests, which are similar and equal to one's own. "Welfare (positive) rights entail the right to receive basic goods such as education, medical care, and police protection, as well as a duty on the part of others such as the government to provide these social goods" (Brannigan & Boss, 2001, p. 33).

As opposed to welfare rights, liberty (negative) rights involve the right to noninterference from any person or governmental entity when pursuing one's legitimate interests (Brannigan & Boss, 2001). "Liberty or negative rights include autonomy, privacy, freedom of speech, and freedom from harassment, confinement, unwanted medical treatment, or participation in experiments without our informed consent" (p. 33). The liberty rights of every person include a fundamental right to health without prejudice; around the world and in the United States, these are emphasized over welfare rights, except in cases of elders and the poor.

Informed Consent

Considerations of **informed consent** fall within the overview of respect for autonomy, or self-direction (Beauchamp & Childress, 2012; Veatch, 2003). Although nurses often facilitate informed consent and have a role in terms of patient advocacy, the actual responsibility for ensuring informed consent historically has belonged to the physician. However, with the increased numbers of advanced practice nurses and the increased complexity of nurses' roles, informed consent has become more of a direct ethical issue for nurses. A liberally applied concept of informed consent includes the following rule: "[M]eaningful information must be disclosed even if the clinician does not believe it [the information] will be beneficial" (Veatch, 2003, p. 75). This definition is in contrast to the rule applied under the Hippocratic Oath, which allowed for healthcare professionals to withhold information if they believed it would harm or upset a patient.

A patient's signature on a consent form proves neither that a patient read the form nor that the patient understands what is written on it (Veatch, 2003). It would be impossible to inform each patient of everything about a procedure. In an attempt to deal with this reality, two standards are often applied. The first is the reasonable person standard, which states the healthcare professional will disclose information any reasonable person would want to know. The second is the subjective standard of disclosure, which is based on the subjective interests of a particular patient rather than a hypothetical reasonable person. The ideal standard, therefore, adjusts what a reasonable person would want to know with what the healthcare professional knows is of interest for the patient to know.

Patient Self-Determination Act

The **Patient Self-Determination Act (PSDA)**, enacted in 1991, was designed to facilitate the knowledge and use of advance directives (Koch, 1992). Under the act, healthcare providers must ask patients if they have advance directives and provide patients with advance directive information according to patients' wishes. This act provides nurses with a good opportunity to take an active role in facilitating the moral rights of patients in terms of end-of-life decision making. In addition to responding to patients' direct questions about advance directives and end-of-life options, nurses would do well to "listen" for the subtle cues that patients give, such as signs of their anxieties and uncertainty about end-of-life care. Part of a nurse's compassionate practice entails listening intently and genuinely to patients' voices and attempting to alleviate patients' suffering and fears in regard to end-of-life decision making.

Advance Directives

An **advance directive** is "a written expression of a person's wishes about medical care, especially care during a terminal or critical illness" (Veatch, 2003, p. 119). Said another way, individuals lose control over their lives when they lose their decision-making capacity, and advance directives become instructions about health care for the future (Devettere, 2000). Advance directives may be self-written instructions or may be prepared by someone else as instructed by the patient.

The two main types of advance directives are (1) a living will and (2) a durable power of attorney. A **living will** is a formal legal document that provides written directions concerning medical care to be provided in specific circumstances (Beauchamp & Childress, 2012; Devettere, 2000). The living will gained recognition in the 1960s, but the Karen Ann Quinlan case in the 1970s brought significant public attention to the living will and subsequently prompted legalization of the document. Although the onset of living wills was a good beginning, today living wills are inadequate, unsound, and do not hold up legally in court. One reason for the inadequate living wills is the vague language, with only instructions for unwanted treatments, and a lack of legal penalties for people who choose to ignore living wills. Living wills might be legally questionable regarding their authenticity. The most reliable legal advance directive document is the **durable power of attorney,** a written directive in which a designated person is allowed to make either general or healthcare decisions for a patient (Devettere, 2000).

Often, families and healthcare professionals experience fear about making wrong decisions regarding a patient who is incapacitated. Advance directives help to reduce emotional stress, but at the same time can produce ethical dilemmas.

Social Justice
Definition and Theories of Social Justice

A Sicilian priest first used the term **social justice** in 1840, and then in 1848, the term was popularized by Antonio Rosmini-Serbati (Novak, 2000). Since then, social justice has been defined as (Center for Economic and Social Justice, n.d.):

> A virtue that guides us in creating those organized human interactions we call institutions. In turn, social institutions, when justly organized, provide us with access to what is good for the person, both individually and in our associations with others. Social justice also imposes on each of us a personal responsibility to work with others to design and continually perfect our institutions as tools for personal and social development. (Section 3, *Defining Social Justice*)

A large portion of the use of the term has been related more to competing powers of social systems and regulative principles on an impersonal basis, such as "high unemployment," "inequality of incomes," "lack of a living wage," and "social injustice" (Novak, 2000, p. 1). The term is also related to the question of what makes the common good for everyone (Brannigan & Boss, 2001). People who take a communitarian approach put the common good of the community over individual freedoms.

John Rawls (1971), a social contract and justice theorist, viewed fairness and equality as being under a **veil of ignorance.** This idealistic concept means that if people had a veil to conceal their own or others' economic, social, and class standing, each person would likely make justice-based decisions from a position free from all biases and would view the distribution of resources in unprejudiced ways. Under the veil, people would view social conditions neutrally because they could not anticipate what their own position might be at the time the veil is lifted. The not knowing or ignorance of persons about their own position means they cannot gain any type of advantage for themselves by their choices. This "ignorance" principle is a just view because of the application of the two principles of equality and justice: (1) everyone should be given equal liberty no matter what adversities exist for people, and (2) differences should be recognized among people by making sure the least advantaged people are given fair opportunity for improvements (Rawls, 1971).

Nozick (1974) presented the idea of an entitlement system, meaning if individuals could pay for insurance, only then were they entitled to health care. A just and fair system would be essential to rewarding people who contribute to the system. A decade later, Daniels (1985) further explored Rawls's concept of justice in his own book on the liberty principle. In his liberty view, every person should have equal opportunity, equal health care, and reasonable access to healthcare services; therefore, he recommended national healthcare reform.

Allocation and Rationing of Healthcare Resources

The cost of health care is spiraling out of control worldwide; therefore, deciding how to allocate healthcare resources is at the forefront of people's concerns. The unfortunate and troublesome experiences with healthcare reimbursements are played out through narratives on the front page of almost every newspaper. A central question that healthcare professionals, economists, and politicians have asked themselves for years is: What makes up a just and equitable healthcare system? The question continues to be unanswered.

The health care of people in the United States is not the best in the world. As of a 2013 report, the United States ranked 11th of 11 countries in five different areas: (1) overall ranking of health care, (2) cost-related problem with access, (3) efficiency, (4) equity, and (5) healthy lives (Davis, Stremikis, Squires, & Schoen, 2014). The United States ranked 9th out of 11 in overall access to care. The U.S. government's second major goal in Healthy People 2010 was to eliminate health disparities (National Center for Health Statistics, 2012). This remains a major goal in Healthy People 2020, yet the disparities continue to occur without much, if any, improvement in the health of people in the United States (Office of Disease Prevention and Health Promotion, 2014). Inequalities in health care commonly exist because of complex differences in socioeconomic status, racial and ethnic backgrounds, education levels, and healthcare access. These differences underlie many of the current health issues.

As healthcare costs increase, resources become more limited for people. Distributive justice has become a critical issue in the healthcare system. Guidelines in how scarce resources are distributed must be clearly delineated. Guiding questions for members of society involve the ethical concerns always present in distributive justice.

- Does every person have a right to health care?
- Is health care a right or a privilege that must be earned?
- How should resources be distributed so everyone receives a fair and equitable share of health care?
- Should healthcare rationing ever be considered as an option in the face of scarce healthcare resources? If so, how?

There might never be clear and concise answers to these complex questions. Brannigan and Boss (2001) outlined criteria for when rationing should be considered. The criteria include standards of distribution by market or according to people who could afford to pay; social worth; medical needs; age; a first-come, first-served basis; and randomization. From the 1990s to the present, systems of managed care have been operating in the United States as one strategy to improve the use of services based on needs and to maximize health and well-being while reducing overall healthcare costs to individuals (Sugarman, 2000). However, the public has responded very poorly to managed care. Some people have labeled managed care as an ethical disaster. Before such complaints are made, healthcare professionals and nurses need to address the sources of the problems.

Enormous travesties occurred with the Medicaid and Medicare systems from 1965 to 1990. The U.S. federal government made big money available based on the autonomous practice of physicians—meaning that physicians could redirect large amounts of money from taxpayers to the care of sick people through Medicaid and Medicare (Sugarman, 2000). This period is often referred to as the good old days or the golden years, when physicians were not required to justify or show evidence for their medical care for sick people. Since 1990, times have changed, and criticism is plentiful. No matter what healthcare system is in place, physicians and the public will give unfavorable remarks. Engelhardt (1996), a bioethicist, commented on the healthcare system of the era before 1990.

> Concepts of adequate care are not discoverable outside of particular views of the good life and of proper medical practice. In nations encompassing diverse moral communities, an understanding of what one will mean by an adequate level or a decent minimum of health care will need to be fashioned, if it can indeed be agreed to, through open discussion and by fair negotiation. (p. 400)

KEY COMPETENCY 14-3

Examples of Applicable *Nurse of the Future: Nursing Core Competencies*

Professionalism:

Attitudes/Behaviors (A8b) Values and upholds altruistic and humanistic principles

Source: Massachusetts Department of Higher Education. (2010). *Nurse of the future: Nursing core competencies* (p. 15). Retrieved from http://www.mass.edu/currentinit /documents/NursingCoreCompetencies.pdf

CRITICAL THINKING QUESTION ✳

Think about the questions posed in this section in relation to the distribution of scarce healthcare resources using Rawls's "veil of ignorance." Then, answer the same questions taking your own circumstances into account. Do you come up with the same answers to the questions? Explain your rationale. ✳

Promoting open dialogue for expressing moral views in the community and in institutions, negotiating policy change for better allocation and an improved healthcare system, and maintaining a firm commitment to better patient health outcomes are just a few ways that nurses can assist with supporting good health for the common good of the community.

Ethics and Organ Transplantation

A persistently looming social allocation issue is the scarce resources in organ transplantation. As of April 2015, almost 123,400 people in the United States were awaiting organs for transplant (OPTN, n.d.a). In the United States, those in need of organs are placed on a national list according to each person's level of need for the organ. Three ethical issues are involved with organ transplantation: (1) the moral acceptability of transplanting an organ from one person to another, (2) organ procurement, and (3) allocation of the organs.

The first ethical issue is in the form of a question: "Is performing transplants 'playing God'?" (Veatch, 2003, p. 136). The phrase "playing God" became quite common during the birth of bioethics from 1947 to the 1970s, as organ transplantation procedures, genetics, and human reproduction technologies emerged. Many people view transplantations as an unacceptable option for treatment because of their religious or cultural beliefs, or just basic beliefs, such as the association that the human heart has with romance and as the "seat of the soul" (p. 137).

The second ethical issue is procurement of organs. **Organ procurement** is the obtaining, transferring, and processing of organs for transplantation through systems, organizations, or programs. In some countries, but not the United States, a common practice is the salvaging of organs without the consent of the patient or family member based on the notion that organs, once the person is dead, become the property of the state or country. In the United States, however, the rights and self-determination of each person dictate when and if the donation and salvaging of organs will occur. Adults in the United States express their wishes regarding organ donation through a required response, usually upon admission to hospitals or consent to treatments. People can decline or willingly agree to donate their organs, and they can allow a relative to be their designated surrogate. Donor cards are legal documents used along with other documentation in the organ donation process in the United States. A donor card gives permission for the use of a person's bodily organs in the event of death. People can "opt in" by signing a donor card to become a potential donor of one or more organs in the event of their death. Advance directives are also legal documents used to express one's desires about organ donation.

The third ethical issue, **organ allocation**, continues to be one of the most debated issues in health care today because of the scarcity of donor organs. The OPTN (n.d.b) tries to ensure a balanced allocation and ethical decision based on two concepts: (1) justice and (2) medical utility. Justice is the "fair consideration of candidates and medical needs," and medical utility is an effort to "increase the number of transplants performed and the length of time patients and organs survive" (OPTN, n.d.b, para. 1).

Because of the assurance of fair distribution of organs by OPTN, social merit should never be a reason to deny or allocate an organ to someone. For those needing an organ because of diseases associated with lifestyle-related behaviors, such as smoking, the harmful use of alcohol and other drugs, an unhealthy diet, and physical inactivity, some people have questioned whether restricted or rationed access to treatment and resources could be a justified ethical choice. Another view of social merit relates to those who feel they are justifiably more deserving of an organ than are others due to their perceived importance and power in terms of society or monetary net worth (Butts, 2016a). When patients are involved in a transplantation process, nurses should provide a balanced caring and fairness approach (see **Box 14-1**).

One primary role for nurses is to assist with attempting to eliminate health disparities. Education programs with substantive content that target particular populations provide a beginning role for nurses, who function on a broad community level. Other roles for nurses include encouraging patients and families to express their feelings and attitudes about donations and transplantations, especially in regard to ethical issues involving death and dying; supporting, listening, and maintaining confidentiality with patients and families; assisting in monitoring patients for organ needs; continually being aware of inequalities and injustices in the healthcare system, which can affect the care of patients; and assisting in the care of surgical organ transplant and donation patients and their families.

BOX 14-1 BALANCED CARING AND FAIRNESS APPROACH FOR NURSES

Nurses are ethically obligated to provide care with a balanced caring and fairness approach and work toward assisting to eliminate health disparities. Strategies to achieve this balanced approach include:

- Encourage patients and families to express their feelings and attitudes about ethical issues involving end of life, organ donation, and organ transplantation.
- Support, listen, and maintain confidentiality with patients and families.
- Assist in monitoring patients for organ needs.
- Be continually mindful of inequalities and injustices in the healthcare system and how the nurse might help balance the care.
- Assist in the care of patients undergoing surgery for organ transplant as well as donation patients and their families.
- Provide educational programs for particular target populations at a broader community level.

Death and End-of-Life Care

Defining Death

The last words of the great composer Frédéric Chopin were, "The earth is suffocating…. Swear to make them cut me open, so that I won't be buried alive" (Australian Museum, 2009). In the 1700s and 1800s, especially in Europe, there was widespread fear of premature burial or being buried alive because of the inadequate methods for detecting when a person was dead and because of actual accounts of people being buried alive (Bondeson, 2001). "Buried alive" stories trace back to those days. One example of this type of story is when a body was exhumed for some reason, and claw marks were found on the inside of the coffin lid (Mappes & DeGrazia, 2001). Because of the widespread fear, a variety of special safety coffins were invented with detailed devices to help the dead, once they were buried, to communicate with others above the ground (Australian Museum, 2009). The devices included such things as a rope extending to the surface of the ground with a bell on the other end, a speaking tube from the coffin to the outside world, a shovel, and food and water. In addition to a law that prevented premature burial, funeral home attendants even went to the extent of having their employees monitor dead bodies for any signs of life during the "wait" time before burial.

For several centuries, when a person became unconscious, physicians or other people would palpate for a pulse, listen for breath sounds with their ears, look for condensation on an object when it was held close to the body's nose, and check for fixed and dilated pupils (Mappes & DeGrazia, 2001). In 1819, fear was reduced when the stethoscope was invented because physicians could listen with greater certainty for a heartbeat through a magnified listening device. In 1903, Willem Einthoven, a Dutch physician, discovered the existence of the electrical properties of the heart with his invention of the electrocardiograph, which provided sensitive information about whether the electrical activity of the heart was functioning. The artificial respirator of the 1950s brought about more uncertainty regarding death as physicians kept patients alive in the absence of a natural heartbeat (Australian Museum, 2009). By the 1960s, when transplants were being performed, it was becoming apparent that a diagnosis of death would not depend necessarily on the absence of a heartbeat; rather, the definition of death would need to include brain death criteria in the future.

The first attempt to redefine death was made in the United States by the Harvard Medical School ad hoc committee in 1968. The definition was based on the committee members' attempt to identify reliable clinical criteria for respirator-dependent patients who had no brain function (Youngner & Arnold, 2001). Then, in 1981, the President's Commission members sanctioned a definition of death, which included brain death, and recommended its adoption by all states. The 1981 definition led to the **Uniform Determination of Death Act (UDDA)**, in which death is defined as follows:

> An individual who has sustained either (1) irreversible cessation of circulatory and respiratory functions or (2) irreversible cessation of all functions of the entire brain, including the brain stem, is dead. A determination of death must be made in accordance with accepted medical standards. (President's Commission, *Defining Death*, 1981; as cited in Mappes & DeGrazia, 2001, p. 318)

Since this definition was adopted, criteria for brain death have been integrated in almost every state but have been continually debated. Veatch (2003) contributed a provocative notion to the debate on the definition of death in terms of the loss of full moral standing of human beings. This statement triggers the question as to when humans should be treated as full members of the human community. Although almost every person has reconciled the thought that some persons have full moral standing and others do not, there is continued controversy about when full moral standing ceases to exist and what characteristics qualify the cessation of full moral standing. Losing full moral standing, to some philosophers, is equivalent to ceasing to exist. Presently, various groups have proposed and debated the following four conceptions of death since the enactment of the UDDA in 1981 (Munson, 2004, pp. 692–693):

- *Traditional:* A person is dead when he is no longer breathing and his heart is not beating (cardiopulmonary).
- *Whole-brain:* Death is regarded as the irreversible cessation of all brain functions … no electrical activity in the brain, and even the brain stem is not functioning (brain death).
- *Higher brain:* Death is considered to involve the permanent loss of consciousness. Someone in an irreversible coma would be considered dead, even though the brain stem continued to regulate breathing and heartbeat (persistent vegetative state).
- *Personhood:* Death occurs when an individual ceases to be a person. This can mean loss of features essential to personal identity or for being a person.

With whole-brain death, a patient physically can survive for an indeterminate period of time with a mechanical ventilator. With higher brain death, a patient lives in a persistent vegetative state indefinitely but without the need for mechanical ventilation. It is because of these situations that the question exists regarding when a person should be treated as one who has full moral standing within the human community. Society, physicians, and nurses have had difficulty in defining death using the UDDA definition, which includes the traditional and the whole-brain concepts. However, the greatest difficulty has been when they have tried to incorporate the concepts of higher brain death and personhood death (Munson, 2004). No definite criteria for either of these concepts—higher brain or personhood—have been established for defining death. The debate continues, and questions continue about when life begins, when life ends, and what it is that ceases to exist when someone is dead (Benjamin, 2003; Veatch, 2003).

Euthanasia

Most people do not want prolonged agony and suffering before their death and would like to keep their emotional, financial, and social burdens to a minimum and their dignity intact. However, dying the "good death" is not always possible (Munson, 2004). *Euthanasia*, meaning "good death" in Greek, has come to mean "easy death" and has developed a strong appeal in recent years. A patient might ponder options of euthanasia if suffering and pain become too much for the person to bear. There are two major types of euthanasia: active and passive. **Active euthanasia** occurs when a person takes an action to end a life (including one's own life). Active euthanasia can include a lethal dose of medication, such as in PAS. **Passive euthanasia** means a person allows another person to die by not acting to stop death or prolong life. An example of this type of euthanasia is withholding treatment necessary to prevent death at a point in time.

Euthanasia also is recognized by the categories of voluntary and nonvoluntary (Brannigan & Boss, 2001). **Voluntary euthanasia** occurs when a person with a sound mind authorizes another person to take his or her life or to assist in achieving death. This type of euthanasia also includes the taking of one's own life. **Nonvoluntary euthanasia** occurs when persons are not able to express their decision about death. A blending of these types of euthanasia can occur, such as voluntary active, nonvoluntary active, voluntary passive, and nonvoluntary passive.

A vigorous debate in the United States continues about whether there is a real moral difference between active euthanasia, such as the intentional taking of someone's life, and passive euthanasia, such as withholding or withdrawing life-sustaining treatments (Brannigan & Boss, 2001; Jonsen, Veatch, & Walters, 1998). The action versus omission distinction many times causes nurses and physicians to ponder this troublesome question: "Is there a moral difference between actively killing and letting die?"

Rational Suicide

The thought of morally accepting the act of a person's committing **rational suicide** weighs heavily on the hearts of most people, even today. The very connection of the terms *rational* and *suicide* seems a contradiction (Engelhardt, 1996; Finnerty, 1987). However, suicide is an enormous public health crisis.

Worldwide, there are more than 800,000 suicides each year (World Health Organization, 2014). In a 2010 report, the annual occurrence of suicide in the United States was 38,364, which is an average of 105 suicides per day (Centers for Disease Control and Prevention, 2012). Rational suicide is a self-slaying and is categorized as voluntary active euthanasia. In this category, the person has made a reasoned choice of rational suicide, which seems to make sense to others at the time. The person contemplating rational suicide has a realistic assessment of life circumstances, is free from severe emotional distress, and has a motivation that would seem understandable to most uninvolved people within the person's community (Siegel, 1986).

Endorsing any suicide seems so contradictory to good healthcare practice because nurses and mental health professionals have been intervening for years to prevent suicide. Many times, nurses' responses are guided by their cultural, religious, and personal beliefs. Autonomy and beneficence need to be considered when nurses are deciding about interventions to provide for persons who are planning rational suicide. Interventions become unique to each situation and can include everything from being asked to provide information regarding the Hemlock Society to being asked about lethal injections. Because nurses are closely involved with end-of-life decision making, the issue of nurses' responsibility with voluntary active euthanasia is increasingly a common dilemma.

> **CRITICAL THINKING QUESTIONS** *
>
> If the nurse knows of a plan for rational suicide, would the nurse be obligated to intervene? If so, what actions could the nurse take at this point? Does a nurse have the right to try to stop a person from committing rational suicide (to act in the best interest of the patient)? Is a nurse supposed to support the person's autonomous decision to commit rational suicide, even when that decision is morally and religiously incompatible with the nurse's perspective? *

Palliative Care

Palliative care is providing comfort rather than curative measures for terminally ill patients. Nurses are actively involved in meeting the palliative needs of dying patients. In the last decade, the palliative care movement has become quite organized through official associations and organizations. The World Health Organization (n.d.) defined palliative care as follows:

> An approach that improves the quality of life of patients and their families facing the problem associated with life-threatening illness, through the prevention and relief of suffering by means of early identification and impeccable assessment and treatment of pain and other problems, physical, psychosocial, and spiritual. (para. 1)

When a patient chooses to receive this type of care, nurses need to understand they do not hasten or prolong death for these patients; they provide relief of pain and suffering and attempt to allow the patient to die with dignity. Patients or patients' families may choose to forgo, withhold, or withdraw treatment. Some patients have a do-not-resuscitate order, which is a written physician's order placed in the patient's chart in an attempt to ensure that no resuscitative measures are initiated when a patient's cardiopulmonary functions cease. Usually there is one of three reasons for the decision to initiate a do-not-resuscitate order: (1) there is no medical benefit that can come from cardiopulmonary resuscitation (CPR), (2) the person had a very poor quality of life before CPR, or (3) the person's life after CPR is anticipated to be very poor (Mappes & DeGrazia, 2001).

Rule of Double Effect

The **rule of double effect** is defined narrowly in health care as the use of high doses of pain medication to lessen the chronic and intractable pain of terminally ill patients even if doing so hastens death (Quill, 2001). The first group to define the rule of double effect was the Roman Catholic Church in medieval times. When the rule is applied, nurses need to be aware that the harmful effect, or the hastening of death, can be foreseen but is not the intended outcome of their actions. According to Quill (2001), critical aspects of the rule are as follows:

- The act must be good or at least morally neutral.
- The agent must intend the good effect and not the evil effect (which can be "foreseen" but not intended).
- The evil effect must not be the means to the good effect.
- There must be a "proportionally grave reason" to risk the evil effect. (p. 167)

Nurses might have conflicting moral values concerning the use of high doses of pain medications, such as morphine sulfate. In times when nurses feel uncomfortable, they need to explore their attitudes and opinions with their supervisor and, when appropriate, in clinical team meetings. In the *Code of Ethics for Nurses with Interpretive Statements*, the ANA (2015) supports nurses to reach a good resolution through considered decisions. Decisions related to withholding and withdrawing life-sustaining interventions, foregoing nutrition and hydration, and palliative care are examples of decisions that are commonly recognized as requiring careful consideration. In addition, the ANA directs nurses to provide interventions aimed at pain relief and other care congruent with palliative care standards; however, the nurse "may not act with the sole intent to end life" (Provision 1.4, p. 3).

The Greek philosopher and scientist Aristotle (Aristotle, 2005; Broadie, 2002) labeled a considered judgment as **practical wisdom**, or *phronêsis*, which is a notion he believed requires calculated intellectual ability, contemplation, and deliberation.

Refusing or Forgoing Treatment

Well-informed patients with decision-making capacity have the autonomous right to refuse or forgo recommended treatments (Jonsen, Siegler, & Winslade, 2002). When a person elects to forgo treatment, most of the time there is no ethical or legal backlash. The courts uphold the right of competent patients to refuse treatment (Jonsen et al., 2002; Mappes & DeGrazia, 2001). Even so, it is of the utmost importance that healthcare professionals make certain the patient's decision is noncoercive and autonomous, and the decision has been made based on the patient's mentally competent decision-making capacity (Mappes & DeGrazia, 2001). Although nurses and other healthcare professionals might have the assurance of the patient's autonomous and competent decision making, sometimes the patient's decision is difficult to accept. Refusal of medical treatments can occur at any time in life, whether at the end of life or not, such as when patients refuse treatment based on religious or cultural beliefs.

Deciding for Others

When patients are no longer able to make competent decisions, families can experience problems in trying to determine a progressive right course of action. The ideal situation is for patients to be autonomous decision makers, but when autonomy is no longer possible, decision making falls to a surrogate (Beauchamp & Childress, 2012). The surrogate, or proxy, either is chosen by the patient, is court appointed, or has other authority to make decisions.

There are three standards for surrogate decision making (Beauchamp & Childress, 2012; Veatch, 2003). The **standard of substituted judgment** is used to guide medical decisions that involve formerly competent patients who no longer have any decision-making capacity. This standard is based on the assumption that incompetent patients have the exact same rights as competent patients to make judgments about their health care (Buchanan & Brock, 1990). Surrogates make medical treatment decisions based on how the surrogates believe that patients would have decided were the patients still competent and able to express their wishes. In making decisions, the surrogates use their understanding of the patients' previous overt or implied expressions of their beliefs and values (Veatch, 2003). Before losing competency, the patient could have either explicitly informed the proxy of treatment wishes by oral or written instruction or implicitly made clear treatment wishes through informal conversations with the proxy.

Decisions based on the **pure autonomy standard** are made on behalf of an incompetent person and are based on decisions the formerly competent person made. This type of decision also is called the principle of autonomy extended, meaning a person's autonomy continues to be honored even when the person cannot exercise autonomy through normal channels. The **best interest standard** is based on the goal of the surrogate's doing what is best for the patient or what is in the best interest of the patient (Veatch, 2003). This standard is applied when the patient the proxy or surrogate represents has never been competent, such as a child.

Withholding and Withdrawing Treatment

People in society and healthcare professionals have accepted and ethically justified withholding and withdrawing treatments that have been deemed as futile care, or possibly extraordinary. When a treatment has no physiologic benefit for a terminally ill person, the treatment is known as **medical futility** (Beauchamp & Childress, 2012). These types of medical treatments can include CPR, medications, mechanical ventilation, artificial feeding and fluids, hemodialysis, chemotherapy, and other life-sustaining technologies. Futility issues need to be discussed among nurses, physicians, family members, and patients when possible. A court-appointed proxy or family surrogate can be the spokesperson and decision maker for the patient. Nurses need to ensure that an appropriate decision-making process between the healthcare team and the decision makers for the patient takes place for all involved people to express feelings and concerns (Ladd, Pasquerella, & Smith, 2002).

Three Legal Cases

Three cases generated landmark decisions about withholding and withdrawing treatments. These court rulings led to decisions that set a precedent, such as right to die, right to privacy, and right to receive or refuse treatment. Additionally, some of the court rulings brought new recognition, expansion, and progress to some concepts. The President's Commission defined death, which led to the UDDA in 1981. The Quinlan case contributed to the definition of the term *persistent vegetative state* and the development of advance directives. The Cruzan case established conditions for withdrawing treatments and the expansion of advance directives for health care.

Case 1: Karen Ann Quinlan.   In 1975, Karen Ann Quinlan's case reaffirmed a person's right to privacy by choosing the right to die, discontinue mechanical ventilation, and make decisions to receive or refuse any treatment (Jonsen et al., 1998). However, once the New Jersey physicians removed Karen Ann Quinlan from the mechanical ventilator, she continued to breathe. Karen Ann Quinlan's continuance to live, once unplugged, alerted ethicists and physicians to rethink her definition of brain death, because they realized she was not brain dead because her lower brain's vital functioning enabled her to continue to breathe. Instead, she was in a persistent vegetative state.

A few years before the Karen Ann Quinlan case, Jannett and Plum (1972) had already coined the term **persistent vegetative state** and defined it as a patient condition with severe brain injury and coma that has progressed to a state of wakefulness without detectable awareness. Then, in 1994, the Multi-Society Task Force on persistent vegetative state defined in more detail persistent vegetative state as:

> ...a clinical condition of complete unawareness of the self and the environment, accompanied by sleep-wake cycles with either complete or partial preservation of hypothalamic and brain-stem autonomic functions. The condition may be transient, marking a stage in the recovery from severe acute or chronic brain damage, or permanent, as a consequence of the failure to recover from such injuries. The vegetative state can also occur as a result of the relentless progression of degenerative or metabolic neurologic diseases or from developmental malformations of the nervous system. The vegetative state can be diagnosed according to the following criteria: (1) no evidence of awareness of self or environment and an inability to interact with others; (2) no evidence of sustained, reproducible, purposeful, or voluntary behavioral responses to visual, auditory, tactile, or noxious stimuli; (3) no evidence of language comprehension or expression; (4) intermittent wakefulness manifested by the presence of sleep–wake cycles; (5) sufficiently preserved hypothalamic and brain-stem autonomic functions to permit survival with medical and nursing care; (6) bowel and bladder incontinence; and (7) variably preserved cranial-nerve reflexes (pupillary, oculocephalic, corneal, vestibulo-ocular, and gag) and spinal reflexes. (p. 1500)

Case 2: Nancy Cruzan.   In 1983, Nancy Cruzan, age 25, lost control of her car on a Missouri road; the accident resulted in a diagnosis of sustained brain injury. She remained in a coma for years. In 1990, the U.S. Supreme Court of Missouri overturned a previous ruling and established three conditions in the ruling: (1) the patient has a right to refuse medical treatment, (2) artificial feeding constitutes medical treatment, and (3) if the patient is mentally incompetent, then each state must document clear and convincing evidence that the patient's desires were for discontinuance of medical treatment (Jonsen et al., 1998).

Case 3: Terri Schiavo.   A more recent case was that of Theresa "Terri" Marie Schiavo, a young woman in a persistent vegetative state for 15 years. She died on March 31, 2005. There were a total of 21 legal suits, but the last few cases involved the request of her husband Michael Schiavo to have her feeding tube discontinued, which also would end her artificial nutrition and hydration. Terri's parents forcefully fought this request. According to Florida law, Michael Schiavo as a spouse and guardian had a legal right to serve as a surrogate decision maker for Terri Schiavo.

In conjunction with this legal right, the standard of substituted judgment served as the ethical standard. Because Terri Schiavo had no written advance directive, her surrogate was charged with making an unbiased substituted judgment about her care. The judgment should be based on an understanding of what she would decide for herself and not the values of the surrogate. Michael Schiavo and other people testified that Terri had stated she did not want to live in a condition in which she would be a burden to anyone else. This evidence served as the basis for many of the court's denials of her parents' requests to continue Terri's artificial nutrition and hydration.

In the *Code of Ethics for Nurses with Interpretive Statements*, Provision 1.4, the ANA (2015) takes the position that nurses ethically support the provision of compassionate and dignified end-of-life care as long as nurses do not have the sole intention of ending a person's life. Before Terri Schiavo died, a special statement concerning the case was released to the press by the president of the ANA on March 23, 2005, which upheld the decision for the right of a patient or surrogate to choose forgoing artificial nutrition and hydration. No matter what the outcome of difficult end-of-life decisions, family members and patients need to feel a sense of confidence that nurses will maintain moral sensitivity and good judgment.

Terminal Sedation

Legally permissible yet ethically controversial, **terminal sedation (TS)** seems to be moving slowly toward a social and an ethical acceptance (Quill, 2001). Quill (2001) defined TS as follows:

> When a suffering patient is sedated to unconsciousness, usually through the ongoing administration of barbiturates or benzodiazepines. The patient then dies of dehydration, starvation, or some other intervening complication, as all other life-sustaining interventions are withheld. (p. 181)

When the word *terminal* is used, there is an understanding among the healthcare team members and family that the outcome, and possibly a desired outcome, is death (Sugarman, 2000). TS has been used in situations when patients severely suffer and need pain relief, which requires being sedated to the point of unconsciousness. The ANA (2015) did not address TS directly in the *Code of Ethics for Nurses with Interpretive Statements*, but does state nurses are to give compassionate care at the end of life. The ANA emphasized that nurses are not to have the sole intent of ending a person's life.

Physician-Assisted Suicide

Moral outrage toward acceptance regarding PAS has occurred in society. **Physician-assisted suicide (PAS)** is defined as "the act of providing a lethal dose of medication for the patient to self-administer" (Sugarman, 2000, p. 213). Five states and one state's county have approved PAS: Oregon, Washington, Vermont, Montana, and California (Volz, Dubois, Rathke, &

BOX 14-2   DID BRITTANY MAYNARD HAVE A RIGHT TO CHOOSE PHYSICIAN-ASSISTED SUICIDE?

Brittany Maynard was 29 years old and married for 1 year when she was diagnosed with aggressive brain cancer and had approximately 6 months left to live. She decided that she did not want her family to watch her suffering with pain during her dying process. After a long discussion with her physicians, her husband, and other family members, she decided to move from California to Oregon to take advantage of the Death with Dignity Act. She opted for physician assisted suicide (PAS), which is a procedure that would allow her to self-administer physician-prescribed barbiturate medications to facilitate her death. She chose to die on November 1, 2014. Before her death, Brittany made a public statement on the right of terminally ill people to end their suffering quickly by emphasizing her own argument that no one could determine when her suffering became intolerable, when her life became unlivable, and at what point her dignity was fading.

1. What ethical issues arise during and after the decision to opt for PAS?
2. What is your opinion of Brittany Maynard's decision to end her life at age 29 years? Please explore your rationale and explain.

Source: Data from Maynard, B. (2014, November 2). My right to die with dignity at 29. Retrieved from http://www .cnn.com/2014/10/07/opinion/maynard-assisted-suicide-cancer-dignity/

Blankinship, 2015), in addition to the mandated ruling in Bernalillo County, New Mexico (Eckholm, 2014). The Oregon Death with Dignity Act (Oregon Health Authority, 1994) was the first law on PAS. With certain restrictions, patients who are near death can obtain prescriptions to end their lives in a dignified way. A case study by Butts (2016b; 2016d) is a recent example of a dying person's exercise of her right to PAS (see **Box 14-2**).

Although the ANA (2015), in the *Code of Ethics for Nurses with Interpretive Statements*, plainly states nurses are not to act with the sole intent of ending a person's life, the Oregon Nurses Association issued special guidelines for nurses that relate to the Death with Dignity Act (Ladd et al., 2002). The guidelines include (1) maintaining support, comfort, and confidentiality, (2) discussing end-of-life options with the patient and family, and (3) being present for the patient's self-administration of medications and during the death. Nurses may not administer the medications themselves, breach confidentiality, subject others to any type of judgmental comments or statements about the patient, or refuse care to the patient.

End-of-Life Decisions and Moral Conflicts

Nurses first must sort out their own feelings about the various types of euthanasia before appropriate guidance and direction can be offered to patients and families. In one Japanese study of 160 nurses, Konishi, Davis, and Toshiaki (2002) studied withdrawal of artificial food and fluid from terminally ill patients. The majority of the nurses supported this act only under two conditions: (1) if the patient requested the withdrawal of artificial food and fluids and (2) if the act relieved the patient's suffering. Nurses agreed that comfort for the patient was a great concern. One nurse in the study stated this: "[Artificial food and fluid] AFF only prolongs the patient's suffering. When withdrawn, the patient showed peace on the face. I have seen such patients so many times" (Konishi et al., 2002). In the same study, another nurse who was experiencing an ethical conflict with the decision to withdraw the artificial food and fluid stated: "Withdrawal is killing and cruel. I feel guilty" (Konishi et al., 2002).

Other end-of-life issues can generate ethical conflicts, as well. Georges and Grypdonck (2002) conducted a literature review on the topic of ethical issues in terms of how nurses perceive their care to dying patients. They outlined some of the moral dilemmas particularly related to nurses and end-of-life care. Some of the ethical issues that nurses experienced were the following:

- Communicating truthfully with patients about death because they were fearful of destroying all hope among the patient and family
- Managing pain symptoms because of fear of hastening death
- Feeling forced to collaborate with other health team members about medical treatments that in nurses' opinions were futile or too burdensome
- Feeling insecure and not adequately informed about reasons for treatment
- Trying to maintain their own moral integrity throughout relationships with patients, families, and coworkers because of feeling that they were forced to betray their own moral values

Although the conscientious nurse has an obligation to provide compassionate and palliative care, the nurse also has a right to withdraw from treating and caring for a patient as long as another nurse has assumed care for the dying patient. When care is such that the nurse perceives it as violating personal morality and values, the professional nurse must seek alternative approaches to achieve patients' goals.

Conclusion

Nurses' involvement with bioethical issues has become more complicated with advances in technology that impact patient care options and trajectories. Nurses must learn to cultivate good professional relationships and avoid being distracted by the stresses of delivering ethical and patient-centered direct or indirect patient care. Practicing ethical nursing care cannot be based merely on intuitive functioning; rather, nurses must understand key ethical concepts and seek active involvement in being valuable members of healthcare teams.

CASE STUDY 14-1 ▪ END-OF-LIFE CARE

Gertrude, an 85-year-old woman, was diagnosed with end-stage renal disease, long-standing adult-onset diabetes, and aortic stenosis. Her renal disease now has led to a terminal condition. Still conscious, she told her youngest daughter she wanted no life-sustaining measures done. The next day, she lost consciousness. Then, her other two daughters arrived at the hospital from out of town. The three daughters argued about the treatment for their mother; the youngest wanted to honor the wishes of her mother and the other two wanted full medical treatment to be initiated. The physician and nurse discussed the treatment options and the futility issue with the family. To avoid further disagreement, the youngest daughter decided to go along with the decision of the other two sisters.

Case Study Questions

1. Explain the reason that the physician and nurse discussed futile treatment with the daughters.

2. Do you believe the mother had a right to choose her course of treatment? Explain.

3. Discuss the end-of-life options the daughters could have chosen for their mother's care had they chosen the "no treatment" option.

4. Discuss the different types of surrogate decision making. Was there a surrogate decision maker in this family? Explain.

5. What specific nursing support and care could you offer to this family and patient?

References

American Nurses Association. (2005, March 23). Press release: The American Nurses Association statement on the Terri Schiavo case. Statement Attributed to Barbara A. Blakeney, MS, RN, President. Retrieved from http://www.nursingworld.org /FunctionalMenuCategories/MediaResources/PressReleases/2005/pr03238523.aspx

American Nurses Association. (2015). *Code of ethics for nurses with interpretive statements*. Silver Spring, MD: Author.

Angeles, P. A. (1992). *The HarperCollins dictionary of philosophy* (2nd ed.). New York, NY: HarperCollins.

Aristotle. (2005). *Nicomachean ethics*. (W. D. Ross, Trans.). Stilwell, KS: Digireads.com Publishing.

Australian Museum. (2009). What is death? Retrieved from http://australianmuseum .net.au/What-is-death

Beauchamp, T. L., & Childress, J. F. (2012). *Principles of biomedical ethics* (7th ed.). New York, NY: Oxford University Press.

Benjamin, M. (2003). Pragmatism and the determination of death. In G. McGee (Ed.), *Pragmatic bioethics* (2nd ed., pp. 193–206). London, England: Bradford Book, MIT Press.

Benner, P., Sutphen, M., Leonard, V., & Day, L. (2010). *Educating nurses: A call for radical transformation*. San Francisco, CA: Jossey-Bass.

Bondeson, J. (2001). *Buried alive: The terrifying history of our most primal fear*. New York, NY: W. W. Norton.

Brannigan, M. C., & Boss, J. A. (2001). *Healthcare ethics in a diverse society*. Mountain View, CA: Mayfield.

Broadie, S. (2002). Philosophical introduction. In S. Broadie & C. Rowe (Eds.), C. Rowe (Trans.), *Aristotle: Nicomachean ethics* (pp. 1–91). New York, NY: Oxford University Press.

Buchanan, A. E., & Brock, D. W. (1990). *Deciding for others: The ethics of surrogate decision making*. New York, NY: Cambridge University Press.

Butts, J. B. (2016a). Adult health nursing ethics. In J. B. Butts & K. L. Rich (Eds.), *Nursing ethics: Across the curriculum and into practice* (4th ed., pp. 219–239). Burlington, MA: Jones & Bartlett Learning.

Butts, J. B. (2016b). Ethical issues in end-of-life nursing care. In J. B. Butts & K. L. Rich (Eds.), *Nursing ethics: Across the curriculum and into practice* (4th ed., pp. 271–313). Burlington, MA: Jones & Bartlett Learning.

Butts, J. B. (2016c). Ethics in professional nursing practice. In J. B. Butts & K. L. Rich (Eds.), *Nursing ethics: Across the curriculum and into practice* (4th ed., pp. 71–121). Burlington, MA: Jones & Bartlett Learning.

Butts, J. B. (2016d). The case of Brittany Maynard: "My right to die." In J. B. Butts & K. L. Rich (Eds.), *Nursing ethics: Across the curriculum and into practice* (4th ed., pp. 449–450). Burlington, MA: Jones & Bartlett Learning.

Center for Economic and Social Justice. (n.d.). Defining economic justice and social justice. Retrieved from http://cesj.org/learn/definitions/defining-economic-justice -and-social-justice/

Centers for Disease Control and Prevention. (2012). Suicide: Facts at a glance. Retrieved from http://www.cdc.gov/violenceprevention/pdf/suicide-datasheet-a .pdf

Chambliss, D. E. (1996). *Beyond caring: Hospitals, nurses, and the social organization of ethics*. Chicago, IL: University of Chicago Press.

Daniels, N. (1985). *Just health care*. Cambridge, England: Cambridge University Press.

Davis, K., Stremikis, K., Squires, D., & Schoen, C. (2014, June 16). Mirror, mirror on the wall, 2014 update: How the U.S. health care systems compares internationally. The Commonwealth Fund. Retrieved from http://www.commonwealthfund.org /publications/fund-reports/2014/jun/mirror-mirror

Devettere, R. J. (2000). *Practical decision making in health care ethics: Cases and concepts* (2nd ed.). Washington, DC: Georgetown University Press.

Eckholm, E. (2014, January 13). New Mexico judge affirms right to 'aid in dying.' Retrieved from http://www.nytimes.com/2014/01/14/us/new-mexico-judge-affirms -right-to-aid-in-dying.html?_r=0

Engelhardt, H. T. (1996). *Rights to health care, social justice, and fairness in health care allocations: Frustrations in the face of finitude: The foundations of bioethics* (2nd ed.). New York, NY: Oxford University Press.

Finnerty, J. L. (1987). Ethics in rational suicide. *Critical Care Nursing Quarterly, 10*(2), 86–90.

Fry, S., & Johnstone, M. J. (2002). *Ethics in nursing practice: A guide to ethical decision making* (2nd ed.). Oxford, England: Blackwell Science.

Georges, J. J., & Grypdonck, M. (2002). Moral problems experienced by nurses when caring for terminally ill people: A literature review. *Nursing Ethics, 9*(2), 155–178.

International Council of Nurses. (2012). *The ICN code of ethics for nurses*. Geneva, Switzerland: Author. Retrieved from http://www.dsr.dk/ser/documents/icncode _english.pdf

Jameton, A. (1984). *Nursing practice: The ethical issues*. Englewood Cliffs, NJ: Prentice Hall.

Jannett, B., & Plum, F. (1972). Persistent vegetative state after brain damage: A syndrome in search of a name. *The Lancet, 1*(7753), 734–737.

Jonsen, A. R., Siegler, M., & Winslade, W. J. (2002). *Clinical ethics* (5th ed.). New York, NY: McGraw-Hill.

Jonsen, A. R., Veatch, R. M., & Walters, L. (1998). *Source book in bioethics*. Washington, DC: Georgetown University Press.

Kelly, C. (2000). *Nurses' moral practice: Investing and discounting self*. Indianapolis, IN: Sigma Theta Tau International.

Koch, K. A. (1992). Patient Self-Determination Act. *Journal of the Florida Medical Association, 79*(4), 240–243.

Konishi, E., Davis, A. J., & Toshiaki, A. (2002). The ethics of withdrawing artificial food and fluid from terminally ill patients: An end-of-life dilemma for Japanese nurses and families. *Nursing Ethics, 9*(1), 7–19.

Ladd, R. E., Pasquerella, L., & Smith, S. (2002). *Ethical issues in home health care*. Springfield, IL: Charles C Thomas.

MacIntyre, A. (1999). *Dependent rational animals*. Chicago, IL: Open Court.

Maes, S. (2003). How do you know when professional boundaries have been crossed? *Oncology Nursing Society News, 18*(8), 3–5.

Mappes, T. A., & DeGrazia, D. (2001). *Biomedical ethics* (5th ed.). Boston, MA: McGraw-Hill.

Massachusetts Department of Higher Education. (2010). *Nurse of the future: Nursing core competencies*. Retrieved from http://www.mass.edu/currentinit/documents/NursingCoreCompetencies.pdf

Maynard, B. (2014, November 2). My right to die with dignity at 29. Retrieved from http://www.cnn.com/2014/10/07/opinion/maynard-assisted-suicide-cancer-dignity/

McKenna, B. G., Smith, N. A., Poole, S. J., & Coverdale, J. H. (2003). Horizontal violence: Experiences of registered nurses in their first year of practice. *Journal of Advanced Nursing, 42*(1), 90–96.

Multi-Society Task Force on PVS. (1994, May 26). Part 2: Medical aspects of persistent vegetative state. *New England Journal of Medicine, 330*(21), 1499–1508.

Munson, R. (2004). *Intervention and reflection: Basic issues in medical ethics* (7th ed.). Victoria, Australia: Wadsworth.

National Center for Health Statistics. (2012). *Healthy people 2010 final review*. Hyattsville, MD: U.S. Department of Health and Human Services. Retrieved from http://www.cdc.gov/nchs/data/hpdata2010/hp2010_final_review.pdf

Novak, M. (2000). Defining social justice. *First Things First, 108*, 11–13.

Nozick, R. (1974). *Anarchy, state and utopia*. New York, NY: Basic Books.

Office of Disease Prevention and Health Promotion. (2014). Healthy people 2020: Topics and objectives. U.S. Department of Health and Human Services. Retrieved from http://www.healthypeople.gov/2020/topicsobjectives2020/default

Oregon Health Authority. (1994). Death with dignity act. Retrieved from https://public.health.oregon.gov/ProviderPartnerResources/EvaluationResearch/DeathwithDignityAct/Pages/index.aspx

Organ Procurement and Transplantation Network. (n.d.a). At a glance. Retrieved from http://optn.transplant.hrsa.gov

Organ Procurement and Transplantation Network. (n.d.b). How organ allocation works. Retrieved from http://optn.transplant.hrsa.gov/learn/about-transplantation/how-organ-allocation-works/

President's Commission for the Study of Ethical Problems in Medicine and Biomedical and Behavioral Research. (1981). *Defining death*. Washington, DC: U.S. Government Printing Office.

Quill, T. E. (2001). *Caring for patients at the end of life: Facing an uncertain future together*. New York, NY: Oxford University Press.

Rawls, J. (1971). *A theory of justice*. Cambridge, MA: Harvard University Press.

Shotton, L., & Seedhouse, D. (1998). Practical dignity in caring. *Nursing Ethics, 5*(3), 246–255.

Siegel, K. (1986). Psychosocial aspects of rational suicide. *American Journal of Psychotherapy, 40*(3), 405–418.

Sokolowski, R. (1991). The fiduciary relationship and the nature of professions. In E. D. Pellegrino, R. M. Veatch, & J. P. Langan (Eds.), *Ethics, trust, and the professions: Philosophical and cultural aspects* (pp. 23–43). Washington, DC: Georgetown University Press.

Stein, L. I., Watts, D. T., & Howell, T. (1990). The doctor–nurse game revisited. *Nursing Outlook, 38*(6), 264–268.

Sugarman, J. (2000). *20 common problems: Ethics in primary care*. New York, NY: McGraw-Hill.

Veatch, R. M. (2003). *The basics of bioethics* (2nd ed.). Upper Saddle River, NJ: Prentice Hall.

Volz, M., Dubois, S., Rathke, L., & Blankinship, D. (2015, October 6). A look at efforts to legalize physicial-assisted suicide. Retrieved from http://www.nytimes.com/aponline/2015/10/06/us/ap-us-right-to-die-california-qa.html

Wildes, K. W. (2000). Moral acquaintances: Methodology in bioethics. Notre Dame, IN: University of Notre Dame Press.

World Health Organization. (2014). Suicide: Key facts. Retrieved from http://www.who.int/mediacentre/factsheets/fs398/en/

World Health Organization. (n.d.). WHO definition of palliative care. Retrieved from http://www.who.int/cancer/palliative/definition/en/

Youngner, S. J., & Arnold, R. M. (2001). Philosophical debates about the definition of death: Who cares? *Journal of Medicine and Philosophy, 26*(5), 527–537.

Zaner, R. M. (1991). The phenomenon of trust and the patient–physician relationship. In E. D. Pellegrino, R. M. Veatch, & J. P. Langan (Eds.), *Ethics, trust, and the professions: Philosophical and cultural aspects* (pp. 45–67). Washington, DC: Georgetown University Press.

CHAPTER 15

Law and the Professional Nurse

Kathleen Driscoll, Kathleen Masters, and Evadna Lyons

Learning Objectives

After completing this chapter, the student should be able to:

1. Discuss the functions and sources of law as they relate to nursing practice.
2. Describe civil proceedings including the nurse's role as an expert witness.
3. Discuss the scope and standards of professional nursing practice.
4. Discuss the elements of malpractice and negligence.
5. Examine the functions of the state boards of nursing.
6. Apply the concept of professional accountability to professional and legal standards in relationship to informed consent, confidentiality, and privacy.
7. Examine the legal aspects of delegation.
8. Examine strategies for avoiding legal problems.

The professions of law and nursing are both devoted to helping patients, clients, and society. A harmonious interaction between the areas of law and nursing is necessary for achieving effective outcomes for both the nurse and the patient. Nurses must understand how the legal system works to be safe and effective practitioners. The advanced state of medical technology creates new legal, ethical, moral, and financial problems for the consumer and the healthcare practitioner. Patients are more aware of their legal rights; hence, nurses must make a concerted effort to practice by the legal and professional standards set forth by federal and state entities.

Law and nursing are both professions devoted to helping patients/clients and society by advocating for healthcare improvements and justice. Law serves as a guiding force for relationships between persons, persons and groups, and groups and other groups. Note the words *guiding* and *force*. For guidance to occur, law must be developed. For implementation to occur, the law must be enforced.

Key Terms and Concepts

» Statutory law
» Lobbyists
» Administrative (or regulatory) law
» Case law
» Civil law
» Tort
» Reasonable standard of care
» Expert witness
» Scope of nursing practice
» Standards of nursing practice
» Professional performance standards

Law evolves by accommodating to changes in society while adhering to the basic principles set forth in a nation's guiding document, which in the United States is the Constitution. Principles set forth in the Constitution include freedom of religion and assembly, freedom from undue interference by government, and the right to trial by jury in criminal cases. Three sources of law are built on the fundamental law of the federal Constitution. They are statutory law, administrative law or regulatory law, and case law. It is important to note that federal law is administered the same way in all states. However, each state might vary on how it interprets and implements laws. Hence, interpretation of legal issues for nurses varies from state to state.

Nursing and healthcare law set forth nursing and health policy goals. A nurse practice act has the goal of protecting the safety of the public who receive nursing care. Each state has statutes that govern the practice of nursing, and although some differences exist from state to state, in general the nurse practice acts define who must be licensed, requirements for licensure, duties of the licensed nurse, and grounds on which the license may be revoked or taken away. This chapter discusses the sources of law and professional and legal accountability in nursing practice.

The Sources of Law

Statutory Law

In a democratic society such as the United States, the people elect representatives to governing bodies that consider proposed legislation. Most states and the federal government have a legislative body that is composed of two houses. The federal government has the House of Representatives and the Senate. Most state legislatures have similar names for their legislative bodies. Together the federal legislative body is termed Congress. Most state legislatures also have inclusive names for their legislative bodies; for example, the combination of two state bodies might carry a designation such as General Assembly.

Statutory law consists of ever-changing rules and regulations created by the U.S. Congress, state legislators, local governments, and constitutional law. The statutes are the rights, privileges, or immunities secured and protected for each citizen by the U.S. Constitution (Fremgen, 2002).

The process of creating legislation is complex. The process can begin with a legislator responding to the interests of a group of persons. A legislator might also initiate action on a problem by convening a group of interested persons or other legislators to consider legislative options for resolving the problem. Interested persons or groups can represent specific concerns. Since the turn of the 21st century, nursing organizations such as the American Nurses Association (ANA) and the American Association of Colleges of Nursing have focused on legislation addressing patient safety, such as specific staffing levels and controlling mandatory overtime. Such organized groups often hire lobbyists rather than relying on group members to promote their interests to legislators.

Lobbyists develop expertise on proposed legislation and learn to present that information to legislators clearly and concisely. Conscientious legislators and their staffs listen to both sides before voting on an issue. On a very important issue, however, organizations also encourage their members to write letters supporting the organization's position or to make an appointment to speak with the legislator or talk with the legislator's staff.

Generally, no action is taken on bills introduced to legislative bodies unless there is a confluence of problems, solutions, and political circumstances that create a climate for passing legislation (Longest, 2002). Many more bills are introduced into Congress and the state legislatures than are passed. Legislative action alone is insufficient for a bill to become law. Congressional bills require the president's signature, and state bills require the signature of the state's governor to be enacted into law. The president and state governors can also choose to veto legislation. This check on legislative power by the executive branch of government is part of the system of balances among the branches of government ensured by the nation's founders.

Administrative Law (Regulations)

Once a bill becomes law, that law is subject to further refinement by federal or state agencies, which are part of the executive branch of government. Enacted statutory law states what Congress or a state legislature wants to accomplish and what activities should occur to accomplish the legislative goal. Federal or state agencies carry out that activity by developing regulations that further define the law and establish the procedures for administering the law. For example, a state nurse practice act might provide that advanced practice nurses develop a formulary of medications they may prescribe. The process for developing the formulary will be done through the rule-making or regulatory process.

The regulatory process is itself governed by statutory law called administrative procedure acts at both federal and state levels. These acts provide that before regulations can be adopted, a published notice of the proposed rules and where they are available must occur. The published notice and availability of the proposed rules provide concerned persons with the opportunity to comment on and suggest changes to the rules before final adoption. When rules are adopted, they become **administrative (or regulatory) law** within a set period of time. Thus, the process has three steps: (1) proposal of regulations, (2) consideration of proposed regulations, and (3) adoption of regulations with or without changes.

Staffs of executive branch agencies develop proposed regulations. In the case of federal regulations, notice of the proposed regulations is provided through a publication called the *Federal Register*. An example is Medicare regulations that describe conditions for healthcare facilities to receive reimbursement. This is a serious concern for hospitals because a high percentage of hospital revenue comes from Medicare reimbursement. Information on federal statutory and administrative law is available at http://thomas.loc.gov. Information on state law can be found at state websites. These can be accessed by entering terms such as *State of Ohio* or *State of California* in an Internet search.

Case Law

Case law is established from court decisions, which can explain or interpret the other sources of law. For example, a court case might explain what the constitution, a statute, or a regulation means. Case law or common law also defines legal rights and obligations. For example, a nurse's obligation to practice as a reasonably prudent nurse is a legal obligation stemming from actual court decisions. Case law is based on precedent, meaning a ruling in one case is subsequently applied to later similar cases. When case law is applied, it must be reviewed by the court to determine if it is still relevant; hence, many case laws are changed and updated over the years. The prevailing ruler over case law is ultimately the state supreme court for state laws and the U.S. Supreme Court for federal statutes. When the judicial branch of government becomes involved, it creates case law. The judicial branch of government is the third component of the balance of power in government at both the federal and state levels.

Classification and Enforcement of the Law

When people choose not to follow the law, courts have the obligation to enforce the law. Enforcers of the law also include police and prosecutors. The Justice Department at the federal level and the attorney general's offices at the state level represent federal and state government interests. Judges are also enforcers of the law. In jury trials, they instruct jurors to apply the facts of a case to the law; in cases in which there is no jury, trial judges both examine the facts and apply the law.

Case law is both civil and criminal. **Civil law** involves relationships between individuals or between individuals and the government. Civil laws are divided into six categories: tort, contract, property, inheritance, family, and corporate law. Criminal law protects the public from the harmful acts of others.

Civil Law

Civil laws that commonly affect nurses include tort and contract laws. Tort law governs acts that result in harm to another. A **tort** is a wrongful act that is committed against another person or property that results in harm. Contract law includes enforceable agreements between two or more persons.

To sue for a tort, a patient must have suffered a mental or physical injury that was caused by the healthcare professional and the patient might recover monetary damages. Torts can be intentional or accidental. According to Fremgen (2002), intentional torts can include assault, battery, false imprisonment, defamation, fraud, and invasion of privacy:

- *Assault:* The threat of bodily harm to another. There does not have to be actual touching (battery) for an assault to take place; for example, threatening to harm a patient or to perform a procedure without the informed consent (permission) of the patient.
- *Battery:* Actual bodily harm to another person without permission. This is also referred to as unlawful touching or touching without consent; for example, performing surgery or a procedure without the informed consent (permission) of the patient.
- *False imprisonment:* A violation of the personal liberty of another person through unlawful restraint; for example, refusing to allow a patient to leave an office, a hospital, or a medical facility when the person requests to leave.
- *Defamation of character:* Damage caused to a person's reputation through spoken or written word; for example, making a negative statement about another nurse's ability.
- *Fraud:* Deceitful practice, such as promising a miracle cure.
- *Invasion of privacy:* The unauthorized publicity of information about a patient; for example, allowing personal information, such as test results for human immunodeficiency virus, to become public without the patient's permission.

An unintentional tort usually occurs when the nurse does not act within the reasonable standards of nursing care. A **reasonable standard of care** means that the nurse must implement the type of care that a reasonably prudent nurse would use in a similar circumstance. Often, unintentional torts result from negligence. Nurses should focus on preventing negligence rather than trying to defend it during a civil case.

The Trial Process for Civil Procedures

Nurses are most often involved in civil cases related to malpractice or negligence. The patient brings the case against the healthcare facility or nurse, who becomes the defendant. If the defendant loses, the plaintiff receives monetary damages as compensation for the injury. For a civil case to be won, the judge or jury must find a preponderance of evidence for the winning side.

Nurses should have a basic understanding of the proceedings involved in a civil trial because this is the type of trial that involves the nursing profession. In a civil case, if the judge or jury finds in favor of the plaintiff, the defendant will be ordered to pay the plaintiff a monetary award. A plaintiff or defendant may appeal the decision to a higher court (Havighurst, Blumstein, & Brennan, 1998). See **Figure 15-1** for an illustration of a civil trial procedure.

Figure 15-1   Example of a civil case flowchart

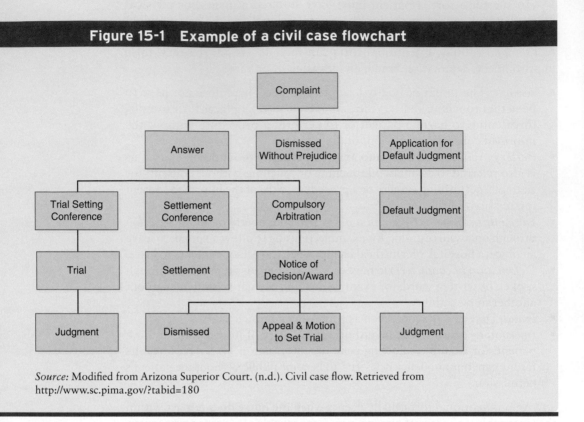

Source: Modified from Arizona Superior Court. (n.d.). Civil case flow. Retrieved from http://www.sc.pima.gov/?tabid=180

Nurses as Expert Witnesses

Nurses with advanced degrees and clinical knowledge are often called as an **expert witness** during civil trials. An expert witness has complex knowledge beyond the general knowledge of most people in the court or on the jury. Most nurses who testify as experts are called to testify as to what the "standard of care" for a patient is in a similar circumstance. Expert witnesses generally do not testify about the exact facts of the case. Instead, they clarify points of knowledge using charts, models, and diagrams.

Criminal Law

Criminal laws protect society from the harmful acts of others. Criminal acts are classified as felonies or misdemeanors. A felony carries a punishment of death or imprisonment in a state or federal facility. Felonies often involve murder, rape, robbery, or practicing without a license. Misdemeanors are less serious and include theft, traffic violations, and disturbing the peace. A nurse's license may be revoked by the state board of nursing if he or she is convicted of a crime.

A nurse selling or stealing drugs results in a criminal case. In a criminal case, society is the plaintiff, and the nurse becomes the defendant. If the nurse defendant loses, the nurse will have restrictions placed on his or her liberty. Restrictions can include a prison term, probation, or treatment in lieu of conviction. In the last situation, the restriction is compliance with a drug treatment program that includes random drug testing. Failure to comply with the treatment program can result in a criminal punishment such as probation or even incarceration. Criminal cases have a higher standard of evidence. Juries must find the defendant guilty beyond a reasonable doubt. The U.S. justice system is based on the premise that people are innocent until proven guilty. Because the plaintiff is claiming that the nurse violated the law, the burden of proof is placed upon the plaintiff to prove that the defendant is liable.

Boards of nursing also act as enforcers of the law when they discipline a nurse for violation of a provision of the law or rules of the state's nurse practice act. Boards use the preponderance-of-evidence standard rather than the higher standard required in criminal cases.

Nursing Scope and Standards

The nurse's duty is to function within the parameters of the **scope of nursing practice** and based on the established standards of the nursing profession. What is the scope of nursing practice? The profession of nursing has one scope of practice that encompasses the full range of nursing practice; however, "the depth and breadth in which individual registered nurses engage in the total scope of nursing practice are dependent on their education, experience, role and the population served" (ANA, 2010, p. 2). The scope of practice describes the who, what, where, when, why, and how of nursing practice.

According to the ANA, "nursing is the protection, promotion, optimization of health and abilities, prevention of illness and injury, facilitation of healing, alleviation of suffering through the diagnosis and treatment of human response, and advocacy in the care of individuals, families, groups, communities, and populations" (2015b, p. 1). The scope of nursing practice has its foundation in the definition of nursing and serves as a basis for the development of regulatory systems, quality improvement systems, reimbursement and financing methodologies, development and evaluation of nursing service delivery systems, certification activities, educational offerings, agency policies, position descriptions, and the establishment of legal standards of care (ANA, 2010).

What are the **standards of nursing practice**? The ANA defines standards of practice as "authoritative statements of the duties of all registered nurses, regardless of role, population, or specialty, are expected to perform competently" (ANA, 2015b, p. 3). ANA standards of practice are broad and are formatted according to the steps of the nursing process, which is the critical thinking tool of nursing. The steps include assessment, diagnosis, outcome identification, planning, implementation, and evaluation. The standards also include competencies expected of the graduate-level prepared nurse and advanced practice registered nurse (RN). Competencies accompany each standard that may be considered evidence of compliance; however, the list of competencies is not exhaustive for each standard, and whether a competency applies is dependent on the patient care circumstances (ANA, 2015b).

A legal nurse consultant or nurse expert scrutinizing a healthcare record at issue in a lawsuit can use these standards to determine whether there is reason to go forward with a malpractice suit. The nurse will also apply the more specialized and specific standards developed by specialty groups in nursing. For example, the Neonatal Nursing Association, the Association of Women's Health, Obstetric and Neonatal Nurses, and the American Association of Critical-Care Nurses have their own standards. Standards come from other sources as well. A good example is the Blood-Borne Pathogen Standard promulgated by the Occupational Safety and Health Administration. This standard is an example of a standard for all healthcare providers, not just nurses. The legal nurse consultant will expect that the nurses documenting in the medical record demonstrate current knowledge and competency based on general and specialized standards in their area of practice.

Standards of nursing practice are critical, but there are also standards that are expectations of a professional. Recognizing these expectations, the ANA elected to add **professional performance standards** to its 1991 standards document. Professional performance standards relate to how the nurse functions according to the standards of practice, completes the nursing process, and addresses other contemporary practice concerns. These standards address ethics, culturally congruent practice, communication, collaboration, leadership, education, evidence-based practice and research, quality of practice, professional practice evaluation, resource utilization, and environmental health (ANA, 2015b, pp. 5–6). Because the healthcare environment and the role of the professional nurse evolve over time in response to research, societal needs, and expectations, the ANA's professional performance standards have evolved since their initial publication. Practice and professional standards are also reflected in state practice acts and rules.

One of the standards applicable to this particular chapter topic is professional performance Standard 15. This standard indicates that the nurse is required to evaluate his or her own and others' nursing practice in relation to professional practice standards, guidelines, relevant statutes, rules, regulations, organizational policies, and procedures. Examples of competencies associated with this standard include that the nurse will engage in self-reflection and self-evaluation to identify areas for professional growth and will ensure that nursing practice is consistent with regulatory requirements pertaining to licensure (ANA, 2015b, p. 81).

Many state boards of nursing have used the Standards of Practice and Standards of Professional Performance to guide the development of their state nurse practice act or regulation. State boards of nursing also often defer to the professional standards when interpretation of practice is required (ANA, 2012, p. 30). ANA standards may be used by boards of nursing to develop scope of practice statements for licensure and to expand scope statements for advanced practice nurses; make decisions about new practices and procedures; define new categories of licensure, recognition, and certification; determine appropriateness and level of discipline; and define state accreditation of nursing educational programs (ANA, 2012, pp. 30–31).

Evidence of Standards of Care Used in Court

Standards of practice and professional performance are often used in nursing negligence and malpractice decisions as well as board of nursing actions. Standards are used to establish the standard of care, which is the level of care for which a nurse should be held accountable; this, in turn, is used by legal authorities to determine what should or should not have been done for a patient (ANA, 2012, p. 31). The following list includes types of evidence of standards of care that are often used in court:

- *Statutes:* Common law rules that mandate certain conduct. An example of a statute as evidence of the standard of care is child abuse reporting requirements. These statutes clearly state what a healthcare provider must do when child abuse is suspected.
- *Agency regulations:* Federal and state administrative agencies promulgate rules and regulations that also can affect the standard of care.
- *Accreditation standards:* The Joint Commission standards have been recognized in some court cases as evidence for standard of care.
- *Facility documents:* These might include policies, procedures, job descriptions, and professional nursing guidelines.
- *Manufacturer's instructions:* In regard to medical equipment or a medication involved in an injury, manufacturer instructions can be examined as standards of care.
- *Nursing literature:* This includes textbooks and journal articles.
- *Expert testimony:* Expert witnesses provide testimonial evidence relevant to duty and standard of care.

It is important to remember that nurses cannot be held as negligent if, when an incident happens, they were performing based on standards of practice. It would be up to their employer to accept liability on their behalf. However, when nurses fail to follow the standards of practice, it can result in claims of malpractice or negligence.

KEY COMPETENCY 15-1

Examples of Applicable *Nurse of the Future: Nursing Core Competencies*

Professionalism:

Knowledge (K2) Describes legal and regulatory factors that apply to nursing practice

Skills (S2a) Uses recognized professional standards of practice

Attitudes/Behaviors (A2a) Values professional standards of practice

Source: Massachusetts Department of Higher Education. (2010). *Nurse of the future: Nursing core competencies* (p. 13). Retrieved from http://www.mass.edu/currentinit/documents/NursingCoreCompetencies.pdf

KEY COMPETENCY 15-2

Examples of Applicable *Nurse of the Future: Nursing Core Competencies*

Professionalism:

Knowledge (K2) Describes legal and regulatory factors that apply to nursing practice

Skills (S2b) Implements plan of care within legal, ethical, and regulatory framework of nursing practice

Attitudes/Behaviors (A2b) Values and upholds legal and regulatory principles

Source: Massachusetts Department of Higher Education. (2010). *Nurse of the future: Nursing core competencies* (p. 13). Retrieved from http://www.mass.edu/currentinit/documents/NursingCoreCompetencies.pdf

Malpractice and Negligence

The public generally has a very positive view of nurses. Nurses are expected to be of good moral and ethical character because the public has a great deal of trust for nurses. Furthermore, the privilege of obtaining a nursing license is often overlooked as an opportunity, and the right to practice nursing is frequently perceived as an "incidental entitlement" after completing a nursing education (Clevette, Erbin-Rosenmann, & Kelly, 2007). The nurturing aspect of nursing supports a "goodwill" profile with little, if any, intention of wrongdoing, but it is worth mentioning that obtaining or maintaining the license to practice nursing is not viewed as a right, but rather as a privilege.

Most nurses are very familiar with the terms *negligence* and *malpractice*. What is the difference between the two? **Negligence** is defined as the failure to act as a reasonably prudent person would have acted in a specific situation (Finkelman, 2006). Can a nurse be brought to court for negligence? Yes. A finding of negligence occurs when the nurse owes a duty to a patient and breaches an ordinary standard of care known by laypersons, and the patient is harmed. An example would be the nurse leaving the side rail down on the bed of a 2-month-old infant. An ordinary person would know that leaving the side rail down is unsafe. Nurses can be both negligent and guilty of malpractice. Findings of either malpractice or negligence result in the nurse being liable to compensate the harmed person. A malpractice lawsuit requires an expert witness, whereas a negligence lawsuit does not.

Malpractice requires that the harm be foreseeable only by the nurse because a person without professional education would not know that harm could occur. An example is a nurse giving potassium to a patient who has not urinated postoperatively. With no route for excretion, potassium could build up in the body and cause a cardiac arrest. A layperson would not be expected to know this information. Another example is a nurse administering a patient's daily dose of Lanoxin without checking the apical pulse and without checking the digoxin level. The patient becomes bradycardic followed by a full cardiac arrest. Upon inspection of the patient's digoxin level, the nurse discovers that the patient was experiencing digitalis toxicity. A layperson would not know to check the apical pulse and digoxin level prior to administering Lanoxin; however, a professional nurse knows that failure to do so prior to Lanoxin administration is a breach of the professional standard of care.

Malpractice is professional negligence. A nurse found liable in a malpractice suit will be found to have a duty of care to the patient bringing the suit, to have breached the duty of care by not adhering to the expected standard of care, and because of his or her action or inaction proximately caused physical, financial, or emotional injury to the patient. If the patient has survived, the patient will bring a malpractice suit. If the patient has not survived, the family will bring a wrongful death suit. In a wrongful death suit, the elements of malpractice will still need to be present: duty, breach of duty, and harm because the standard of care was not followed. Damages are primarily awarded for the purpose of compensation to help restore the injured party. Damages may be awarded in one or more of four categories: general damages for pain and suffering and any permanent disability, special damages for losses and expenses such as cost of medical care related to the injury, emotional damages if there is also apparent physical harm, and punitive or exemplary damages if it can be shown that there was conscious disregard for patient safety (Guido, 2014, p. 78).

CRITICAL THINKING QUESTION✳

What does "reasonable and prudent" mean as it relates to standards of care?✳

Thus, malpractice is the failure of a professional to use such care as a reasonably prudent member of the profession would use under similar circumstances, which leads to harm. The reasonable and prudent nurse is defined as "a similarly educated and experienced nurse who has average intelligence, judgment, foresight, and skill and who would have responded to the same situation, case, facts, or emergency in the same or similar manner" (ANA, 2012, p. 31).

To summarize, according to Guido (2014, p. 70), to be successful in a malpractice case, the plaintiff must prove the following elements:

- Duty owed to the patient
- Breach of the duty owed the patient
- Foresceability
- Causation
- Injury or harm
- Damages

The U.S. Department of Health and Human Services (2003) conducted a study to determine the types of malpractice acts commonly reported to the National Practitioners Data Bank. The results of the study indicated about 1 out of 50 malpractice reports were made for nurses. The nursing specializations included in this study were RN, nurse anesthetist, nurse–midwife, nurse practitioner, advanced practice nurse, and licensed vocational nurse/licensed practical nurse (LPN) (Bolin, 2005). The types of malpractice codes reported are listed in **Table 15-1**.

A question that often comes up with nurses is who is ultimately responsible for the malpractice or negligence: the nurse or the employing institution? **Respondeat superior** is the doctrine that indicates the employer might also be responsible if the nurse was functioning in the employee role at the time of the incident (Grossman, 2005). This implies that both the healthcare organization and the nurse can be sued.

A frequent question about legal issues from practicing nurses is "Should I carry my own malpractice insurance even though I am covered under my employer's insurance?" The answer is "Never leave home without it!" Nurses are rarely individually sued. Malpractice insurance of the facility for which the nurse works will most often cover damages. Nurses, however, can and should purchase malpractice insurance to avoid the risk of losing their personal assets.

TABLE 15-1 Malpractice Act or Omission Codes

Diagnosis	Failure, wrong, improper performance, unnecessary, delay, lack of informed consent
Anesthesia	Failure to properly assess, monitor, test, and use equipment; improper choice; intubation; positioning; and failure to obtain informed consent
Surgery	Failure to perform, improper positioning, foreign body, wrong body part, improper performance, unnecessary surgery, delay, improper management, and lack of informed consent
Medication	Wrong med, dosage, improper administration, improper technique, and lack of informed consent
IV and Blood	Failure to monitor, wrong solution, wrong type, improper administration, and management
Obstetrics	Improper delivery, delay in delivery, failure to properly manage, delay, abandonment
Treatment	Wrong treatment, improper instruction, improper performance, failure to supervise, failure to refer or seek consult
Monitoring	Failure to monitor, failure to respond and report
Equipment/ Product	Improper maintenance, improper use, failure to instruct patient, malfunction or failure
Miscellaneous	Breach of confidentiality, injury to third parties, improper behavior, breach of institutional policies

Source: U.S. Department of Health and Human Services. (2003). *Survey of the national practitioner's data bank.* Washington, DC: Author.

The nurse might be in a situation in which he or she is viewed as practicing as a nurse and harm occurs. An example might be poor advice given to a friend in failing to recommend further assessment by a healthcare provider when a child is injured in a fall. In addition, nurses should carry their own malpractice insurance because there is a difference and separation between the nurse's liability for a wrongdoing and his or her employer's liability. The nurse uses his or her own judgment within the context of the scope and standards of practice (ANA, 2015b). Thus, the nurse needs to have his or her own insurer that will pay for the nurse's defense and pay damages if necessary.

Nurses must be accountable for their actions while providing patient care. The nurse has a duty to practice competently and possess knowledge, skills, and abilities required for lawful, safe, and effective practice. Malpractice and negligence are not intentional actions or inactions.

CRITICAL THINKING QUESTIONS ✳

What measures are taken when a nurse is summoned to court for a legal action? Is a nurse more responsible than a doctor in the situation if both were involved with the patient's care? ✳

They are careless actions or inactions that are more likely to occur in stressful circumstances or because the nurse has not maintained knowledge and competency in an area of practice. Montgomery (2007) examined basic principles of human error and sleep physiology and evaluated the evidence for potential effects of fatigued healthcare workers and workload on medical errors. The researchers conducted the study in a pediatric intensive care unit, which is a highly complex environment in which fatigue and excessive workload might allow errors to occur. The results indicated that nursing fatigue and workload have documented effects on increasing intensive care unit errors, infections, and cost. Specific environmental factors such as distractions and communication barriers were also associated with greater errors. The researchers concluded that fatigue, excessive workload, and the pediatric intensive care environment could adversely affect the performance of physicians and nurses working in this type of setting.

Prevention requires learning how to manage stress and adhering to current standards of care. Nurses should learn to leave their personal life stresses at the door of their workplace. They should resist the temptation to self-medicate their stresses with alcohol or other drugs. When they find themselves doing so, they should seek help before their professional practice is affected.

Nurses should also seek to practice in work environments that encourage examination of incidents that might have caused or do cause harm to patients. Often, systems in which the nurse works can be changed to make the environment safer for both nurses and patients. The Institute of Medicine (IOM) recommends changing systems to lower the risk of practice errors in several reports. These include *To Err Is Human: Building a Safer Health System, Crossing the Quality Chasm: A New Health System for the 21st Century*, and *Keeping Patients Safe: Transforming the Work Environment of Nurses* (IOM, 1999, 2001, 2004). Changing systems is not the sole solution. Patterns of substandard practice still require the facility to either help the nurse improve practice or make a complaint to the state board of nursing so that disciplinary action can remove the nurse from being in a position to harm patients through either revocation, suspension, or a monitored practice improvement program.

KEY COMPETENCY 15-3

Examples of Applicable *Nurse of the Future: Nursing Core Competencies*

Professionalism:

Knowledge (K3) Understands the professional standards of practice, the evaluation of practice, and the responsibility and accountability for the outcome of practice

Skills (S3a) Demonstrates professional comportment

Attitudes/Behaviors (A3a) Recognizes personal capabilities, knowledge base, and areas for development

Source: Massachusetts Department of Higher Education. (2010). *Nurse of the future: Nursing core competencies* (p. 13). Retrieved from http://www.mass.edu/currentinit /documents/NursingCoreCompetencies.pdf

Nursing Licensure

History of Licensure

Nursing has evolved on a track parallel with other healthcare professions. The education of nurses particularly parallels the education of doctors of medicine. Both disciplines first experienced apprenticeship education followed by gradual evolution to education within educational institutions.

CRITICAL THINKING QUESTION ✳

You have been asked by a charge nurse on a medical-surgical unit to discuss the importance of the legal system for nurses. What are the important aspects regarding law and nursing that you will include in your presentation? ✳

Even today, a critical piece of this education remains the opportunity for clinical practice in healthcare facilities. Increasingly, however, understanding of human physiology has been refined to examination at the cellular and molecular levels. Advances in diagnostic and treatment technology have also occurred. These changes have bred the need for an increasing knowledge base at both the foundational and specialization levels of education in both nursing and medicine (Kalisch & Kalisch, 1995).

Licensure was not always a requirement for nursing practice. In fact, the acknowledged founder of modern nursing, Florence Nightingale, did not believe nurses should be recognized by a government body (Kalisch & Kalisch, 1995). Members of the fields of medicine and nursing eventually thought otherwise. An increasing knowledge base led to increasing risk for patients. Evidence of a basic education with recognized components led to nurses first being registered and later being licensed. The term *registered nurse* is of historical vintage and reflects the period of permissive licensure for nurses. Permissive licensure meant anyone could practice nursing, but only a person with a recognized foundation of nursing education could use the title "registered nurse." During this time, which in some states spanned 60 years, from the first to the sixth decade of the 1900s, the education of nurses primarily took place in hospital schools of nursing. Because hospitals were not recognized as institutions of higher learning, state licensure boards set the standards for nursing education. Boards of nursing continue to be involved in program accreditation today—despite the advent of accreditation bodies for nursing education. The advent of practical nursing education (known as vocational nursing in some states) was another reason for the change from permissive to mandatory licensure. Permissive licensure provides for title recognition. Mandatory licensure provides for a scope of practice. Two levels of nursing practice necessitated defining a scope of practice.

Today there are also advanced practice nurses who have specified scopes of practice under the titles nurse practitioner, nurse–midwife, nurse anesthetist, and clinical specialist. Nursing licensure boards contrast with medical boards in that they license or certify at multiple levels rather than a single basic level. A student of medicine obtains board certification by passing a professional examination that then allows the physician to practice in a specialty area; there is only one level of licensure. Nurse licensure boards require that nurses with a master's degree in a particular area pass a certification exam generated by a recognized nursing professional organization prior to being recognized as advanced practice nurses.

Nurses initially licensed in one state can acquire licensure in another state through a process called endorsement. Endorsement requires verification that the nurse's license has not been disciplined in another state. Previous discipline might or might not preclude licensure by endorsement, depending on the circumstances of the discipline. The nurse seeking endorsement also must meet licensure requirements in the endorsing state. Criminal background checks and continuing education requirements are two examples of such requirements.

In the late 1990s, the National Council of State Boards of Nursing (NCSBN) developed the Nurse Licensure Compact. The compact is a statutory agreement between and among states to permit nurses who are residents of one state to have the privilege of practicing in another state without acquiring a license in the second state. The nurse does become subject to the provisions of the law and rules of the second state. In this respect, compact state nurses enjoy the same privileges provided by a state driver's license. Drivers in one state can travel through others subject to the vehicular laws of other states. If, however, the driver becomes a resident of another state, the driver must obtain a license in that state. In the case of the compact, until all states adopt the compact, the nurse will have to determine whether the state in which he or she seeks to practice requires licensure by endorsement or is a member of the compact. A major advantage of the compact is the facilitation of practice in border areas of states.

The NCSBN (2015) generates the initial licensure exam for both the LPN and RN. Initial licensure measures competence at a minimal level to ensure safe practice. Clearly, the changing nature of practice demands acquisition of knowledge consistent with continuing competence. The content of the NCLEX-RN test plan is organized into four major client needs categories: safe and effective care environment, health promotion and maintenance, psychosocial integrity, and physiologic integrity. The categories that relate to the legal aspects of nursing are found primarily under the category of safe and effective care. The related content includes the following:

- Advance directives
- Advocacy
- Client rights
- Confidentiality and information security
- Delegation
- Ethical practice
- Informed consent
- Legal rights and responsibilities
- Safe use of equipment

Although it has never been clearly demonstrated that continuing education translates into continuing competence in nursing, many states do require continuing education for licensure renewal. It has been argued that conscientious nurses would undertake continuing education voluntarily, and mandatory continuing education adds only reluctant nurses to program attendance with perhaps little impact on the reluctant nurses' competence. Current competence is also of concern for nurses reentering practice. Mandatory refresher courses seem desirable but have the drawback of high cost for persons who might be reentering practice for economic reasons. Ideally, the burden of maintaining competence rests with the nurse, and the organization where the nurse practices should provide and support opportunities for the nurse to maintain competence.

The Function and Composition of Boards of Nursing

The statutory law governing nursing practice in all states and territories of the United States is known as the Nurse Practice Act. Boards of nursing are the state or territorial agencies that administer the law. Members of boards of nursing represent various types of nursing expertise and various geographic areas within the state or territory. A recent trend has been for boards to include consumer members to represent the public. Board members are generally appointed by the governor of the state or territory.

The overriding obligation of all board members is to protect the safety of the public by initially and continuously licensing only competent nurses. Board members direct the activities of the agency by providing direction to the executive director of the board, who in turn directs the activities of board staff. Board staffs can be as few as 2 or as many as 50 or more, depending on the number of licensees in the state or territory. Boards set standards of practice and delegation and often standards for nursing education through the rule-making process. Other board rules govern the disciplinary process and programs such as alternative programs for drug and alcohol abuse and practice intervention improvement.

Boards meet at regularly scheduled intervals during the year to act on disciplinary matters, approve nursing education programs, and review and update the nurse practice act and regulations governing practice as nursing practice evolves. A trend among nursing boards has been to assume the legal oversight of other types of healthcare providers as well, including nursing assistants, dialysis technicians, community health workers, and medication technicians.

Discipline of Nurses

In legal terms, licensure is a privilege not a right. Not surprisingly, a privilege can be withdrawn or withheld from a person if the behavior of the person does not merit the privilege. Thus, a board of nursing holds legal authority to discipline a nurse who holds a license or to act to withhold licensure from a person seeking initial licensure within a state or territory.

In recent years, boards of nursing have moved to bar from initial licensure persons who have been convicted of, who have pled guilty to, or who had a judicial finding of guilt for felonies involving potential or actual physical harm to persons. Examples of such felonies include murder, robbery, kidnapping, rape, sexual battery, or sexual imposition. Because a large proportion of board disciplinary actions is related to alcohol and substance abuse, boards are concerned about previous histories of drug abuse and drug treatment.

Uncontrolled psychiatric illness is also often associated with incompetent practice and substance abuse. Persons with a history of drug-related and psychiatric health problems seeking initial licensure in a state may be allowed to practice but are required to enter into an agreement to be monitored for a period of time under a set of prescribed conditions to ensure that they are safe practitioners. The monitoring would not constitute a disciplinary action. However, if monitoring conditions are violated or the person's practice is unsafe, the board can consider the full range of disciplinary actions. According to Clevette and colleagues (2007), common disciplinary categories reviewed by boards of nursing include the following:

- Substandard nursing practice not involving medications including verbal abuse, using force to administer medications, or failing to respond to changes in patient condition
- Destruction or alteration of patient records including fraudulent charting and/or signatures and/or replacement of records with intent to mislead or deceive
- Physical patient abuse, such as when a nurse hits, strikes, or performs similar physical acts of aggression involving physical contact
- Failure to follow policy such as violation of an employer's policy statements
- Medication "errors," including inaccurate documentation, discarding meds and charting them as given, wrong dosages, wrong route, wrong time, and/or incorrect medication technique
- Controlled substance violations or chemical dependency including diversion of drugs from facility or patient for self-use or sale, prescription fraud, doctor-shopping to obtain prescriptions, or practicing under the influence
- Impaired mental or physical competency; for example, practice negatively affected by mental or physical incapacity
- Inappropriate management decision such as when a supervisor or manager makes a decision contrary to acceptable nursing standards such as permitting practice without a license
- Practice beyond the authorized scope such as administering medications without a physician's order
- Sexual misconduct including nurse and client communication or contact of a sexual nature or convictions related to sexual misconduct not with clients but related to the practice of nursing
- Patient or employer abandonment such as leaving or not arriving for a patient care assignment
- Unethical actions with a rational relationship to nursing practice, including actions not directly related to nursing care such as falsification of licensure or employment applications, diversion of third-party payments, embezzlement, or distribution of a controlled substance
- Actions demonstrating poor judgment, including irrational behavior not described under the other categories

What are the differences between nursing disciplinary action by a board of nursing and legal ramifications set forth by state and federal laws?✳

Boards of nursing have a number of disciplinary choices: denying a license, imposing a fine, issuing a reprimand, placing restrictions on a license, and suspending or revoking a license. Boards must follow a designated process before taking action against a license. First, the board must receive a complaint. Complaints are investigated by board staff. If board staff conclude that the evidence merits action against the nurse's license, a consent agreement might be offered. This procedure is a disciplinary action that bypasses the hearing process, and the nurse agrees to conditions placed on his or her license. An example would be a period of suspension with random drug testing and treatment for drug abuse. Compliance with the agreement would lead to returning to practice with a person in the workplace assigned to report on the nurse's practice at regular intervals. The nurse might also be expected to provide evidence of attendance at a support group for persons with addictions. Consent agreements must be approved by the state's board of nursing before being implemented.

In the absence of a consent agreement, the nurse receives a notice of opportunity for a hearing. When a timely response requesting a hearing is not received, the board members decide the disciplinary action at a subsequent board meeting. Hearings might be conducted by a board or a hearing examiner. In both instances, board members must make the final decision with respect to action against a nursing license.

Reasons for disciplinary action are described in nurse practice acts. Some common examples include conviction of a misdemeanor in the course of practice, conviction of any felony, self-administering a prescription medication without a prescription, impairment of ability to practice safely because of habitual or excessive use of drugs or alcohol, and assaulting or causing harm to a patient.

Professional Accountability

RNs are expected to engage in professional role activities appropriate to their level of educational preparation and position and are accountable to self, peers, patients, families, and ultimately society for their actions (ANA, 2015a). Some specific responsibilities for which nurses are accountable with direct links to the law are informed consent, privacy and confidentiality, and delegation.

Informed Consent

There are two components to **informed consent**—the patient must be fully informed and there must be voluntary consent. The practitioner is required to communicate the following information to the patient in terms that the patient can understand:

- A brief but complete explanation of the patient diagnosis and proposed treatment or procedure
- The name and qualifications of the person who will perform the procedure or treatment
- Information related to available alternatives to the recommended treatment
- Information related to possible complications of the treatment or procedure
- An explanation related to the patient's right to refuse treatment without having care discontinued (Guido, 2014)

The American Medical Association (2007) states that informed consent is more than simply getting a patient to sign a written consent form. It is a process of communication between a patient and physician that results in the patient's authorization or agreement to undergo a specific medical intervention. In the communication process, the physician providing or performing the treatment and/or procedure (not a delegated representative) should disclose and discuss with the patient the required information. This communication process is both an ethical obligation and a legal requirement spelled out in statutes and case law in all 50 states.

Informed consent cases are a type of malpractice suit. An informed consent case can be brought by a patient when a risk of a procedure occurs that should have been divulged but was not or when alternatives to the procedure were not provided that the patient would have chosen had he or she known the particular risk. Informed consent cases arise with invasive procedures and complicated treatment regimens such as those for cancer. Central to informed consent is ensuring that the patient is capable of comprehending the information; otherwise, the consent is invalid.

Information components of informed consent include explanation by the physician of the nature of the procedure, its risks, its benefits, and alternatives to the procedure, including the risks and benefits of the alternatives. The information to be provided is generally described as what is material to the patient's decision to go forward with the procedure, decline the procedure, or select an alternative to the proposed procedure. Material risks are expected serious risks such as death, hemorrhage, infection, or any other risk that would seriously compromise the functioning of a person, such as a stroke or paralysis. Failure to meet these standards of disclosure puts the physician at risk for a malpractice suit resulting from failure to provide informed consent if the undisclosed risk occurs and the patient is harmed (*Nickell v. Gonzalez*, 1985). In a leading case that helped establish this type of malpractice suit, the physician did not inform the patient of the risk of paralysis with back surgery (*Canterbury v. Spence*, 1972). In an Ohio case, a patient's incapability to express himself because of temporary aphasia led to the signing of a consent form for a procedure that in his individual case put him at high risk for a stroke, and a stroke occurred (*Greynolds v. Kurman*, 1993). In a California case (*Truman v. Thomas*, 1980), a physician was sued for failing to warn the patient of the risks of not consenting to a diagnostic test.

Are there differences in the responsibility related to informed consent for the nurse and physician? If so, what are the differences? ✳

The standards used for determining whether consent information is sufficient vary from state to state. The first is the medical standard—what are regarded as material risks in the medical community. The second is what a reasonable patient would need to know. The third is what a particular patient needs to know. The first errs in favor of the medical community. The second is considered objective because it provides a standard favoring the patient community. The third is clearly subjective and essentially leaves physicians in the dark as to what information to give patients.

Is there a role for nurses when informed consent is required? The nurse is responsible for facilitating informed consent for patient care as a part of providing patient-centered care (Quality and Safety Education for Nurses, n.d.). When a nurse obtains a signature on a hospital or ambulatory facility consent form, that interaction provides an opportunity to ascertain whether the patient has questions about a procedure. When a conversation reveals that the patient has misconceptions about the procedure or its risks and benefits, the nurse should contact the physician so that additional communication regarding the procedure can occur. The advocacy role of the nurse in this situation is not a legally defined role. It falls in the realm of professional performance standards and a code of ethics responsibility to collaborate with other healthcare providers and the patient to ensure appropriate care. The legal role of the nurse in the informed consent process is acting as a witness to the patient's signature.

Privacy and Confidentiality

Privacy is the right of a person to be free from unwanted intrusion into his or her personal affairs. To receive appropriate health care, however, a person often must disclose very personal information. Sexual activity and acknowledgment of alcohol or drug abuse are examples of such personal information. Because of the stigma attached to mental illness, patients might also be reluctant to disclose a family or personal history of mental illness. To fulfill their social contract to provide nursing care, nurses must often gather such sensitive information from patients. Thus, the nurse, along with other caregivers, has the obligation to keep healthcare information confidential. Privacy is the right of the patient. **Confidentiality** is the obligation of all healthcare providers.

The *Code of Ethics for Nurses with Interpretive Statements* addresses privacy and confidentiality under provision 3, "The nurse promotes, advocates for, and strives to protect the health, safety, and rights of the patient" (ANA, 2015a, p. 9); specifically, the nurse has a duty to maintain the confidentiality of all patient information. It is noteworthy that, although not the norm, the "duty to maintain confidentiality is not absolute and may be limited, as necessary, to protect the patient or others parties, or by law or regulation such as mandated reporting for safety or public health reasons" (ANA, 2015a, p. 10). Rules of boards of nursing also spell out the nurse's duty of confidentiality.

In 2000, federal rules protecting patient privacy were issued. The rules affect health plans, healthcare clearinghouses, and healthcare providers who engage in electronic transactions. The rules were a response to concerns that patient privacy would be compromised without legal standards for the scope of information that could be shared. The rules required all of these groups (called entities) to be in compliance with the rules by April 14, 2003, with the exception of small health plans. The small health plan compliance date was April 14, 2004. The rules were promulgated by the U.S. Department of Health and Human Services under provisions of the Health Insurance Portability and Accountability Act (HIPAA) of 1996.

The rules assure patients that only necessary information will be shared with groups such as insurers and third-party intermediaries who administer insurance plans by engaging in functions such as claims processing and membership tracking. The rules also ensure access to patient records by patients themselves, although a reasonable period of time might be needed to copy those records, and the patient might be charged for the cost of copying and sending records. The rules prohibit patient information from being shared for marketing purposes without the patient's consent. The rules require employee training on the provisions of the rules for employees of all healthcare employers.

Health Insurance Portability and Accountability Act (HIPAA) protection of patient privacy highlights the traditional value placed on patient privacy by the healthcare professions. Nurses should remember that conversations in healthcare facilities about patients should occur only among healthcare providers. Elevators and cafeterias are not appropriate sites for such discussions. Specific healthcare information should be shared with family members only with the express permission of the patient. Generally, medical records cannot be sent to anyone without written consent except when the record is subpoenaed.

Each nurse needs to be aware of and follow the policies and procedures related to oral, written, or electronic patient-identifiable data set up by the healthcare organization regarding issues where the nurse practices; however, some key areas affected by these privacy regulations include:

- Patients must be informed of their privacy rights.
- Patients must be informed as to who will see their records and for what purpose.
- Patients have the right to inspect and obtain a copy of their medical records.
- Valid authorization to release health information must contain certain information, such as a copy of the signed authorization given to the patient,

---

KEY COMPETENCY 15-4

Examples of Applicable *Nurse of the Future: Nursing Core Competencies*

Systems-Based Practice:

Knowledge (K5a) Understands that legal, political, regulatory, and economic factors influence the delivery of patient care

Skills (S5a) Provides care based upon current legal, political, regulatory, and economic requirements

Attitudes/Behaviors (A5a) Appreciates that legal, political, regulatory, and economic factors influence the delivery of patient care

Attitudes/Behaviors (A5b) Values the need to remain informed of how legal, political, regulatory, and economic factors impact professional nursing practice

Source: Massachusetts Department of Higher Education. (2010). *Nurse of the future: Nursing core competencies* (p. 20). Retrieved from http://www.mass.edu/currentinit /documents/NursingCoreCompetencies.pdf

in understandable language, that also includes information about how the patient may revoke authorization.

- Although information might be used for research purposes to assess outbreak of a disease, all individual identifiable data must be removed.
- Personal data may not be used for marketing (Finkelman, 2006).

Persons who violate HIPAA may incur fines, and there are multiple cases of nurses being dismissed from employment due to violations of this act. Nurses should access the medical records of patients only when they are members of the team responsible for their care. Accessing the medical records of friends or family members constitutes a HIPAA violation. See **Figure 15-2** for a flowchart illustrating the HIPAA Privacy and Security Rule Complaint Process.

Figure 15-2   HIPAA Privacy and Security Rule Complaint Process

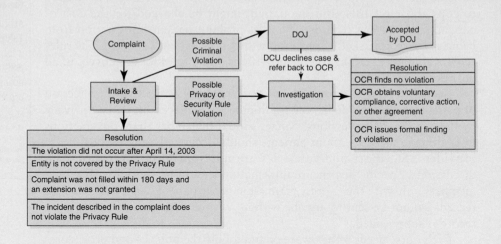

Source: U.S. Department of Health and Human Services. (n.d.). HIPAA privacy and security rule complaint process. Retrieved from http://www.hhs.gov/ocr/privacy/hipaa/enforcement /process/index.html

Delegation

Delegation in nursing practice is viewed in both a legal and an ethical context. In both contexts, the primary premise is that nurses are accountable and responsible for their delegation of nursing activities and that those assignments must be consistent with state practice acts, organizational policy, and standards of nursing practice (ANA, 2015a, p. 17). Delegation is addressed again by the ANA as a standard of professional performance in Standard 16. This standard requires that the nurse use appropriate resources to plan, provide, and sustain evidence-based nursing services that are safe, effective, and fiscally responsible. In order to meet this standard, one of the competencies generally required of the nurse is the delegation of elements of care in accordance with applicable legal and policy parameters (2015b, p. 82).

As licensed professionals, RNs are responsible for providing safe, competent, and effective care for patients in a variety of healthcare settings. In each setting, RNs work beside other licensed professionals and delegate tasks to these other licensed professionals as well as unlicensed assistive personnel (UAP) to give efficient care to patients. The ANA and the NCSBN define delegation as "the process for a nurse to direct another person to perform nursing tasks and activities" (ANA & NCSBN, 2006, p. 1). Delegation can be direct (i.e., verbal instructions) or indirect (i.e., tasks verified by hospital policy) in the healthcare setting (Trappen, Weiss, & Whitehead, 2004). The RN or nurse manager judges which staff member is competent to perform an assigned duty; however, some permitted tasks might depend on the organization or institution or the state of practice.

In terms of accountability, nurses must take responsibility for their actions and the actions of others involved in the delegation process. When allegations of unethical, illegal, and inappropriate conduct occur, nurses "must answer to patients, nursing employers, the board of nursing, and the court system when the quality of patient care provided is compromised" (ANA, 2005, p. 4). Therefore, it is important for RNs and nurse managers to be knowledgeable of the delegation guidelines within each state's nurse practice act, the facility's job descriptions, and the scope of practice of other licensed and unlicensed personnel.

Delegation is part of the language of management. Work might be within the job description of a healthcare worker, but this does not automatically make delegation of a particular task appropriate. The nurse making an assignment is acting as a manager of care. The nurse must carefully select the person to whom a task is assigned because ultimately the nurse as manager is accountable for whether the task is accomplished and whether the desired outcome is achieved. For example, complete independence in caring for a complex critical care patient would not be an appropriate assignment for a newly licensed RN. LPNs cannot shoulder complete responsibility for acting on the assessment of a newly admitted patient. UAP may take blood pressures, but they should do so with clear parameters established for communicating deviance from those parameters.

Certain activities cannot be delegated. An advanced practice nurse may delegate the drawing of blood to a nursing assistant but cannot delegate the decision for the types of lab tests to be performed. Only the advanced practice nurse can make the judgment as to what tests are necessary. Furthermore, the advanced practice nurse could not delegate the blood draw to a nursing assistant if the nursing assistant had not learned the proper technique for drawing blood and had not received sufficient supervision in carrying out the procedure to determine the nursing assistant's competence.

UAP cannot delegate a task delegated to them by a nurse because that would be engaging in the practice of nursing without a license. Similarly, a nurse cannot delegate a task if the nurse does not know how to do the task. That would be delegating beyond the nurse's scope of practice.

The nurse delegating any task must provide supervision to the unlicensed person. This means determining the competence of the person to carry out the task properly. If the unlicensed person does not properly carry out the task, the unlicensed person should not again be delegated the task until further education ensures that the person has reached a level of competence; however, demonstrated competence does not eliminate the supervisory role of the nurse.

The five rights of delegation as outlined jointly by the ANA and the NCSBN in 2006 are as follows:

- *The right task:* One that is delegable for a specific patient
- *The right circumstances:* An appropriate patient setting, available resources, and consideration of other relevant factors
- *The right person:* Delegating the right task to the right person to be performed on the right person
- *The right direction and communication:* A clear, concise description of the task, including objectives, limits, and expectations
- *The right supervision and evaluation:* Appropriate monitoring, intervention, and, as needed, feedback.

Keeping this rights mantra in mind helps the nurse to delegate care according to the legal standard of acting as a reasonable and prudent nurse would do in similar circumstances. However, authority to delegate specific tasks may vary by state, so licensed nurses must check the jurisdiction's statutes and regulations.

Barriers to Delegation

Nurses face many challenges when trying to delegate to others. Contributing factors leading to delegation barriers "range from not having had educational opportunities to learn how to work with others effectively to not knowing

---

KEY COMPETENCY 15-5

Examples of Applicable *Nurse of the Future: Nursing Core Competencies*

Leadership:

Knowledge (K6) Understands the principles of accountability and delegation

Skills (S6b) Assigns, directs, and supervises ancillary personnel and support staff in carrying out particular roles/functions aimed at achieving patient care goals

Attitudes/Behaviors (A6a) Recognizes the value of delegation

Attitudes/Behaviors (A6b) Accepts accountability for nursing care given by self and delegated to others

Source: Massachusetts Department of Higher Education. (2010). *Nurse of the future: Nursing core competencies* (p. 18). Retrieved from http://www.mass.edu/currentinit /documents/NursingCoreCompetencies.pdf

the skill level and abilities of nursing assistive personnel to simplify the work pace and turnover of patients" (ANA & NCSBN, 2006, p. 4). In addition, the scope of nursing practice is changing, and the tasks performed by UAP are increasing in complexity. This can make many nurses apprehensive in delegating tasks because of a fear of endangering their own licensure. Because of the nursing shortage, many inexperienced nurses are being placed at the helm who are not yet knowledgeable about how to communicate effectively and how to use the institution's resources efficiently. Ultimately, barriers that lead to ineffective delegation place a strain on the quality of patient care.

In 2005, Kalisch conducted a qualitative study to examine the care missed on medical-surgical units. By interviewing 107 RNs, 15 LPNs, and 51 nursing assistants from two hospitals in the United States, Kalisch (2006) found that the following activities were frequently missed: "ambulation, turning, feedings, patient teaching, discharge planning, emotional support, hygiene, intake and output documentation, and surveillance" (p. 307). Several factors contributed to why hospital employees missed these important measures; ineffective delegation was cited as one of the major factors. Kalisch (2006) discovered that many nursing assistants were not present during routine nursing reports, and the nurses did not relay report information to the nursing assistants. "Even when nursing assistants received report, there was a lack of collaborative planning for patient care" (Kalisch, 2006, p. 310).

In addition, many nurses had difficulty retaining accountability. "Many nurses considered the work delegated to nursing assistants as no longer the RN's responsibility" (Kalisch, 2006, p. 310). This is a major misconception, because according to state nurse practice acts, the nurse remains accountable for the care given to the patient. Another problem was that many staff members did not feel that it was their job to perform a particular task. "Nurses stated that certain tasks such as vital signs were the nursing assistant's responsibility, and if the nursing assistant did not complete these tasks, it was the 'fault' of the nursing assistant, not the nurse" (Kalisch, 2006, p. 310). Hospitals and institutions have policies and procedures that help define which tasks can be delegated. State nurse practice acts define the scope of practice and specify what nurses can delegate. These documents are clear that the nurse retains responsibility for the task delegated.

Kalisch (2006) also cites that many nurses had difficulty with conflict management: "Many nurses reported limited authority and influence over the nursing assistants and expressed reluctance to confront nursing assistants who did not 'do their job'" (p. 310). In several cases, staff members tried to avoid confrontation and had difficulty engaging in conflict management to strive for a solution. "If delegates are resistant, the delegator may simply choose to do the task him- or herself to avoid confrontations; instead, the situation should be reevaluated from the UAP's point of view" (Quallich, 2005, p. 122). In some cases, UAP might lack the confidence or knowledge to perform a task; however, if

UAP refuse to perform a task as a way to defy authority, guidelines for delegation should be clearly reinstituted. If a nurse lacks confidence and does not trust the abilities of other staff members, delegation is also unlikely to occur. "Similarly, delegation will be unsuccessful if the only tasks that are delegated are those that are time-consuming or unpleasant; this approach risks exhausting staff that are otherwise capable" (Quallich, 2005, p. 122).

Regardless of the institution, delegation involves a strict chain of command among employees. Nurses sometimes might experience feelings of guilt about those to whom they delegate tasks. The RN also might worry about being labeled as lazy when delegating a task to other employees. "But working in an organizational hierarchy should not result in the delegator taking on disproportionate amounts of responsibility in order to respect the feelings of other delegatees" (Quallich, 2005, p. 122). Some nurses might also feel that they should show loyalty to other nurses and should delegate to student and graduate nurses only. However, this loyalty or discrimination is not cost-efficient and only acts as another delegation barrier; if a nurse refuses to delegate a task as instructed by the employer, the nurse may actually face disciplinary actions by the employer (Haslauer & Jones, 2003). If a nurse has concerns regarding the implementation of a task or activity, it is important to document concerns for patient safety and to inform the employer. After nursing staff become comfortable with their skill at delegation, the next challenge is making sure they have the skills necessary to assess the competence of their UAP for individual tasks.

Delegation Decision-Making Tree

In 1997, the NCSBN developed a delegation decision-making tree that identifies several steps nurses can take to help them make delegation decisions. In 2006, the ANA and the NCSBN published a joint paper on the topic of delegation that includes the ANA principles of delegation and the NCSBN decision-making tree. The decision-making tree is a useful tool or "grid that may be used by staff education specialists to provide orientation and education to staff nurses and UAP" (Kleinman & Saccomano, 2006, p. 168).

Conclusion

Preventing legal problems intentionally runs as a theme through this chapter. In summary, prevention requires consistently following the nursing process—the decision-making process of nursing in all nursing care situations. Because nurses act as managers of care, following management principles also reduces the risk of legal problems. This is especially true with delegation of care, an activity that predictably will increase as care systems adjust to the nursing shortage.

Communication with patients, families, nursing staff, and other healthcare providers also reduces the risk of legal problems. In addition, the nurse should tailor risk prevention by being aware of the law and rules that affect the nurse's particular practice situation. Nurses holding administrative positions should know the laws and rules affecting their area of practice. In turn, they should educate nursing staff regarding their responsibilities to provide nursing care based on current law and practice standards in the setting. The practice of nursing is never static. Practice is a continuous quest involving adaptation to the current healthcare environment with a commitment to making that environment as safe as possible for the patients for whom nurses care.

Nurses are generally law-abiding citizens who have a positive relationship and respect for their profession. However, a clear understanding of the legal system and strategies for avoiding legal problems is essential. Nurses have a duty to be knowledgeable about the regulation of nursing practice. A diagram depicting the model of professional nursing practice regulation is available at www.nursingworld.org/modelofpracticeregulation. The model depicts a triangle with four layers encapsulated within a circle. The four layers of the triangle include a foundation composed of the scope of practice, standards of practice, code of ethics, and specialty certification. Layer two of the triangle, nurse practice act and rules and regulations, rests on the first layer of the triangle. The third layer is composed of institutional policies and procedures. The final layer is self-determination of the nurse. The triangle is surrounded by quality, safety, and research. Grounding nursing practice in the components of the regulation model will assist the nurse to provide high-quality care for patients as well as assist the nurse to avoid claims of malpractice or issues resulting in disciplinary action related to nursing licensure.

CASE STUDY 15-1 ▪ DELEGATION

As the nurse on the medical-surgical unit, you are responsible for the care of eight acute patients. You have two nursing assistants working with you on this shift. Both of the nursing assistants have worked on the unit for several years. To provide adequate care for all of the patients under your care, it is necessary to delegate some of the nursing care to the nursing assistants working with you. You request that the first nursing assistant check the vital signs for Mr. Martin and you request that the second nursing assistant assess Ms. Smith's level of pain because you have recently administered pain medication.

Case Study Questions

1. Is the delegation of the assignment to the first nursing assistant in the case study appropriate? Why or why not?

2. Is the delegation of the assignment to the second nursing assistant in the case study appropriate? Why or why not?

Classroom Activity 1

A mock trial is a fun way to explore some of the concepts in this chapter. Assign roles to students and use a graduation gown for the judge to increase the realism. Make up your own case or use one already prepared, such as the excellent mock trial presented in *Nurse Educator* by Haidinyak (2006).

References

American Medical Association. (2007). *Informed consent*. Chicago, IL: Author.

American Nurses Association. (2005). Principles for delegation [Brochure]. Retrieved from http://www.healthsystem.virginia.edu/internet/e-learning/principlesdelegation.pdf

American Nurses Association. (2010). *Social policy statement: The essence of the profession*. Silver Spring, MD: Author.

American Nurses Association. (2012). *The essential guide to nursing practice: Applying ANA's scope and standards in practice and education*. Silver Spring, MD: Author.

American Nurses Association. (2015a). *Code of ethics for nurses with interpretive statements*. Silver Spring, MD: Author.

American Nurses Association. (2015b). *Nursing: Scope and standards of practice* (3rd ed.). Silver Spring, MD: Author.

American Nurses Association & National Council of State Boards of Nursing. (2006). Joint statement on delegation. Retrieved from https://www.ncsbn.org/Delegation_joint_statement_NCSBN-ANA.pdf

Arizona Superior Court. (n.d.). Civil case flow. Retrieved from http://www.sc.pima.gov/?tabid=180

Bolin, J. N. (2005). When nurses are reported to the national practitioner's data bank. *Journal of Nursing Law, 10*(3), 141–148.

Canterbury v. Spence, 464 F.2d 772 (D.C. Cir. 1972).

Clevette, A., Erbin-Rosenmann, M., & Kelly, C. (2007). Nursing licensure: An examination of the relationship between criminal convictions and disciplinary actions. *Journal of Nursing Law, 11*(1), 5–8.

Finkelman, A. W. (2006). *Leadership and management in nursing*. Upper Saddle River, NJ: Pearson Prentice Hall.

Fremgen, B. F. (2002). *Medical law and ethics*. Upper Saddle River, NJ: Prentice Hall.

Greynolds v. Kurman, 91 Ohio App.3d 389 (1993).

Grossman, S. C. (2005). *The new leadership challenge*. Philadelphia, PA: F. A. Davis.

Guido, G. W. (2014). *Legal and ethical issues in nursing* (6th ed.). Upper Saddle River, NJ: Pearson.

Haidinyak, G. (2006). Try a mock trial. *Nurse Educator, 31*(3), 119–123.

Haslauer, S., & Jones, D. (2003, Winter). Delegation: Concept, art, skill, process. *Arkansas State Board of Nursing Update*, 22–24.

Havighurst, C., Blumstein, J. F., & Brennan, T. A. (1998). *Health care law and policy: Readings, notes and questions* (2nd ed.). Westbury, NY: Foundation Press.

Institute of Medicine. (1999). *To err is human: Building a safer health system*. Washington, DC: National Academy Press.

Institute of Medicine. (2001). *Crossing the quality chasm: A new health system for the 21st century*. Washington, DC: National Academy Press.

Institute of Medicine. (2004). *Keeping patients safe: Transforming the work environment of nurses*. Washington, DC: National Academy Press.

Kalisch, B. J. (2006). Missed nursing care: A qualitative study. *Journal of Nursing Care Quality, 21*(4), 306–313.

Kalisch, P. A., & Kalisch, B. J. (1995). *The advance of American nursing* (3rd ed.). Philadelphia, PA: Lippincott.

Kleinman, C. S., & Saccomano, S. J. (2006). Registered nurses and unlicensed assistive personnel: An uneasy alliance. *Journal of Continuing Education in Nursing, 37*(4), 162–170.

Longest, B. B. (2002). *Health policymaking in the United States* (3rd ed.). Chicago, IL: Health Administration Press.

Massachusetts Department of Higher Education. (2010). *Nurse of the future: Nursing core competencies*. Retrieved from http://www.mass.edu/currentinit/documents /NursingCoreCompetencies.pdf

Montgomery, V. L. (2007). Effect of fatigue, workload, and environment on patient safety in the pediatric intensive care unit. *Pediatric Critical Care Medicine, 8*(Suppl. 2), 11–16.

National Council of State Boards of Nursing. (2015). *NCLEX-RN test plan*. Chicago, IL: Author.

Nickell v. Gonzalez, 17 Ohio St.3d 136, 477 N.E.2d 1145 (1985).

Quality and Safety Education for Nurses. (n.d.). Evidence-based practice. Retrieved from http://qsen.org/competencies/pre-licensure-ksas/#evidence-based_practice

Quallich, S. A. (2005). A bond of trust: Delegation. *Urologic Nursing, 25*(2), 120–123.

Trappen, R. M., Weiss, S. A., & Whitehead, D. K. (2004). *Essentials of nursing leadership and management* (3rd ed., pp. 91–103). Philadelphia, PA: F. A. Davis.

Truman v. Thomas, 27 Cal. 3d 285, 611. P2d (1980).

U.S. Department of Health and Human Services. (2003). *Survey of the national practitioner's data bank*. Washington, DC: Author.

U.S. Department of Health and Human Services. (n.d.). HIPAA privacy and security rule complaint process. Retrieved from http://www.hhs.gov/ocr/privacy/hipaa /enforcement/process/index.html

APPENDIX A

Standards of Professional Nursing Practice

American Nurses Association (2015)

Standards of Practice

Standard 1   Assessment: The registered nurse collects pertinent data and information relative to the healthcare consumer's health or the situation.

Standard 2   Diagnosis: The registered nurse analyzes assessment data to determine actual or potential diagnoses, problems, and issues.

Standard 3   Outcomes Identification: The registered nurse identifies expected outcomes for a plan individualized to the healthcare consumer or the situation.

Standard 4   Planning: The registered nurse develops a plan that prescribes strategies to attain expected, measurable outcomes.

Standard 5   Implementation: The registered nurse implements the identified plan.

Standard 6   Evaluation: The registered nurse evaluates progress toward attainment of goals and outcomes.

Standards of Professional Performance

Standard 7   Ethics: The registered nurse practices ethically.

Standard 8   Culturally Congruent Practice: The registered nurse practices in a manner that is congruent with cultural diversity and inclusion principles.

Standard 9   Communication: The registered nurse communicates effectively in all areas of practice.

Standard 10 Collaboration: The registered nurse collaborates with healthcare consumer and other key stakeholders in the conduct of nursing practice.

Standard 11 Leadership: The registered nurse leads within the professional practice setting and the profession.

Standard 12 Education: The registered nurse seeks knowledge and competence that reflects current nursing practice and promotes futuristic thinking.

Standard 13 Evidence-Based Practice and Research: The registered nurse integrates evidence and research findings into practice.

Standard 14 Quality of Practice: The registered nurse contributes to quality nursing practice.

Standard 15 Professional Practice Evaluation: The registered nurse evaluates one's own and others' nursing practice.

Standard 16 Resource Utilization: The registered nurse utilizes appropriate resources to plan, provide, and sustain evidence-based nursing services that are safe, effective, and financially responsible.

Standard 17 Environmental Health: The registered nurse practices in an environmentally safe and healthy manner.

Source: American Nurses Association. (2015). *Nursing: Scope and standards of practice* (3rd ed., pp. 53–84). Silver Spring, MD: Author. © 2015 By American Nurses Association. Reprinted with permission. All rights reserved.

APPENDIX B

Provisions of Code of Ethics for Nurses

American Nurses Association (2015)

Provision 1: The nurse practices with compassion and respect for the inherent dignity, worth, and unique attributes of every person.

Provision 2: The nurse's primary commitment is to the patient, whether an individual, family, group, community, or population.

Provision 3: The nurse promotes, advocates for, and protects the rights, health, and safety of the patient.

Provision 4: The nurse has authority, accountability, and responsibility for nursing practice; makes decisions; and takes action consistent with the obligation to promote health and to provide optimal care.

Provision 5: The nurse owes the same duties to self as to others, including the responsibility to promote health and safety, preserve wholeness of character and integrity, maintain competence, and continue personal and professional growth.

Provision 6: The nurse, through individual and collective effort, establishes, maintains, and improves the ethical environment of the work setting and conditions of employment that are conducive to safe, quality health care.

Provision 7: The nurse, in all roles and settings, advances the profession through research and scholarly inquiry, professional standards development, and the generation of both nursing and health policy.

Provision 8: The nurse collaborates with other health professionals and the public to protect human rights, promote health diplomacy, and reduce health disparities.

Provision 9: The profession of nursing, collectively through its professional organizations, must articulate nursing values, maintain the integrity of the professions, and integrate principles of social justice into nursing and health policy.

The ICN Code of Ethics for Nurses

International Council of Nurses (2012)

The ICN Code of Ethics has four principal elements that outline the standards of ethical conduct.

1. Nurses and people
   - The nurse's primary responsibility is to people requiring nursing care.
   - In providing care, the nurse promotes an environment in which the human rights, values, customs and spiritual beliefs of the individual, family and community are respected.
   - The nurse ensures that the individual receives accurate, sufficient and timely information in a culturally appropriate manner on which to base consent for care and related treatment.
   - The nurse holds in confidence personal information and uses judgment in sharing this information.
   - The nurse shares with society the responsibility for initiating and supporting action to meet the health and social needs of the public, in particular those of vulnerable populations.
   - The nurse advocates for equity and social justice in resource allocation, access to health care and other social and economic services.
   - The nurse demonstrates professional values such as respectfulness, responsiveness, compassion, trustworthiness and integrity.
2. Nurses and practice
   - The nurse carries personal responsibility and accountability for nursing practice, and for maintaining competence by continual learning.
   - The nurse maintains a standard of personal health such that the ability to provide care is not compromised.
   - The nurse uses judgment regarding individual competence when accepting and delegating responsibility.

- The nurse at all times maintains standards of personal conduct which reflect well on the profession and enhance its image and public confidence.
- The nurse, in providing care, ensures that the use of technology and scientific advances are compatible with the safety, dignity, and rights of people.
- The nurse strives to foster and maintain a practice culture promoting ethical behavior and open dialogue.

3. Nurses and the profession
   - The nurse assumes the major role in determining and implementing acceptable standards of clinical nursing practice, management, research and education.
   - The nurse is active in developing a core of research-based professional knowledge that supports evidence-based practice.
   - The nurse is active in developing and sustaining a core of professional values.
   - The nurse, acting through the professional organization, participates in creating a positive practice environment, and maintaining safe, equitable social and economic working conditions in nursing.
   - The nurse practices to sustain and protect the natural environment and is aware of its consequences on health.
   - The nurse contributes to an ethical organizational environment and challenges unethical practices and settings.

4. Nurses and co-workers
   - The nurse sustains a respectful and collaborative relationship with co-workers in nursing and other fields.
   - The nurse takes appropriate action to safeguard individuals, families and communities when their health is endangered by a co-worker or any other person.
   - The nurse takes appropriate action to support and guide co-workers to advance ethical conduct.

Source: International Council of Nurses. (2012). *The ICN code of ethics for nurses.* Geneva, Switzerland: Author. Retrieved from http://www.icn.ch/images/stories/documents/about/icncode_english.pdf

GLOSSARY

Access to care: Living in rural areas presents unique concerns related to gaining entry into the healthcare system. As finances influence the closing of many rural hospitals, more communities find themselves struggling to find primary care providers who will work in those areas.

Accountability measures: Evidence-based care processes closely linked to positive patient outcomes.

Active euthanasia: Taking action to end a life (including one's own life). It can include a lethal dose of medication, such as in physician-assisted suicide.

Administrative (or regulatory) law: Governed by statutory law called administrative procedure acts at both federal and state levels, this law provides that before regulations can be adopted, a published notice of the proposed rules and where they are available must occur. The published notice and availability of the proposed rules provide concerned persons with the opportunity to comment on and suggest changes to the rules before final adoption. Thus, the process has three steps: (1) proposal of regulations, (2) consideration of proposed regulations, and (3) adoption of regulations with or without changes.

Advance directive: A written expression of a person's wishes about medical care, especially care during a terminal or critical illness.

Advanced beginner: Stage 2 of Benner's model, in which the student is able to formulate principles that dictate action. For example, the student would grasp the rationale behind why different medications require different injection techniques.

Age-related changes: Changes in cognition, vision, and hearing that occur as one ages. Research has demonstrated that teaching is not as effective if it does not accommodate for these cognitive and sensory changes.

American Journal of Nursing (AJN): The first nursing journal, developed by Mary Adelaide Nutting, Lavinia Dock, Sophia Palmer, and Mary E. Davis in October 1900. Through the American Nurses Association and the journal, nurses then had a professional organization and a national journal with which to communicate with each other.

American Nurses Association (ANA): The only full-service professional organization representing the nation's 2.9 million registered nurses through its 54 constituent member associations. It advances the nursing profession by fostering high standards of nursing practice, promoting the rights of nurses in the workplace, projecting a positive and realistic view of nursing, and lobbying the Congress and regulatory agencies on healthcare issues affecting nurses and the public.

Andragogy: Learner-focused education for people of all ages. It was initially defined as "the art and science of helping adults learn."

Assumptions: Describe concepts or connect two concepts and represent values, beliefs, or goals. When challenged, they become propositions.

Autonomy: One's ability to self-rule and to generate personal decisions independently.

Barton, Clara: The founder of the American Red Cross, who convinced Congress to ratify the Treaty of Geneva in 1882.

Basic dignity: Intrinsic, or inherent, and dwells within all humans, with all humans being ascribed this moral worth.

Benchmarking: An attribute or achievement that serves as a standard for other providers or institutions to emulate.

Beneficence: The actions taken by nurses to benefit patients and to facilitate their well-being.

Best interest standard: Based on the goal of the surrogate doing what is best for the patient or what is in the best interest of the patient.

Bioethics: A specific domain of ethics that is focused on moral issues in the field of health care.

Bolton, Frances Payne: This congressional representative from Ohio is credited with the founding of the Cadet Nurse Corps through the Bolton Act of 1945. By the end of World War II, more than 180,000 nursing students had been trained through this act, and advanced practice graduate nurses in psychiatry and public health nursing had received graduate education to increase the numbers of nurse educators.

Breckinridge, Mary: Founder of the Frontier Nursing Service.

Brewster, Mary: Establisher of the Henry Street Settlement in 1893 and a colleague of Lillian Wald. She quit medical school and devoted the remainder of her life to "visions of a better world" for the public's health.

Brown Report: Also know as *Nursing for the Future*, authored by Esther Lucille Brown in 1948 and sponsored by the Russell Sage Foundation.

This report was critical of the quality and structure of nursing schools in the United States. It became the catalyst for the implementation of educational nursing program accreditation through the National League for Nursing.

Burnout: Progressive, involves disengagement and withdrawal, and is characterized by physical, emotional, or mental exhaustion.

Care bundle: A small set of evidence-based interventions for a defined population of patients and care setting.

Career management: A planned logical progression of one's professional life that includes clearly defined goals, objectives, and a plan for achievement.

Case law: Established from court decisions, which might explain or interpret the other sources of law.

Case management: A current nursing model of nursing care delivery, relying on clinical pathways to evaluate care. The critical pathway refers to expected outcomes and interventions that the collaborative practice team establishes. The professional nurse is responsible for initiating and updating the plan of care, care map, or clinical pathway used to consistently guide and evaluate client care.

Chadwick Report: A major figure in the development of the field of public health in Great Britain, Edwin Chadwick drew attention in a well-known report to the cost of the unsanitary conditions that shortened the life span of the laboring class and the threats to the wealth of Britain. One consequence of his report was the establishment of the first board of health, the General Board of Health for England, in 1848.

Civil law: The law of civil or private rights, as opposed to criminal law.

Clinical judgment: An interpretation or conclusion about a patient's needs, concerns, or health problems, and/or the decision to take action (or not), use or modify standard approaches, or improvise new ones as deemed appropriate by the patient's response or the use of the clinician's experience and knowledge in assessment, diagnosis, planning, intervention, and evaluation.

Clinical nurse leader (CNL): An advanced generalist role prepared at the master's level of education.

Clinical practice guidelines: Standards developed to guide clinical practice and represent an effort to put a large body of evidence into a manageable form.

Clinical reasoning: The processes by which nurses and other clinicians make their judgments, including both the deliberative process of generating alternatives, weighing them against the evidence, and choosing the most appropriate, and those patterns that might be characterized as engaged, practical reasoning.

Cochrane Library: A collection of databases that contain high-quality, independent evidence to inform healthcare decision making.

Collaborative critical pathway: Expected outcomes and interventions that the collaborative practice team establishes, emphasizing interdisciplinary collaboration.

Compassion fatigue: Acute condition resulting from stress that may present itself over involvement in patient care.

Competent: Stage 3 of Benner's model, characterized by the ability to analyze problems and prioritize. The nurse has a solid grasp of the rules and principles. The nurse at this stage has had experience in a variety of clinical situations and is able to draw on prior knowledge and experience.

Complementary and alternative medicine: An approach that combines conventional medicine with less conventional options; an approach used instead of conventional medicine.

Complex adaptive systems (CASs): A collection of individual agents that are free to act in ways not totally predictable and whose actions are interconnected so that one action changes the context for other agents or units.

Composite measures: Combination of the results of related measures into a single percentage rating, calculated by adding up the number of times recommended evidence-based care was provided to patients and dividing this sum by the total number of opportunities to provide this care.

Concept: A term or label that describes a phenomenon. The phenomenon described may be either empirical or abstract.

Concept mapping: Method used to organize and link information about a patient's health problems so that the nurse can see relationships among a patient's problems and plan interventions that can address more than one problem.

Conceptual model: A set of concepts and statements that integrates the concepts into a meaningful configuration.

Confidentiality: The obligation of the nurse, along with other caregivers, to keep healthcare information private. To fulfill their social contract to provide nursing care, nurses must often gather sensitive information from patients. Privacy is the right of the patient.

Consumerism: The concept of consumers having more control of their healthcare experiences.

Continuous quality improvement (CQI): A structured organizational process that involves personnel in planning and implementing the continuous flow of improvements in the provision of quality health care that meets or exceeds expectations.

Core measures: Standardized performance indicators that allow for comparison across healthcare organizations.

Critical thinking: The ability to think in a systematic and logical manner, solve problems, make decisions, and establish priorities in the clinical setting. It is the competent use of thinking skills and abilities to make sound clinical judgments and safe decisions.

Cultural competence: The ability to interact effectively with people of different cultures. It comprises awareness of one's own worldviews, attitude toward cultural differences, knowledge of different cultural practices, and cross-cultural skills.

Culture of safety: An atmosphere in which focus is on what went wrong, rather than who made the error.

Cumulative Index to Nursing and Allied Health Literature (CINAHL): The authoritative resource for nursing and allied health professionals, students, educators, and researchers.

Database: A collection of electronic data of individual records that are systematically organized, indexed, and cross-referenced. It allows for the rapid collection, organization, manipulation, and analysis of data.

Deaconesses: Female servants who did the work of God by ministering to the needs of others. Nursing was most influenced by Christianity with the beginning of these female servants. This role in the church was considered a forward step in the development of nursing, and in the 1800s would strongly influence the young Florence Nightingale.

Delano, Jane A.: Director of nursing in the American Red Cross, she initiated a national publicity campaign to recruit young women to enter nurses' training.

Delegation: The process by which responsibility and authority for performing a certain task are transferred to another individual.

Deontology: Refers to actions that are duty based, not based on their rewards, happiness, or consequences. One of the most influential philosophers for this way of thinking was Immanuel Kant, a German philosopher from the 1700s.

Dignity: The innate right of a person to be valued and respected.

Disaster preparedness: Plans designating response during an emergency and often coordinated by local, state, and federal groups. Firefighters, police officers, and healthcare professionals are part of response teams.

Dix, Dorothea Lynde: A Boston schoolteacher, who became aware of the horrendous conditions in prisons and mental institutions. For the rest of her life, she stood out as a tireless zealot for the humane treatment of the insane and imprisoned. She had exceptional savvy in dealing with legislators.

Dock, Lavinia Lloyd: Became a militant suffragist, linking women's roles as nurses to the emerging women's movement in the United States.

Doctor of nursing practice (DNP): This practice degree encompasses any form of nursing intervention that influences healthcare outcomes for individual patients, management of care for individuals and populations, administration of nursing and health organizations, and the development and implementation of health policy. This practice degree is not the same as the research doctoral degree, and graduates are prepared to blend clinical, economic, organizational, and leadership skills and to use science in improving the direct care of patients, care of patient populations, and practice that supports patient care.

Durable power of attorney: A written directive providing a designated person with the legal authority to make either general or healthcare decisions for another person.

EBSCO Publishing: An electronic journal service available to both academic and corporate subscribers. It aggregates access to electronic journals from various publishers.

Educational Resource Information Center (ERIC): A national information system supported by the U.S. Department of Education, the National Library of Education, and the Office of Educational Research and Improvement. It provides access to information from journals included in the Current Index of Journals in Education and Resources in Education Index.

Electronic health record (EHR): Represents multiple systems that are interfaced to share data and networked to support information management and communication within a healthcare organization.

Email: A method of composing, sending, receiving, and storing messages over electronic communication systems; the most common use of the Internet.

Environment: One of the four concepts of the metaparadigm of nursing; the surroundings within which the person exists.

Error: The failure of a planned action to be completed as intended or the use of a wrong plan to achieve an aim with the goal of preventing, recognizing, and mitigating harm.

Ethic of care: An approach that emphasizes personal relationships and relationship responsibilities. Important concepts in this approach are compassion, empathy, sympathy, concern for others, and caring for others.

Ethical comportment: Good conduct born out of an individualized relationship with the patient that involves engagement in a particular situation and entails a sense of membership in the relevant professional group.

Ethical dilemma: A situation in which an individual is compelled to make a choice between two actions that will affect the well-being of a sentient being and both actions can be reasonably justified as being good, neither action is readily justifiable as good, or the goodness of the actions is uncertain. One action must be chosen, thereby generating a quandary for the person or group who must make the choice.

Ethical principlism: A popular approach to ethics in health care. Involves using a set of ethical principles that are drawn from the common or widely shared conception of morality. The four principles that are most commonly used in bioethics are autonomy, beneficence, nonmaleficence, and justice.

Ethics: The study of ideal human behavior and ideal ways of being. The approaches to this and the meanings of related concepts have varied over time among philosophers and ethicists. As a philosophical discipline of study, it is a systematic approach to understanding, analyzing, and distinguishing matters of right and wrong, good and bad, and admirable and deplorable as they exist along a continuum and as they relate to the well-being of and the relationships among sentient beings.

Evidence-based practice: The provision of high-quality patient care based on research evidence and knowledge rather than tradition, myths, hunches, advice from peers, outdated textbooks, or even what the nurse learned in school 5, 10, or 15 years ago. According to the *Nurse of the Future: Nursing Core Competencies*, the Nurse of the Future will identify, evaluate, and use the best current evidence coupled with clinical expertise and consideration of the patient's preferences, experience, and values to make practice decisions.

Expert: The final stage in Benner's model. The nurse has moved beyond a fixed set of rules. There is an internalized understanding grounded in a wealth of experience as well as depth of knowledge. The expert is always learning and always questioning using subjective and objective knowing.

Expert witness: Someone who has complex knowledge beyond the general knowledge of most people in the court or on the jury.

Family-centered care (FCC): An extension of patient-centered care that widens the circle of concern to include those persons who are important in the patient's life.

Fenwick, Ethel: Led the effort to form the British Nurses' Association to unite British nurses and to mandate registration as evidence of systematic training.

Formation: A process that occurs over time that denotes the development of perceptual abilities, the ability to draw on knowledge and skilled know-how, and a way of being and acting in practice and in the world.

Frontier Nursing Service: The first organized midwifery service in the United States. It served isolated Appalachian communities on horseback until World War II.

Global aging: In the post–World War II era, fertility rates have increased as death rates decreased in both developed and developing countries, leading to the aging of the world's population at an unprecedented rate.

Goldmark Report: A significant report, also known as *Nursing and Nursing Education in the United States,* that was released in 1922 and advocated the establishment of university schools of nursing to train nursing leaders.

Goodrich, Annie: First dean of the Army School of Nursing.

Greek era: The periods of Greek history in classical antiquity, lasting ca. from 750 B.C. (the archaic period) to 146 B.C. (the Roman conquest). It is generally considered to be the seminal culture that provided the foundation of Western civilization. Time of Hippocrates, father of medicine. In Greek society, health was considered to result from a balance between mind and body.

Health: One of the four concepts of the metaparadigm of nursing; the health–illness continuum within which the person falls at the time of the interaction with the nurse.

Health Belief Model (HBM): This model was originally developed to predict the likelihood of a person following a recommended action and to understand the person's motivation and decision regarding seeking health services.

Health Insurance Portability and Accountability Act (HIPAA): Enacted by the U.S. Congress in 1996. It was intended to improve the efficiency and effectiveness of the healthcare system by encouraging the development of a health information system. Several areas are addressed by the act, including simplifying healthcare claims, developing standards for data transmission, and implementing privacy regulations.

Health literacy: The ability to read, understand, and act on health information.

Health Source: The Nursing/Academic Edition provides more than 550 scholarly full-text journals, including more than 450 peer-reviewed journals focusing on many medical disciplines, including nursing and allied health.

Healthcare transparency: Making available to the public information on the healthcare system's quality, efficiency, and consumer satisfaction with care, so that patients and families can make informed decisions when choosing care and to influence the behavior providers, payers, and others to achieve better outcomes.

Henry Street Settlement: An independent nursing service in New York City where Lillian Wald lived and worked. This later became the Visiting Nurse Association of New York City, which laid the foundation for the establishment of public health nursing in the United States.

Idealism: A belief system containing these assumptions: The world is evolving. There is more than meets the eye. The social world is created.

Reality is a conception perceived in the mind. Thinking is dynamic and constructive.

Incivility: Bullying that can include behaviors such as criticism, humiliation in front of others, undervalued efforts, and teasing.

Informed consent: Mandates to the physician or independent healthcare practitioner the separate legal duty to disclose needed material facts in terms that patients can reasonably understand so that they can make an informed choice. Meaningful information must be disclosed even if the clinician does not believe that the information will be beneficial.

Integrity: Acting consistently with personal values and the values of the profession. In a healthcare system often burdened with constraints and self-serving groups and organizations, threats to this can be a serious pitfall for nurses.

International Council of Nurses (ICN): Founded in 1899 by nurses from several countries, such as Ethel Fenwick of Great Britain, Lavinia Dock of the United States, Mary Agnes Snively of Canada, and Agnes Karll of Germany, who advocated for the creation of national nursing organizations that would allow women to self-govern the profession.

Interprofessional healthcare team: Those who are directly involved in a patient's care such as physicians, nurses, and family members, but also those who provide support services who contribute to the patient's care.

Journaling: The process by which one sits down quietly on a daily or regular basis to think and record one's thoughts and ideas in writing. Recording clinical experiences that were meaningful or troubling to you is a recommended way to help enhance and develop reasoning skills.

Just culture: Approach to errors that balances not blaming individuals and not tolerating careless or egregious behavior.

Justice: The fair distribution of benefits and burdens. In regard to principlism, it most often refers to the distribution of scarce healthcare resources.

Learning domains: Three categories include cognitive, psychomotor, and affective.

Licensure: The granting of permission to perform professional actions that may not be legally performed by persons who do not have this permission.

Listservs: Group emails that provide an opportunity for people with similar interests to share information.

Living will: A formal legal document that provides written directions concerning medical care that is to be provided in specific circumstances.

Lobbyists: People who develop expertise on proposed legislation and present to legislators that information clearly and concisely.

Malpractice: The failure of a professional to use such care as a reasonably prudent member of the profession would use under similar circumstances, which leads to harm.

Mance, Jeanne: Founder of the *Hôtel Dieu de Montréal* in 1645.

Medical futility: When a treatment has no physiologic benefit for a terminally ill person.

MEDLINE: The largest biomedical literature database that provides authoritative medical information on medicine, nursing, dentistry, veterinary medicine, the healthcare system, and preclinical sciences.

Mentoring: A relationship between two nurses in which the more experienced nurse provides leadership and guidance to the nurse with less experience, often referred to as the "mentee."

Metaparadigm: The most global perspective of a discipline; acts as an encapsulating unit, or framework, within which the more restricted structures develop.

Mindfulness: Keeping attention focused in the present, resulting in the ability to see salient aspects of the clinical situation and take decisive action to prevent harm.

Models of patient care delivery: A framework for nurses to deliver care to a specific group of patients. Nurses are leaders and managers within various models of patient care delivery. The methods might differ significantly from one organization to another.

Moral reasoning: Pertains to making decisions about how humans ought to be and act.

Moral right: The right to perform certain activities (1) because they conform to the accepted standards or ideas of a community (or of a law, or of God, or of conscience), or (2) because they will not harm, coerce, restrain, or infringe on the interests of others, or (3) because there are good rational arguments in support of the value of such activities.

Moral suffering: Can be experienced when nurses attempt to sort out their emotions when they find themselves in situations that are morally unsatisfactory or when forces beyond their control prevent them from influencing or changing these perceived unsatisfactory moral situations. It can occur because nurses believe that situations must be changed to bring well-being to themselves and others or to alleviate the suffering of themselves and others.

Morals: Specific beliefs, behaviors, and ways of being based on personal judgments derived from one's ethics. They are judged to be good or bad through systematic ethical analysis.

Negligence: The failure to act as a reasonably prudent person would have acted in a specific situation.

Never events: Unexpected, serious, and often preventable adverse events in health care.

Nightingale, Florence: She was identified as a true "angel of mercy," having reformed military health care in the Crimean War and having used her political savvy to forever change the way society views the health of the vulnerable, the poor, and the forgotten. She is perhaps one of the most written about women in history.

Nonmaleficence: Refraining from action that might harm others. The injunction to "do no harm" is often paired with beneficence, but a difference exists between the two principles. Beneficence requires taking action to benefit others.

Nonvoluntary euthanasia: Occurs when persons are not able to express their decision about death.

Novice: The first stage of Benner's model, characterized by a lack of knowledge and experience. In this stage, the facts, rules, and guidelines for practice are the focus. Rules for practice are context free, and the student's task is to acquire the knowledge and skills.

Nursing: (1) Attention to the full range of human experiences and responses to health and illness without restriction to a problem-focused orientation, (2) integration of objective data with an understanding of the subjective experience of the patient, (3) application of scientific knowledge to the processes of diagnosis and treatment, (4) provision of a caring relationship that facilitates health and healing, and (5) one of the four concepts of the metaparadigm of nursing; the nursing actions themselves.

Nursing ethics: Sometimes viewed as a subcategory of the broader domain of bioethics, just as medical ethics is a subcategory of bioethics. However, controversy continues about whether nursing has unique moral problems in professional practice.

Nursing faculty shortage: This shortage is limiting student capacity in nursing programs across the nation.

Nursing informatics (NI): The synthesis of computer science, information science, and nursing science in the organization and comprehension of data that directs nursing practice.

Nursing process: The tool by which all nurses can become equally proficient at critical thinking. The nursing process contains the following criteria: (1) assessment, (2) diagnosis, (3) planning, (4) implementation, and (5) evaluation.

Nursing-sensitive measures: Patient-related processes or outcomes—or structural variables that serve as proxies to these processes and outcomes—that reflect the nurse-quality relationship.

Nursing shortage: Because of the growing complexity of health care, limited educational opportunities for students, the aging of the population, and the overall growth of the population, a shortfall in the number of registered nurses has occurred that will continue to worsen.

Organ allocation: A method used by the Organ Procurement and Transplantation Network to assure a balanced allocation of organs and ethical decision regarding organ allocation based on the concepts of justice and medical utility.

Organ procurement: The obtaining, transferring, and processing of organs for transplantation through systems, organizations, or programs.

Osborne, Mary D.: Supervisor of public health nursing for the state of Mississippi from 1921 to 1946. She had a vision for a collaboration with community nurses and granny midwives, who delivered 80% of the African American babies in Mississippi.

Palliative care: Providing comfort rather than curative measures for terminally ill patients.

Paradigm: The lens through which you see the world. They are also philosophical foundations that support our approaches to research.

Passive euthanasia: Occurs when a person allows another person to die by not acting to stop death or prolong life. An example of this type of euthanasia is withholding treatment that is necessary to prevent death at a point in time.

Paternalism: The deliberate overriding of a patient's autonomy. Nurses might decide to act in ways that they believe are for a patient's "own good" rather than allowing patients to exercise their autonomy.

Patient advocacy: The nurse speaks for the patient or maintains the patient's rights in the face of the healthcare system. An advocate is a person who pleads the cause for patients' rights.

Patient-centered care (PCC): According to the *Nurse of the Future: Nursing Core Competencies*, the Nurse of the Future will provide holistic care that recognizes an individual's preferences, values, and needs and respects the patient or designee as a full partner in providing compassionate, coordinated, age and culturally appropriate, safe, and effective care.

Patient education: Any set of planned educational activities designed to improve patients' health behaviors, health status, or both.

Patient handoff: The transfer of responsibility for a patient from one clinician to another.

Patient Self-Determination Act (PSDA): Legislation designed to facilitate the knowledge and use of advance directives.

Patient teaching: Activities aimed at improving knowledge.

Persistent vegetative state: A clinical condition of complete unawareness of the self and the environment, accompanied by sleep-wake cycles with either complete or partial preservation of hypothalamic and brain stem autonomic functions.

Person: One of the four concepts of the metaparadigm of nursing; the individual receiving the nursing.

Personal dignity: Often mistakenly equated with autonomy; judging others and describing behaviors as dignified or undignified are of an evaluative nature.

Personal health record: Data that conform to interoperability standards and are available via a patient portal. The patient manages, shares, and controls this information.

Philosophies: They form the discipline concerned with questions of how one should live; what sorts of things exist and what are their essential natures; what counts as genuine knowledge; and what are the correct principles of reasoning. They set forth the general meaning of nursing and nursing phenomena through reasoning and the logical presentation of ideas. They are broad and address general ideas about nursing. Because of their breadth, they contribute to the discipline by providing direction, clarifying values, and forming a foundation for theory development.

Physician-assisted suicide (PAS): According to Oregon's Death with Dignity Act, "lethal medications, expressly prescribed by a physician for that purpose."

PICO(T): An acronym that assists in the formatting of clinical questions: P = Patient, Population, or Problem; I = Intervention or Exposure or Topic of Interest; C = Comparison or Alternate Intervention (if appropriate); O = Outcome; T = Time or Time Frame. Using this format helps the nurse to ask pertinent clinical questions, focus on asking the right questions, and choose relevant guidelines.

Practical wisdom: A considered judgment or *phronêsis*, which is a notion Aristotle believed, that requires calculated intellectual ability, contemplation, and deliberation.

Privacy: The right of a person to be free from unwanted intrusion into the person's personal affairs.

Professional boundaries: In nursing, they can be thought of in terms of appropriate professional behavior that serves to maintain trust between patients and nurses and to maintain nurses' good standing within their profession.

Professional performance standards: Describes a competent level of behavior in the professional role that includes areas of contemporary practice concerns related to ethics, culturally congruent practice, education, evidence-based practice and research, quality of practice, communication, leadership, collaboration, professional practice evaluation, resource utilization, and environmental health.

Professional portfolio: A print or electronic collection of evidence of work, achievements, and accomplishments related to one's career.

Professional values: Beliefs or ideals that guide interactions with patients, colleagues, other professionals, and the public.

Proficient: Stage 4 of Benner's model. Refers to the professional who is able to grasp the situation contextually and as a whole. Such nurses have a solid grasp of the norms as well as solid experiences that shed light on the variations from the norm. Incorporated into practice is the ability to test knowledge against situations that might not fit and to solve problems with alternative approaches.

Propositions: Statements that describe relationships among events, situations, or actions.

PsycINFO: Contains nearly 2 million citations and summaries of journal articles, book chapters, books, dissertations, and technical reports, all in the field of psychology.

Pure autonomy standard: Decisions made on behalf of an incompetent person based on decisions that the formerly competent person made.

Quality: The degree to which health services for individuals and populations increase the likelihood of desired health outcomes and are consistent with current professional knowledge.

Quality improvement: It focuses on systems, processes, satisfaction, and cost outcomes, usually within a specific organization. According to the *Nurse of the Future: Nursing Core Competencies*, the Nurse of the Future uses data to monitor the outcomes of care processes and uses improvement methods to design and test changes to continuously improve healthcare systems.

Rathbone, William: A wealthy ship owner and philanthropist, he is credited with the establishment of the first visiting nurse service, which eventually evolved into district nursing in the community. He was so impressed with the private duty nursing care that his sick wife had received at home that he set out to develop a "district nursing service" in Liverpool, England.

Rational suicide: Self-slaying that is categorized as voluntary active euthanasia.

Readiness to learn: Patient's evidence of motivation to receive information at a particular time.

Realism: System of thought that contains these assumptions: The world is static. Seeing is believing. The social world is a given. Reality is physical and independent. Logical thinking is superior.

Reasonable standard of care: Refers to the nurse implementing the type of care that a reasonably prudent nurse would use in a similar circumstance.

Reflective thinking: The process of analyzing, making judgments, and drawing conclusions to create an understanding through one's experiences and knowledge and exploring potential alternatives.

Reformation: Religious changes during the Renaissance that influenced nursing perhaps more than any other aspect of society. During this period, the monasteries were abolished. The effects on nursing were drastic: Monastic-affiliated institutions, including hospitals and schools, were closed, and orders of nuns, including nurses, were dissolved.

Respondeat superior: The doctrine that indicates the employer may also be responsible if the nurse was functioning in the employee role at the time of an incident.

Robb, Isabel Hampton: Founder of the Nurses' Associated Alumnae in 1896, which in 1911 officially became known as the American Nurses Association.

Role transition: The transition from nursing student to registered nurse is sometimes described in terms of reality shock.

Roman era: The periods of Roman history in classical antiquity, lasting ca. 146 B.C. (the Roman conquest of Greece) or 31 B.C. (defeat of Mark Antony by Augustus at the Battle of Actium) to ca. A.D. 476 (fall of the Roman Empire). Roman civilization is often grouped into classical antiquity with ancient Greece, a civilization that inspired much of the culture of ancient Rome. The development of policy, law, and protection of the public's health was an important precursor to our modern public health systems.

Rule of double effect: Usually defined narrowly in health care as the use of high doses of pain medication to lessen the chronic and intractable pain of terminally ill patients even if doing so hastens death.

Safety: According to the *Nurse of the Future: Nursing Core Competencies*, the Nurse of the Future will minimize risk of harm to patients and providers through both system effectiveness and individual performance.

Salience: A perceptual stance or embodied knowledge whereby aspects of a situation stand out as more or less important.

Sanger, Margaret: A staunch activist in the early family planning movement, credited with the founding of Planned Parenthood of America. She worked as a nurse on the Lower East Side of New York City in 1912 with immigrant families. She was astonished to find widespread ignorance among these families about conception, pregnancy, and childbirth. After a horrifying experience with the death of a woman from a failed self-induced abortion, she devoted her life to teaching women about birth control.

Scales, Jessie Sleet: She is considered the first African American public health nurse. She provided district nursing care to New York City's African American families and is credited with paving the way for African American nurses in the practice of community health.

Scope of nursing practice: Describes the who, what, where, when, why, and how of nursing practice.

Search engines: They assist in finding specific topics on the Web by compiling a database of Internet sites.

Self-efficacy: An individual's belief that he or she is capable of performing a behavior.

Sentinel events: Unexpected occurrences involving death or serious physical or psychological injury or the risk thereof.

Shattuck Report: A Boston bookseller and publisher who had an interest in public health, organized the American Statistical Society in 1839, and issued a census of Boston in 1845. His census revealed high infant mortality rates and high overall population mortality rates. In his *Report of the Massachusetts Sanitary Commission* in 1850, he not only outlined his findings on the unsanitary conditions, but also made recommendations for public health reform. He also called for services for well-child care, school-age children's health, immunizations, mental health, health education for all, and health planning. The report was revolutionary in its scope and vision for public health.

Snively, Mary Agnes: In 1908, she met in Ottawa with 16 representatives from organized nursing bodies to form the Canadian National Association of Trained Nurses.

Social justice: A virtue that guides us in creating those organized human interactions we call institutions. In turn, social institutions, when justly organized, provide us with access to what is good for the person, both individually and in our associations with others. Social justice also imposes on each of us a personal responsibility to work with others to design and continually perfect our institutions as tools for personal and social development.

Social learning theory: If a person believes that he or she is capable of performing a behavior (self-efficacy) and also believes that the behavior will lead to a desirable outcome, the person will be more likely to perform the behavior.

Social media: Internet-based applications that enable people to communicate and share resources and information.

Socialization: A process by which a person acquires the knowledge, skills, and sense of identity that are characteristic of a profession.

Standard of substituted judgment: Used to guide medical decisions that involve formerly competent patients who no longer have any decision-making capacity.

Standards of nursing practice: Authoritative statements of the duties that all registered nurses, regardless of role, population or specialty, are expected to perform competently.

Statutory law: Consists of ever-changing rules and regulations created by the U.S. Congress, state legislators, local governments, and constitutional law. The statutes are the rights, privileges, or immunities secured and protected for each citizen by the U.S. Constitution.

Stereotypes: A standardized mental picture that is held in common by members of a group and that represents an oversimplified opinion, prejudiced attitude, or uncritical judgment. For example, Nightingale defined nursing as "female work." Nurses need to face the generalizations present in our society and erase the lines that define us.

Team nursing: A model of care used in the United States most frequently in hospitals and in long-term and extended-care facilities. This arrangement evolved after the functional nursing of the 1940s. With this approach, the nursing staff is divided into teams, and total patient care is provided to a group of patients.

Teamwork and collaboration: Interprofessional healthcare relationships that are grounded in reciprocal and respectful recognition and acceptance of each member's unique expertise, power, and sphere of influence and responsibilities that function to achieve shared goals. According to the *Nurse of the Future: Nursing Core Competencies*, the Nurse of the Future will function effectively within nursing and interdisciplinary teams, fostering open communication, mutual respect, shared decision making, team learning, and development.

Telehealth: The use of electronic information and telecommunications technologies to support long-distance clinical health care, patient and professional health-related education, and public health.

Terminal sedation (TS): When a suffering patient is sedated to unconsciousness, usually through the ongoing administration of barbiturates or benzodiazepines. The patient then dies of dehydration, starvation, or some other intervening complication, as all other life-sustaining interventions are withheld.

Theory: An organized, coherent, and systematic articulation of a set of statements related to significant questions in a discipline that are communicated in a meaningful whole.

Tort: Refers to acts that result in harm to another.

Total patient care: The first model of patient care. In this model, the RN has the responsibility for all aspects of care of the patient(s). The RN works directly with the client, other nursing staff, and physicians in implementing a plan of care. The objective of this model is to have one nurse provide all care to the same patient(s) for the entire shift. Currently, this model is practiced in areas such as critical care units or postanesthesia recovery units, where a high level of expertise is required.

Tyler, Elizabeth: African American nurse hired by Lillian Wald in 1906 as evidence of Wald's commitment to cultural diversity. Although unable to visit white clients, she made her own way by "finding" African American families who needed her service.

Unavoidable trust: Zaner's contention that patients, in most cases, have no option but to trust nurses and other healthcare professionals when the patient is at the point of needing care.

Uniform Determination of Death Act (UDDA): Defines death as when an individual who has sustained either (1) irreversible cessation of circulatory and respiratory functions or (2) irreversible cessation of all functions of the entire brain, including the brain stem, is dead.

Utilitarianism: The ethical approach to promote the greatest good that is possible in situations (i.e., the greatest good for the greatest number).

Values: Refer to a group's or individual's evaluative judgments about what is good or what makes something desirable. These judgments refer to what the normative standard should be, not necessarily to how things actually are. They are the principles and ideals that give meaning and direction to our social, personal, and professional life. They are integral to moral reasoning. In nursing, they encompass appreciating what is important for both the profession and nurses personally, as well as what is important for patients.

Values clarification: A process that can occur in a group or individually and helps us understand who we are and what is most important to us. The outcome of values clarification is positive because the outcome is growth.

Veil of ignorance: Refers to concept that if people had a veil to conceal their own or others' economic, social, and class standing, each person would likely make justice-based decisions from a position free from all biases and would view the distribution of resources in unprejudiced ways.

Violence: The exertion of physical force so as to injure or abuse. Objectives toward the prevention of this and abuse are included in *Healthy People 2020*.

Virtues: *Arête* in Greek; refer to excellences of intellect or character.

Voluntary euthanasia: Occurs when persons with a sound mind authorize another person to take their life or to assist them in achieving death. Also, this type can include the taking of one's own life.

Wald, Lillian: A wealthy young woman with a great social conscience, she graduated from the New York Hospital School of Nursing in 1891 and is credited with creating the title "public health nurse."

Wholeness of character: Pertains to knowing the values of the nursing profession and one's own authentic moral values, integrating these two belief systems, and expressing them appropriately. Integrity is an important feature of it.

INDEX

Note: Page numbers followed by *b*, *f*, and *t* indicate material in boxes, figures, and tables respectively.